RENAL DIET COOKBOOK FOR BEGINNERS

201 HEALTHY RECIPES WITH LOW POTASSIUM, LOW SODIUM AND LOW PHOSPHORUS TO STOP KIDNEY DISEASE AND AVOID DIALYSIS

RENAL DIET COOKBOOK FOR BEGINNERS

CONTENTS

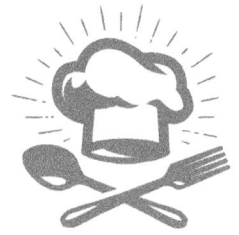

INTRODUCTION

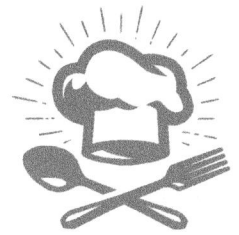

ndividuals with deteriorating kidneys must stick to a renal or kidney diet to lessen up the measure of waste in their blood. These wastes in the blood are the results of diets and liquids that are devoured. When the kidneys aren't performing well, they don't tackle or evacuate waste appropriately and precisely. If that waste remains or is left stuck in the blood, it can adversely influence a patient's electrolyte measures. Following a kidney diet may help advance kidney function and slow the complete kidney failure or dysfunction movement.

A diet is assumed as a renal diet if it lacks sodium, phosphorous, and protein. A renal diet likewise underlines the significance of consuming top-notch protein and restricting the consumption of liquids. A few patients may also need to limit potassium and calcium. Each individual's body is unique, and in this manner, every patient must work with a renal dietitian to think of an appropriately defined diet and well-crafted to the patient's needs.

The renal diet includes deteriorating and diminishing certain nutrients. A high sodium concentration can be destructive to individuals with kidney diseases because their kidneys can't enough dispose of an overabundance of sodium and liquid from the body. As sodium and fluid may rest and settle down in the tissues and circulatory system, it causes increased thirst, swollen legs, hands, face, high pulse, and heart disruptions and attacks. The abundance of liquid in the circulation system can exhaust your heart, making it augmented and feeble, and shortness of breath infers developing fluids in the lungs, making it hard to relax and breathe.

Maintain a crucial distance from table salt and high-sodium garnishes and toppings. Continuously attempt to cook at home, considering that most fast foods are high in sodium—attempt new flavors and herbs instead of salt to diminish and deal with your sodium intake. Attempt to avoid processed foods, if conceivable, because these bundled foods will, in general, be high in sodium. Always

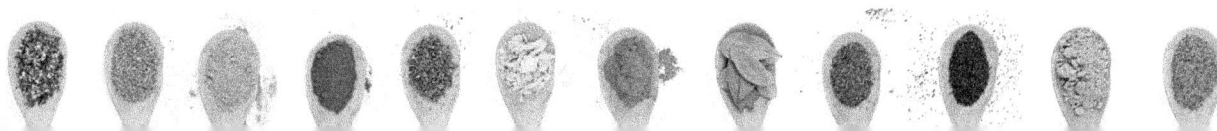

read the labels when shopping and picking foods that are low in sodium. Another route is to wash canned foods like veggies, beans, meats, and fish with water before serving.

If your kidneys cannot tackle potassium quantity, a patient must screen the measure of potassium that enters the body. Ask your primary care physician or dietitian if you have to restrict potassium. Your foods and drink decisions can assist you with bringing down your measures of potassium if necessary.

Salt substitutes can be high in potassium. Peruse the fixing mark. Check with your supplier about utilizing salt derivatives. Put a screening on canned foods before eating. More tips to help keep the degrees of potassium in your blood safe. Pick fresh foods grown from the ground and stay away from salt derivatives or subsidiaries and seasonings with potassium. Phosphorus can be found in numerous nourishments. Along these lines, patients with traded off kidney capacity should work with a renal dietitian to help oversee phosphorus levels.

It's a method for eating that shields your kidneys from further harm. It implies restricting a few ingredients and liquids to limit certain minerals by restrict their development in your body. Simultaneously, you'll need to ensure you get the right amount of protein, calories, nutrients, and minerals. In case you're in early periods of CKD, there might be scarcely any limits on what you can eat. But, as your infection deteriorates and dysfunction of kidneys prosper, you must be progressively cautious about what you consume or intake into your body.

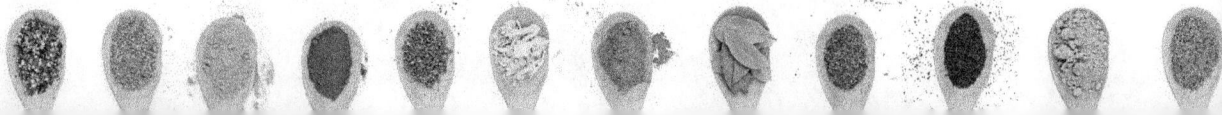

CHAPTER 1

WHAT IS KIDNEY DISEASE

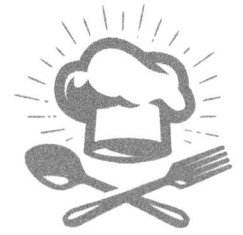

The kidneys maintain the fluids and water levels in the body. If you consume a lot of excess water, it is released out of the body by the kidneys. In the case of dehydration, more water is retained inside. All of this can happen if the kidneys are working properly. It can lead to toxic buildup in the body, damaging kidneys and other organs and disturbing the natural metabolism.

Most people are born with a kidney on each side of the body that simultaneously purifies the blood and supports each other in their renal function. Even when one kidney loses 40 percent of its renal function, the other kidney can hide this damage until properly checked and tested. This is why patients do not come to know about renal disease until there is enough damage done. If any of the kidneys lose its renal function below 25 percent, it must raise the alarms, which is highly dangerous. Individuals whose renal function decreases to only 15 percent would require an external treatment or dialysis.

Chronic kidney disease is a slow-moving disease and does not cause many complaints in the initial stages. The group of chronic kidney disease diseases includes several kidney diseases. The renal function decreases for several years or decades. With the help of timely diagnosis and treatment can slow down and even stop kidney disease progression.

In international studies of renal function in many people, it was found that almost every tenth kidney was found to have impaired kidney function to one degree or another.

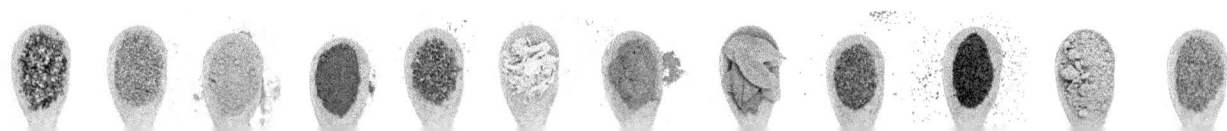

COMMON CAUSES OF CHRONIC KIDNEY DISEASE

Diabetes - in the case of this disease, various organs are damaged, including the kidneys and heart and blood vessels, nerves, and eyes. With long-term diabetic kidney damage, many patients increase blood pressure and need to be treated accordingly.

High blood pressure (hypertension, primary arterial hypertension) - during hypertension, blood pressure cannot be controlled. It begins to exceed the limits of the norm (more than 140/90 mm Hg). If this condition is permanent, it can cause chronic kidney disease, brain stroke, or myocardial infarction.

Glomerulonephritis is a disease that occurs due to a breakdown in the immune system. The kidneys' filtration function disrupts immune inflammation. The disease can affect only the kidneys and spread to the entire body (vacuities, lupus nephritis). Glomerulonephritis is often accompanied by high blood pressure.

Many other conditions can cause chronic kidney disease, for example, hereditary diseases. Due to which many cysts appear in the kidneys, polycystic kidney disease damages renal tissue's functioning and develops renal failure. Other hereditary diseases of the kidneys are much fewer common problems caused by obstructions in the kidneys, and urine excretion - such as congenital malformations of the ureter, kidney stones, tumors, or enlargement of the prostate gland in men repeated urinary tract infections or pyelonephritis.

Does everyone have chronic kidney disease?

Chronic kidney disease can evolve at any age. The greatest risk of getting sick is in people who have one or more of the following risk factors:

- Diabetes
- High blood pressure
- Family members have kidney disease
- Age over 50
- Long-term consumption of drugs that can damage the kidneys
- Overweight or obesity

DIAGNOSE WITH CHRONIC KIDNEY DISEASE

There are two simple tests that your family doctor can prescribe to diagnose kidney disease.

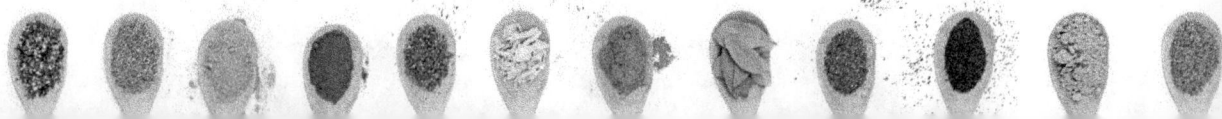

BLOOD TEST:

Glomerular filtration rate (GFR) and serum creatinine level. Creatinine is one of those end products of protein metabolism. The blood level depends on age, gender, muscle mass, nutrition, physical activity, foods before taking the sample (for example, a lot of meat was eaten), and some drugs. Creatinine excretes from the body through the kidneys. Suppose the work of the kidneys slows down, the level of creatinine in the blood plasma increases.

Determining the creatinine level alone is insufficient for diagnosing chronic kidney disease since its value begins to exceed the upper limit of the norm only when GFR decreased by half. The creatinine reading, age, gender, and race of the patient. It shows at what level is the ability of the kidneys to filter. In chronic kidney disease, the GFR indicator indicates the stage of the severity of kidney disease.

URINE ANALYSIS:

The content of albumin in the urine is determined; also, albumin and creatinine values are determined by each other. Albumin is a protein in the urine that usually enters the urine in minimal quantities. Even a small increase in the level of albumin in the urine in some people may be an early sign of incipient kidney disease, especially in those with diabetes and high blood pressure. In normal kidney function, albumin in the urine should be no more than 3 mg/mmol (or 30 mg g). If albumin excretion increases even more, then it already speaks of kidney disease. If albumin excretion exceeds 300 mg g, other proteins are excreted into the urine, and this condition is called proteinuria.

If the kidney is healthy, then albumin does not enter the urine.

In the case of an injured kidney, albumin begins to enter the urine.

After receiving the urine analysis results, the doctor suspects that there is a kidney disease. An additional urine analysis is performed for albumin. If albuminuria or proteinuria is detected again within three months, it indicates chronic kidney disease.

ADDITIONAL EXAMINATIONS

In kidney ultrasound examination: in the diagnosis of chronic kidney disease, it is an examination of the primary choice. Ultrasound examination allows us to assess the kidneys' shape, size, location, and determine possible changes in the kidney tissue and other abnormalities that may interfere with the kidneys' normal functioning. Ultrasound examination of the kidneys does not require special training and has no risks for the patient.

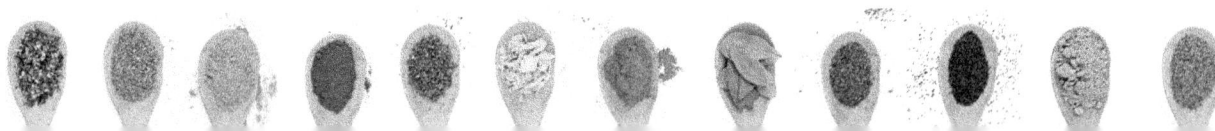

If necessary, and if a urological disease is suspected, an ultrasound examination of the urinary tract can be prescribed (as well as a residual urine analysis). An ultrasound examination of the prostate gland can be prescribed for men and referred to a urologist for a consultation. If a gynecological disease is suspected, a woman is referred for consultation with a gynecologist.

You need to know about the examination with a contrast agent. If you have chronic kidney disease, diagnostic tests such as magnetic resonance imaging, computed tomography, and angiography are used to diagnose and treat various diseases and injuries. In many cases, intravenous and intra-arterial contrast agents (containing iodine or gadolinium) are used, making it possible to see the organs or blood vessels under study.

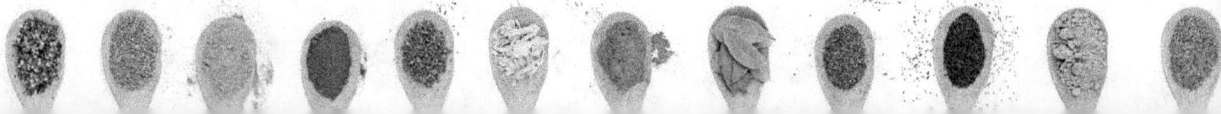

CHAPTER 2

HOW DOES KIDNEY WORK

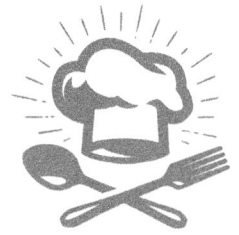

The kidneys are found in the body's dorsal wall on the spine's sides. They are brown, weigh about 150 grams each, and are about 12 centimeters long, 6 centimeters wide, and 3 centimeters thick. In the upper part, each kidney has an endocrine gland attached (it produces vital substances inside the body) called the adrenal gland.

The kidneys are the cleaners where the blood is filtered and cleaned. They produce urine, which contains water, toxins, and salts that the blood has been collecting throughout the body, and that has to be eliminated. They also intervene in other activities such as reproduction because they have sex hormones; regulate the amount of phosphorus and calcium in the bones; they control the tension in the blood vessels, and manufacture substances involved in blood clotting.

Renal insufficiency appears when only 5 percent of the total kidney or nephron filters work. The kidney's basic unit is the nephron, of which there are about 1 million in each organ. Each nephron forms a component that acts as a filter, the glomerulus, and a transport system, the tubule.

Some of the blood that reaches the kidneys is filtered by the glomerulus and passes through the tubules. Various excretion and reabsorption processes occur that give rise to the urine that is eventually removed.

The renal blood flow (RBF or amount of blood reaching the kidney per minute) is approximately adult 1.1 liters per minute. The 0.6 liters plasma enter the glomerulus through the arterioles. The 20 percent is filtered, an operation called renal glomerular filtration.

Therefore, the renal glomerular filtrate is the volume of plasma filtered by the kidneys per unit of time. The amount of filtered plasma per day is 135 to 160 liters. To prevent fluid loss, between 98

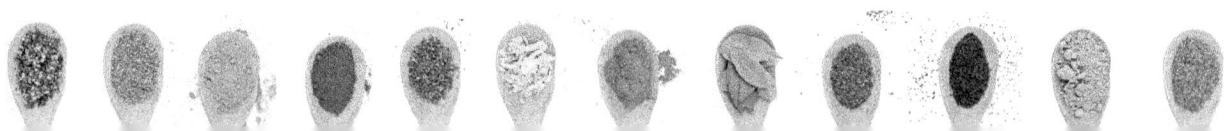

percent and 99 percent of the renal glomerular filtration rate is reabsorbed by the tubules, resulting in the amount of urine removed from between one and two liters per day.

When a kidney disorder occurs, it means that one or more of the renal functions are altered. But not all functions are changed in the same proportion. If two-thirds of the nephrons cease to function, significant changes may not occur because the remaining nephrons adapt. Changes in hormonal production may go unnoticed. Then, renal glomerular filtration calculation is the only way to detect the decrease in the number of nephrons that continue to function.

Chronic renal failure or uremia is the kidneys' inability to produce urine or fabricate low quality ("like water") since it has not been removed enough toxic waste. Although some patients continue to urinate, most cannot. However, the important thing is not the quantity but the composition or quality of the urine.

Chronic kidney disease slowly worsens over time. In the early stages, it may be asymptomatic. Damage of function usually takes months to occur. When the person realizes, he is usually already with the functioning of the kidneys completely compromised.

Early symptoms of chronic renal failure usually also frequently occur in other diseases and may be the only signs of renal failure until it is advanced.

Symptoms may include:

- General malaise and fatigue
- Generalized itching (itching) and dry skin
- Headaches
- Unintentional Weight Loss
- Loss of appetite
- Nausea

Other symptoms that may appear, especially when kidney function worsens, include:

- Abnormally light or dark skin
- Bone pain
- Drowsiness and confusion
- Difficulty concentrating and reasoning
- Numbness in hands, feet, and other body areas
- Muscle spasms or cramps
- Bad breath
- Easy bruising, bleeding, or bloody stools
- Excessive thirst
- Frequent hiccups

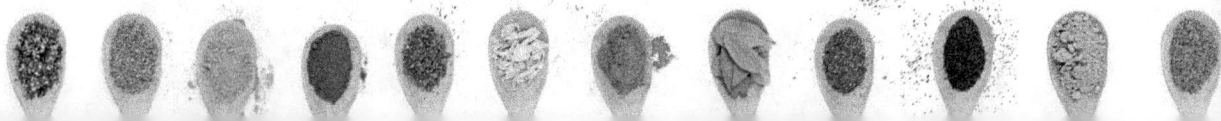

- Low level of sexual interest and impotence
- Interruption of the menstrual period (amenorrhea)
- Sleep disorders
- Swelling of hands and legs (edema)
- Vomiting, usually in the morning

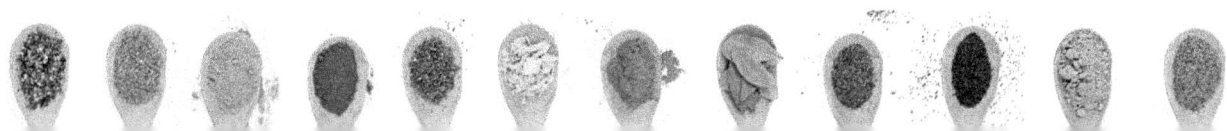

CHAPTER 3

UNDERSTANDING THE DIFFERENT TYPES OF KIDNEY FAILURE

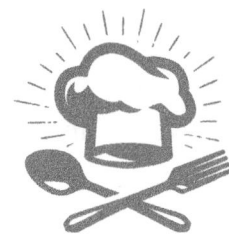

Kidney failure happens when your kidneys lose the capacity to channel waste from your blood adequately. Numerous variables can meddle with your kidney well-being and ability, such as dangerous presentation to natural toxins or certain drugs, certain intense and ceaseless infections, extreme drying out, and kidney injury. Your body gets over-burden with poisons if your kidneys can't do their standard employment. This can prompt kidney failure, which can be perilous whenever left untreated.

Somebody with kidney failure will possess a couple of symptoms of the disease. Once in a while, no symptoms are available. Potential symptoms incorporate a diminished measure of urination, swelling of your legs, lower legs, and feet from the maintenance of fluids brought about by the failure of the kidneys to wipe out water wastes, unexplained brevity of breath, over the top sleepiness or fatigue, steady sickness, confusion, and pain in your chest, seizures, and even outcome in extreme lethargies.

There are five types of kidney failure:

ACUTE PRE-RENAL KIDNEY FAILURE:

Deficient bloodstream to the kidneys can cause acute pre-renal kidney failure. The kidneys can't channel poisons from the blood without enough bloodstream. This sort of kidney failure can, as a rule, be restored once your primary care physician decides the reason for the diminished bloodstream.

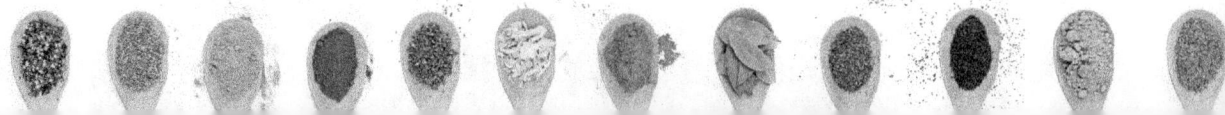

ACUTE INTRINSIC KIDNEY FAILURE:

Acute inborn kidney failure can result from direct injury to the kidneys. Causes also incorporate poison, over-burden, and ischemia, a cut of oxygen supply to the kidneys. The ischemia might be the consequence of serious dying, stun, renal vein deterrent, and glomerulonephritis.

CHRONIC PRE-RENAL KIDNEY FAILURE:

When there isn't sufficient blood streaming to the kidneys for an all-encompassing timeframe, the kidneys start to fade and lose the capacity to work.

CHRONIC POST-RENAL KIDNEY FAILURE:

A long-haul blockage of the urinary tract averts urination. This causes pressure and inevitable kidney harm.

CHRONIC NATURAL KIDNEY FAILURE:

This happens when there's long haul harm to the kidneys because of characteristic kidney diseases. Natural kidney illness creates direct injury to the kidneys, for example, serious draining or absence of oxygen.

Different conditions can meddle with urine and potentially lead to kidney failure, including kidney stones, an expanded prostate, and blood clumps inside your urinary tract. It harms your nerves that control your bladder and some different things that may prompt kidney failure to incorporate blood or around your kidneys contamination.

If your kidneys are harmed or going towards harm at any spot, they may not function just as they should. If your kidneys' damage keeps on deteriorating and your kidneys are less ready to carry out their responsibility, you have chronic kidney diseases. Kidney failure is the last phase of an interminable kidney ailment. This is the reason kidney failure is likewise called end-stage renal disease, or ESRD for short.

SOME KIDNEY DISEASES

PYELONEPHRITIS:

Bacteria may contaminate the kidney. It can cause back pain and fever. A spread of microorganisms from untreated bladder contamination is the most widely recognized reason for pyelonephritis.

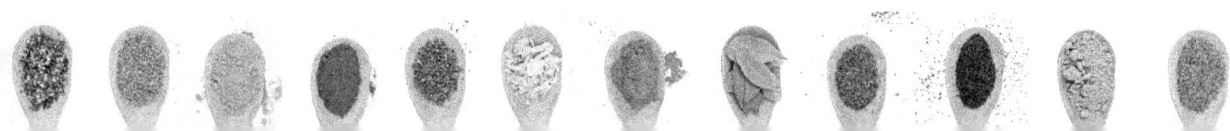

KIDNEY STONES (NEPHROLITHIASIS):

It is minerals in urine structure some crystals, which may develop sufficiently enormous to block urine passageway. It's viewed as one of the most deteriorating conditions. Most kidney stones pass alone. However, some are excessively huge and should be dealt with.

GLOMERULONEPHRITIS:

An overactive resistant framework may assault the kidney, causing aggravation and a little harm. Blood and protein in the urine are basic issues that happen with glomerulonephritis. It can likewise extend up to kidney failure.

NEPHROTIC DISORDER:

Damage to the kidneys makes them spill a lot of protein into the urine. Edema might be a symptom of this disease.

POLYCYSTIC KIDNEY MALADY:

A hereditary condition bringing about huge sores in the two kidneys that obstruct their functioning.

ACUTE RENAL FAILURE:

An unexpected decline in how well your kidneys work. Lack of hydration, a blockage in the urinary tract, or kidney harm can cause acute renal failure, which might or might not be reversed.

CHRONIC RENAL FAILURE:

A long-lasting fractional loss of how well your kidneys work. The most widely recognized causes are diabetes and hypertension.

END-STAGE RENAL DISEASE (ESRD):

Complete loss of kidney functioning and proper structure, as a rule, because of dynamic chronic kidney disorder. Individuals with ESRD require standard dialysis for endurance.

PAPILLARY NECROSIS:

Severe harm to the kidneys can cause lumps of kidney tissue to sever inside and obstruct the kidneys. If that goes untreated, the subsequent damage can prompt all-out kidney failure.

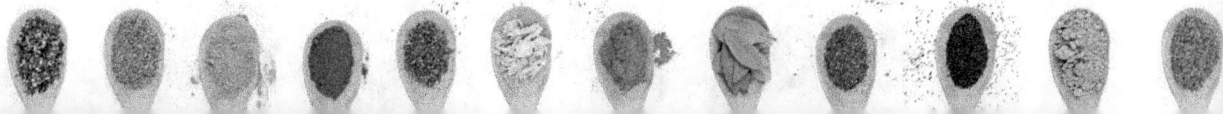

DIABETIC NEPHROPATHY:

High glucose from diabetes logically harms the kidneys, in the end, causing interminable kidney diseases. Protein in the urine may likewise result in this disease to happen.

HYPERTENSIVE NEPHROPATHY:

Kidney harm brought about by hypertension. Chronic renal failure may be the result.

KIDNEY CANCER:

Renal cell carcinoma is the most widely recognized disease influencing the kidney. Smoking is the most well-known reason for kidney cancer.

INTERSTITIAL NEPHRITIS:

Infections of the connective tissue inside the kidney, frequently causing acute renal failure. Unfavorably susceptible responses and medication reactions are common causes.

MINIMAL CHANGE DISEASE:

A type of Nephrotic disorder in which kidney cells look practically normal under the magnifying lens or microscope. The condition can cause significant leg swelling. Steroids are utilized to treat these minimal change diseases.

NEPHROGENIC DIABETES INSIPIDUS:

The kidneys lose the capacity to formulate the urine, as a consequence, because of some drug habits or irregularities. Although it's once in a while risky, diabetes insipidus causes thirst and frequent urination.

RENAL CYST:

Separated kidney cysts regularly occur as an individual's age grows, and they never cause an issue. Complex growths and masses can be destructive.

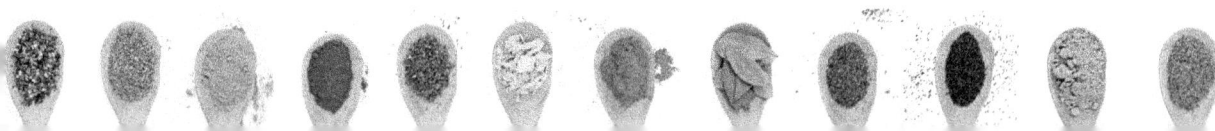

CHAPTER 4

UNDERSTANDING IF YOUR KIDNEYS HAVE FAILED

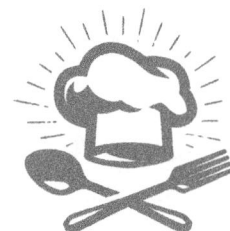

A kidney disease diagnosis can seem devastating at first. The news may come as a shock for some people who may not have experienced any symptoms. It's important to remember that you can control your progress and improvement through diet and lifestyle changes, even when a prognosis is serious. Taking steps to improve your health can make a significant effort to slow kidney disease progression and improve your life quality.

FOCUS ON WEIGHT LOSS

Losing weight is one of the most common reasons for going on a diet. It's also one of the best ways to treat kidney disease and prevent further damage. Carrying excess weight contributes to high toxicity levels in the body by storing toxins instead of releasing them through the kidneys. Eating foods high in trans fats, sugar, and excess sodium contributes to obesity, affecting close to one-third of North Americans and continues to rise in many other countries, where fast foods are becoming easier to access and less expensive. Losing weight is a difficult cycle for many, who often diet temporarily only to return to unhealthy habits after reaching a milestone, which results in gaining the weight back, thus causing a harmful yo-yo diet effect.

There are some necessary and easy changes you can make to shed those first pounds, which will begin to take the pressure off the kidneys and help you onto the path of regular weight loss:

- Drink plenty of water. If you can't drink eight glasses a day, try adding unsweetened natural sparkling water or herbal teas to increase your water intake.

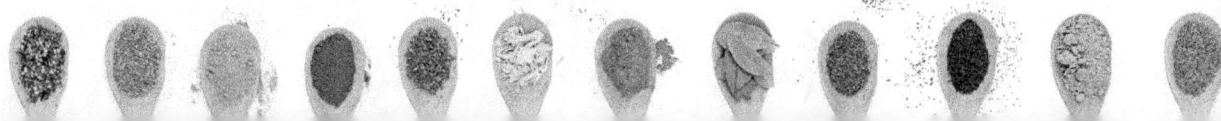

- Limit the sugar and carbohydrates you consume. This doesn't require adapting to a ketogenic or low-carb diet – you'll notice a significant change after ditching soda and reducing the bread and pasta by half.
- Take your time to eat and avoid rushing. If you need to eat in a hurry, grab a piece of fruit or a small portion of macadamia nuts. Avoid sugary and salty foods as much as possible. Choose fresh fruits over potato chips and chocolate bars.
- Create a shortlist of kidney-friendly foods that you enjoy and use this as your reference or guide when grocery shopping. This will help you stock up on snacks, ingredients, and foods for your kitchen that work well within your renal diet plan, at the same time reducing your chances of succumbing to the temptation of eating a bag of salted pretzels or chocolate.

Once you make take a few steps towards changing the way you eat, it will get easier. Making small changes at first is the key to success and progress with a new eating and living way. If you are already in the habit of consuming packaged foods – such as crackers, chips, processed dips, sauces, and sodas, for example – try cutting down on one or two items at a time, and over some time, gradually eliminate and cut down other items. Slowly replace these with fresh foods and healthier choices so that your body has a chance to adapt without extreme cravings that often occur during sudden changes.

QUIT SMOKING AND REDUCE ALCOHOL

It's not easy to quit smoking or using recreational drugs, especially where there has been long-term use and the effects have already impacted your health. At some point, you'll begin to notice a difference in the way you feel and how your body changes over time. This includes chronic coughing related to respiratory conditions, shortness of breath, and a lack of energy. Smoking inevitably catches up with age and contributes to cancer, premature aging, and kidney damage. The more toxins we consume or add to our body, the more challenging it becomes for the kidneys to work efficiently, which eventually slows their ability to function.

For most people, quitting "cold turkey" or all at once is not an option because of the withdrawal symptoms and increased chances of starting again. However, this method can work if applied with a strong support system and a lot of determination, though it's not the best option for everyone. Reducing smoking on your own, or switching to e-cigarettes or a patch or medication, can help significantly over time. Setting goals of reduction until the point of quitting can be a beneficial way to visualize success and provide a sense of motivation. The following tips may also be useful for quitting smoking and other habit-forming substances:

- Join a support group and talk to other people who relate to you. Share your struggles, ideas, and thoughts, which will help others and yourself during this process.

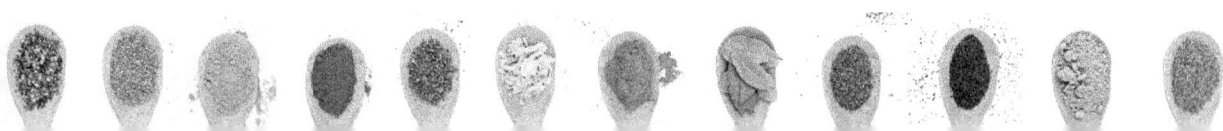

- Track your progress on a calendar or in a notebook, either by pen and paper, or on an application. This can serve as a motivator to display how you've done so far and where you can improve. For example, you may have reduced your smoking from ten to seven cigarettes per day, then increased to nine. This may indicate a slight change that can keep in mind to focus on reducing your intake further, from nine cigarettes to seven or six per day, and so on.
- Be aware of stressors in your life that cause you to smoke or use substances. If these factors are avoidable, make every effort to minimize or stop them from impacting your life. This may include specific people, places, or situations that can "trigger" a craving or make you feel more likely to use than usual. If there are situations that you cannot avoid, such as family, work, or school-related problems, consult with a trusted friend or someone you can confide in who can be present with you during these instances.
- Don't be afraid to ask for help. Many people cannot quit on their own without at least some assistance from others. Seeking a counselor or medical professional's guidance and expertise to better yourself can be one of the most important decisions you make to improve the quality of your life.

GETTING ACTIVE

Staying active and regular exercise is essential ways to keep fit and healthy. Regular movement is critical, and training is different for everyone, depending on their abilities and options. Fortunately, there are unlimited ways to customize an exercise routine or plan that can suit any lifestyle, perhaps low impact to start, or if you're ready, engage in a more vigorous workout. For many people experiencing kidney disease, one of the significant struggles is losing weight and living a sedentary life.

The movement is generally minimal, and exercise is usually not commonly practiced. Smoking, eating processed foods, and not getting the required nutrition can further impair the body so that exercise is seen as a hurdle and a challenge that is best avoided. Making lifestyle changes is not something that should be done all at once, but over some time – especially during the early stages of renal disease – so that the condition's impact is minimized over time and becomes more manageable.

Where can you begin if you haven't exercised at all or for an extended period? For starters, don't sign up for a marathon or engage in any strenuous activities unless it is safe to do so. Start slow and take your time. Before taking on any new movements, always talk to your doctor to rule out any impact this may have on other existing conditions, such as blood pressure and respiratory diseases, as well as your kidneys. Most, if not all, physicians will likely recommend exercise as part of the treatment plan but may advise beginning slowly if your body isn't used to exercise.

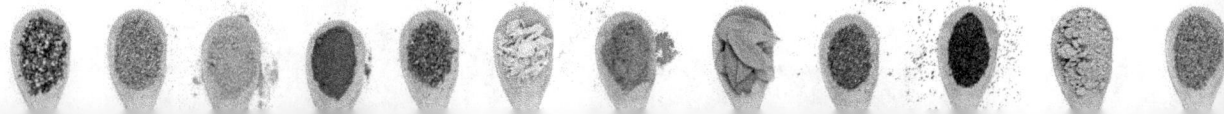

Simple techniques to introduce exercise into your life require a commitment. This can begin with a quick 15-minute walk or jog and a 10-or 15-minute stretch in the morning before starting your day. There are some easy, introductory techniques to consider, including the following:

- Take a walk for 10 to 15 minutes each day, at least three or four days each week. If you find it difficult at first, due to cramping, respiratory issues, or other conditions, walk slowly and breathe deeply. Make sure you feel relaxed during your walks. Find a scenic path or area in your neighborhood that is pleasant and gives you something to enjoy, such as a beautiful sunset or forested park.
- Stretch for five minutes once a day. This doesn't mean you need to do any intricate yoga poses or specific techniques. Moving your ankles, wrists, and arms in circles and standing every so often (if you sit often), and twisting your torso can help release stress, improve your blood flow, lower blood pressure, and help your body transport nutrients areas in need of repair.
- Practice breathing long, measured breaths. This will help prepare you for more endurance-based exercise, such as jogging, long walks, cycling, and swimming. Count to five on each inhale and exhale. Practice moving as you breathe, sync, or coordinate your body's movements with your breathing. If you have difficulty with the respiratory system, take it slow and don't push yourself. If you feel weak or out of breath, stop immediately and try again later or the following day at a slower pace.
- Start a beginner's yoga class and learn the fundamentals of various poses and stretches. It is helpful to arrive early and speak with the instructor, who can provide guidance on which modifications work best if needed. They can also give tips on approaching certain poses or movements that can be challenging for beginners so that you feel more comfortable and knowledgeable before you start.
- If you smoke, exercise will present more of a challenge on your lungs and respiratory function. Once you become accustomed to a beginner's level and become moderately active, you may notice it takes more effort, which requires an increase in lung capacity and oxygen. Smoking will eventually present a challenge. Where quitting can be a long-term and challenging goal in itself, please make an effort to cut back as much as it takes to allow your body's movements and exercise to continue.

Once you get into a basic routine, there is a wide variety of individual and team activities to consider for your life. Joining a baseball team or badminton club may be ideal. For more solitary options, consider swimming, cycling, or jogging. Many gyms and community centers provide monthly plans and may offer a free trial period to see if their facilities work for you. This is an excellent opportunity to try new classes and equipment to gauge how much you can achieve, even if in the early stages of exercise, so that you can decide whether to pursue dance aerobics, spin classes, and weight training. Some gyms will provide a free consultation with a personal trainer to set a simple plan towards weight loss and strength training goals.

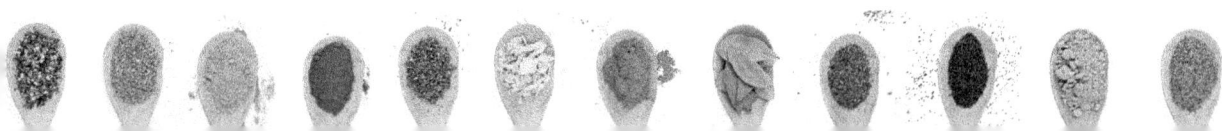

CHAPTER 5

RENAL DIET AND IT BENEFITS

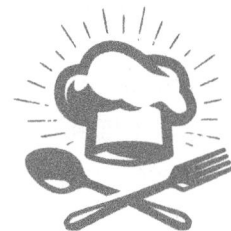

Dietary control, including protein, phosphorus, and sodium limitation, can impact perpetual renal patients by following conventional and nontraditional cardiovascular hazard factors.

Circulatory strain control might be supported by the decrease of sodium consumption and the vegan idea of the eating routine, which is significant for bringing down serum cholesterol and improving the plasma lipid profile.

Protein-limited eating regimens may have likewise calming and against oxidant properties.

The general principles of diet treatment for chronic kidney patients are as follows:

- Limit protein intake to 0.8 gm/kg per kilogram per day for non-dialysis patients. Patients on dialysis need a greater amount of protein to compensate for the possible loss of proteins during the procedure. (1.0 to 1.2 gm/kg daily according to body weight)
- Take enough carbohydrates to provide energy
- Take average amounts of oil—reduction of butter, pure fat, and oil intake.
- Restriction of fluid and water intake in case of swelling (edema)
- Dietary intake of sodium, potassium, and phosphorus limitation
- Take adequate amounts of vitamins and trace elements. A high-fiber diet is recommended.

The details of the selection and modification of the diet for chronic kidney patients are as follows:

HIGH-CALORIE INTAKE

In addition to daily activities to maintain heat, growth, and body weight the body needs calories. Calories are taken with carbohydrates and fats. According to body weight, the daily average

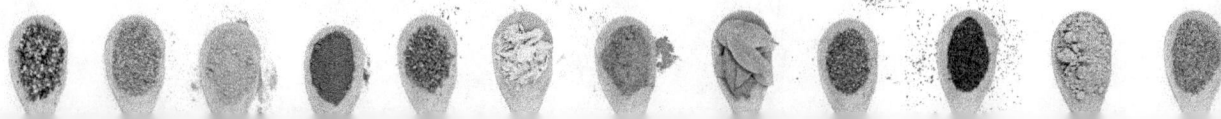

calorie intake of patients suffering from chronic kidney disease is 35-40 kcal/kg. If caloric intake is insufficient, the body uses proteins to provide calories. Such protein distribution may cause harmful effects, such as improper nutrition and increased production of waste materials. Therefore, it is essential to provide sufficient calories to CKD patients. It is essential to calculate the patient's daily calorie requirement based on the ideal body weight, not the current value.

CARBOHYDRATES

Carbohydrates are the primary source of calories required for the body. Diabetes and obesity patients should limit the number of carbohydrates. It is best to use complex carbohydrates that can be obtained from whole grains such as whole wheat or raw rice that can provide fiber. They should constitute a large part of the number of carbohydrates in the diet. The proportion of all other sugar-containing substances should not exceed 20% of the total carbohydrate intake, particularly in diabetic patients. As long as chocolate, hazelnut, or banana desserts are consumed in a limited amount, non-diabetic patients may be replaced with calories, fruit, pies, pastry, cookies, and protein.

OILS

Fats are a source of calories for the body and provide twice as many carbohydrates and proteins. Chronic kidney patients should limit the intake of saturated fat and cholesterol that may cause heart disease. In unsaturated fat, it is necessary to pay attention to the proportion of monounsaturated fat and polyunsaturated fat. Excessive uptake of omega-6 polyunsaturated fatty acids (CFAs) and a relatively high omega-6 / omega-3 ratio are detrimental, while the low omega-6 / omega-3 ratio has beneficial effects. The use of vegetable oils instead of uniform oils will achieve this goal. Trans fat-containing substances such as potato chips, sweet buns, instant cookies, and pastries are extremely dangerous and should be avoided.

RESTRICTION OF PROTEIN INTAKE

Protein is essential for the restoration and maintenance of body tissues. It also helps to heal wounds and fight infection. In patients with chronic renal failure who do not undergo dialysis, protein limitation is recommended to reduce the rate of decrease in renal function and postpone the need for dialysis and renal transplantation. (<0.8 gm/kg daily according to body weight). However, excessive protein restriction should also be avoided due to the risk of malnutrition.

Anorexia is a common condition in patients with chronic kidney disease. Strict protein restriction, low diet, weight loss, fatigue, loss of body resistance, and loss of appetite increase the risk of death. High proteins such as meat, poultry, and fish, eggs, and tofu are preferred. Chronic kidney patients should avoid high protein diets. Similarly, protein supplements or medications such as creatinine

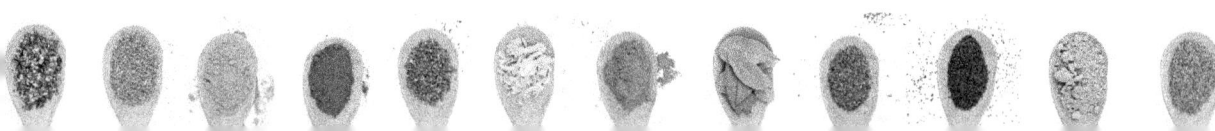

used for muscle development should be avoided unless recommended by a physician or dietician. However, as the patient begins dialysis, daily protein intake should be increased by 1.0 to 1.2 gm/kg body weight to recover the proteins lost during the procedure.

FLUID INTAKE

Why should chronic kidney patients take precautions about fluid intake?

The kidneys are essential in maintaining the correct amount of water in the body by removing excess liquid as urea. In patients with chronic kidney disease, the urea volume usually decreases as the kidney functions deteriorate. Reduction of urea excretion from the body causes fluid retention in the body, resulting in facial swelling, swelling of legs and hands, and high blood pressure. A build-up of fluid in the lungs causes shortness of breath and difficulty breathing. It can be life-threatening if not checked.

What precautions should chronic kidney patients take to control fluid intake?

The amount of fluid taken on a physician's advice should be recorded and monitored to prevent overloading or loss of fluid. The amount of water to be taken for each chronic kidney patient may vary, and this rate is calculated according to the urea excretion and fluid status of each patient.

What is the recommended amount of fluid for patients with chronic kidney disease?

Unlimited edema and water intake can be done in patients who do not have edema and can throw enough urea from the body. It is a common misconception that patients with kidney disease should take large amounts of water and fluids to protect their kidneys. The recommended amount of liquid depends on the patient's clinical condition and renal function.

Patients with edema who cannot appoint sufficient urea from the body should limit fluid intake. To reduce swelling, fluid intake within 24 hours should be less than the amount of urine produced by the daily body.

In patients with edema, the amount of fluid that should be taken daily should be 500 ml more than the previous day's urine volume to prevent fluid overload or fluid loss. This additional 500 ml of liquid will approximately compensate for the fluids lost by perspiration and exhalation.

Why should chronic kidney patients keep a record of their daily weight?

Patients need to record their weight daily to detect fluid increase or loss or to monitor fluid volume in their bodies. Bodyweight will remain constant if the instructions for fluid intake are strictly followed. Sudden weight gain indicates excessive fluid overload due to increased fluid intake in the

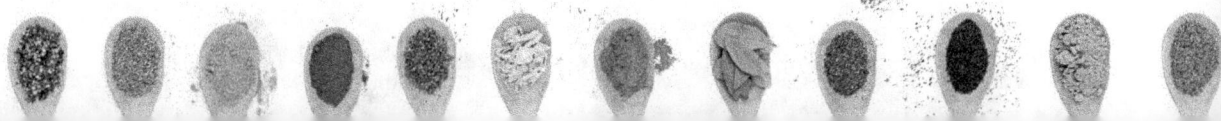

body. Weight gain is a warning that the patient should make more rigorous fluid restriction. Weight loss is usually caused by fluid restriction and the use of diuretics.

USEFUL TIPS FOR RESTRICTING FLUID INTAKE

Reduce salty, spicy, or fried foods in your diet because these foods can increase your thirst and cause more fluid consumption.

Only for water when you are thirsty. Do not drink as a habit or because everyone drinks.

When thirsty, consume only a small amount of water or try ice — sure, taking a little ice cube. Ice stays in the mouth longer than water to give a more satisfying result than the same amount of water. Remember to calculate the amount of liquid consumed. To calculate, freeze the amount of water allocated for drinking in the ice block.

To prevent dry mouth, gargle with water, but do not swallow the water. Dry mouth can also be reduced by chewing gum, sucking hard candies, lemon slices, or mint candies, and using a small amount of water to moisturize your mouth.

Always use small cups or glasses to limit fluid intake. Instead of consuming extra water for medication use, take your medicines while drinking water after meals.

High blood sugar in diabetic patients can increase the level of thirst. It is essential to keep blood sugar under tight control to reduce hunger.

Since the person's thirst increases in hot weather, measures to be in more relaxed environments may be preferred and recommended.

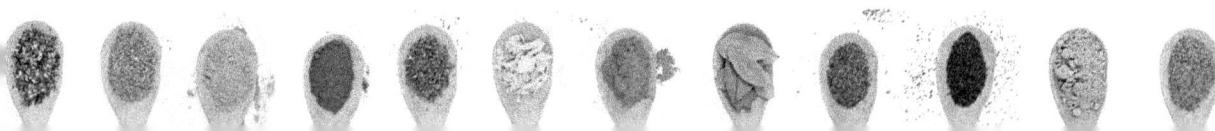

CHAPTER 6

KIDNEY FAILURE TREATMENT

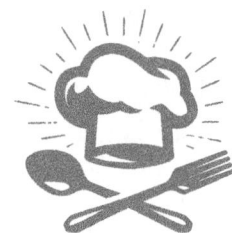

The physician will decide whether you belong to any of the high-risk groups. They're going to run some tests to see if your kidneys are working properly. The following tests may include:

Glomerular filtration rate (GFR) - This test will assess how well the kidneys are functioning and kidney disease level or kidney failure.

Ultrasound or computed tomography (CT) Ultrasound and CT scans will show clear images of your kidneys and urinary tract.

KIDNEY BIOPSY

Your health care provider can remove a piece of tissue from your kidney during a kidney biopsy while you're sleeping. The tissue sample will help the healthcare provider understand what type of kidney disease you have and how much damage has occurred.

URINE TEST

Your doctor may request a sample of urine for albumin testing. Albumin is a protein that can be transmitted to your urine when it damages your kidneys.

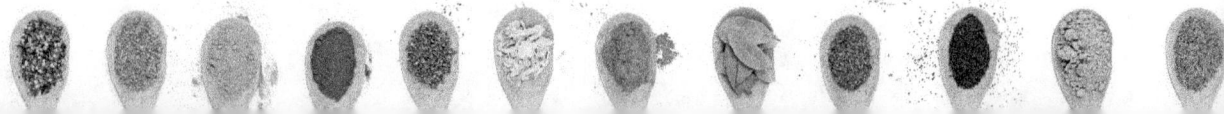

BLOOD CREATININE TEST

Creatinine is a product of waste. Once creatine (a protein in the muscle) is broken down, it will be released into the blood. If your kidneys don't work properly, the creatinine levels in your blood will increase.

With chronic kidney disease, there is no current or permanent treatment. However, some treatment methods or medication can aid control signs and symptoms, delay disease progression, and reduce complications.

Patients suffering from chronic kidney disease need to take a significant number of medications.

TREATMENTS

ANEMIA TREATMENT

Hemoglobin is the material that comes with essential oxygen around the body in red blood cells. If there are low levels of hemoglobin, the patient will have anemia.

Most kidney anemia patients may need blood transfusion. In general, iron supplements must be taken by a person suffering from kidney disease, whether via routine ferrous sulfate tablets or injections.

PHOSPHATE BALANCE

Persons with kidney disease may not be able to extract phosphate from their bodies properly. Patients are guided to decrease their nutritional phosphate intake, like dairy products, red meat, eggs, and fish consumption.

HYPERTENSION

High blood pressure is a widespread problem for patients with chronic kidney failure. It is important to reduce blood pressure to protect the kidneys and then slow down the disease's progression.

SHORTENING SKIN

Antihistamines, such as chlorphenamine, can help relieve itching symptoms.

MEDICINES AGAINST THE DISEASE

If toxins accumulate in the body because the kidneys are not functioning correctly, patients may feel sick (nausea). Medications such as cyclin or metoclopramide help relieve the disease.

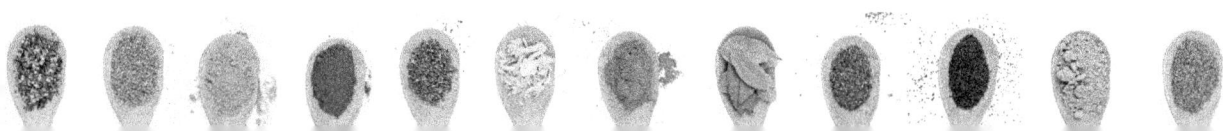

NSAIDS (NON-STEROIDAL ANTI-INFLAMMATORY DRUGS)

NSAIDs, including aspirin or ibuprofen, should be avoided and taken only if a doctor recommends them.

TERMINAL TREATMENT

This is when the kidneys function at less than 10% to 15% of their standard capacity. Measures used to date (diet, medication, and treatments that control the underlying issues) will no longer be available. The kidneys of patients with end-stage renal failure cannot cope with the process of waste and fluid removal: the patient will need dialysis or a kidney transplant to survive.

Most doctors will try to delay dialysis or kidney transplant as much as possible since they carry the risk of potentially serious complications.

RENAL DIALYSIS

A peritoneal dialysis is a treatment option for chronic kidney disease.

There are two main types of renal dialysis. Each class also has subtypes. The two main types are:

Hemodialysis: The blood is pumped from the patient's body and passes through dialysis (an artificial kidney). The patient undergoes hemodialysis approximately three times a week. Each session lasts a minimum of 3 hours.

Experts now identify that more frequent sessions result in a better quality of life for the patient, but modern home dialysis techniques make the regular use of hemodialysis possible.

Peritoneal dialysis: Blood enters the patient's abdomen; in the peritoneal cavity containing an extensive network of small blood vessels. A catheter is implanted in the stomach. The dialysis solution is infused and drained for as long as necessary to eliminate waste and excess fluid.

KIDNEY TRANSPLANT

The kidney donor and recipient must have the same blood type, cell surface proteins, and antibodies to reduce the risk of rejection of the new kidney. The best types of donors are typical brothers or close relatives. When it is impossible to have a living donor, the search for a dead donor must begin.

DRUGS AND MEDICINES

Your doctor will prescribe angiotensin-converting enzymes (ACE) inhibitors, such as lisinopril and ramipril. Or angiotensin receptor blockers (BRA), such as irbesartan and Olmesartan. These are blood pressure drugs that can slow down the progression of kidney disease. Your doctor may

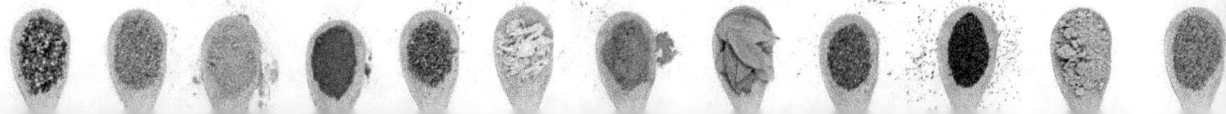

prescribe these medications to help you maintain your kidney function, even if you do not have high blood pressure.

It can also be treated with cholesterol medications (such as simvastatin). These medications can bring down blood cholesterol levels and help to maintain your kidney health properly. Depending on your symptoms observed, your doctor may also prescribe medication to relieve inflammation and treat anemia.

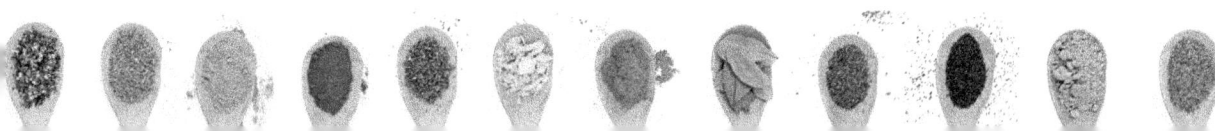

CHAPTER 7

LEARNING TO DEAL WITH KIDNEY FAILURE

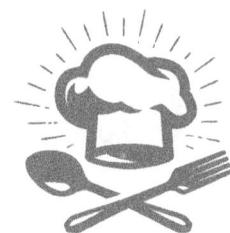

During kidney disease, this is extremely important. They can advise you about sodium, phosphorous, and potassium content of favorite foods and recommend reducing your sodium intake. Your diet will be tailored to you, considering the stage of kidney disease you're in and any other illnesses or diseases you suffer from.

KEEP A FOOD DIARY

You should track what you're eating and drinking to stay within the guidelines and recommendations given to you. Apps such as My Fitness Pal make this extremely easy and even track many of the minerals and levels in foods, including sodium, protein, etc. There are also apps specifically made for kidney disease patients to track sodium, phosphorous, and potassium levels.

READ FOOD LABELS

Some foods have hidden sodium in them, even if they don't taste salty. You will need to cut back on the amount of canned, frozen, and processed foods you eat. Check your beverages for added sodium.

CHECK FOOD LABELS TO AVOID

Potassium chloride, Tetrasodium phosphate, Sodium phosphate, Trisodium phosphate, Tricalcium phosphate, Phosphoric acid, Polyphosphate, Hexametaphosphate, Pyrophosphate, Monocalcium phosphate, Dicalcium phosphate, Aluminum phosphate, Sodium tripolyphosphate, Sodium polyphosphate.

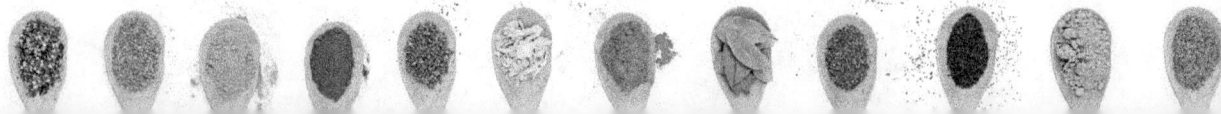

FLAVOR FOODS WITH SPICES AND HERBS RATHER THAN SHOP-BOUGHT DRESSINGS AND CONDIMENTS

These add flavor and variety to your meals and are not packed with sodium; spices also have many health benefits. Stay away from salt substitutes and seasonings that contain potassium. Use citrus fruits and vinegar for dressings and to add flavor.

KEEP UP YOUR APPOINTMENTS WITH YOUR DOCTOR OR NEPHROLOGIST

Let your doctor know if you notice any swelling or changes in your weight.

MONITOR DRINK AND FLUID INTAKE

You have probably been told you need to drink up to eight glasses of water a day. This is true for a healthy body, but for people experiencing the later stages of CKD, these fluids can build up and cause additional problems. The restriction of fluids will differ from person to person. Things to take into consideration are swelling urine output and weight gain. Your weight will be recorded before dialysis begins, and once it's over. This is done to determine how much fluid to remove from your body. If you are undergoing hemodialysis, this will be recorded approximately three times a week. If you are undergoing peritoneal dialysis, your weight is recorded every day. If there is a significant weight gain, you may be drinking too many fluids.

MEASURE PORTION SIZES

Moderating your portion sizes is essential. Use smaller cups, bowls, or plates to avoid giving yourself oversized portions.

Measure your food so you can keep an accurate record of how much you are eating:

- The size of a fist is equal to 1 cup.
- The palm is equal to 3 ounces.
- The tip of your thumb is equivalent to 1 teaspoon.
- A poker chip is equal to 1 tablespoon.

Substitution Tips:

- Use plain white flour instead of whole-wheat/whole-grain
- Use all-purpose flour instead of self-raising,
- Use Stevia instead of sugar,

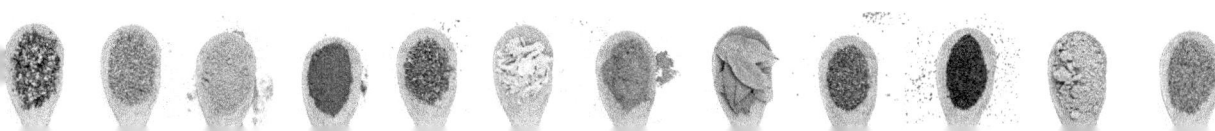

- Use egg whites rather than whole eggs,
- Use soy milk or almond rice instead of cow's milk.

OTHER ADVICE

Be careful when eating in restaurants -ask for dressings and condiments on the side and watch out for soups and cured meats.

- Watch out for convenience foods that are high in sodium.
- Prepare your meals and freeze them for future use.
- Drain liquids from canned vegetables and fruits to help control potassium levels.

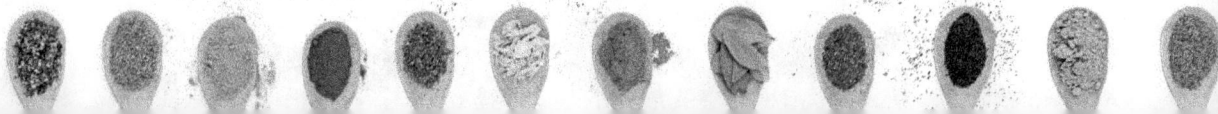

CHAPTER 8

FOODS TO EAT AND TO AVOID

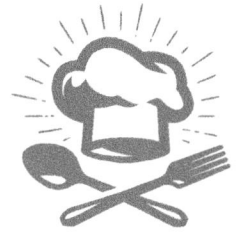

FOOD TO EAT

The renal diet aims to cut down the amount of waste in the blood. When people have kidney dysfunction, the kidneys are unable to remove and filter waste properly. When waste is left in the blood, it can affect the electrolyte levels of the patient. With a kidney diet, kidney function is promoted, and the progression of complete kidney failure is slowed down.

The renal diet follows a low intake of protein, phosphorus, and sodium. It is necessary to consume high-quality protein and limit some fluids. For some people, it is important to limit calcium and potassium.

Promoting a renal diet, here are the substances which are critical to be monitored:

SODIUM AND ITS ROLE IN THE BODY

Most natural foods contain sodium. Some people think that sodium and salt are interchangeable. However, salt is a compound of chloride and sodium. There might be either salt or sodium in other forms in the food we eat. Due to the added salt, processed foods include a higher level of sodium.

Apart from potassium and chloride, sodium is one of the most crucial body's electrolytes. The main function of electrolytes is to control the fluids when they are going out and in the body's cells and tissues.

With sodium:

- Blood volume and pressure are regulated.
- Muscle contraction and nerve function are regulated.

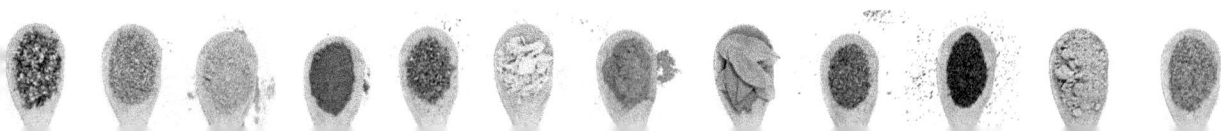

- The acid-base balance of the blood is regulated.
- The amount of fluid the body eliminates and keeps is balanced.

Why is it important to monitor sodium intake for people with kidney issues?

Since the kidneys of kidney disease patients are unable to reduce excess fluid and sodium from the body adequately, too much sodium might be harmful. As fluid and sodium build up in the bloodstream and tissues, they might cause:

- Edema: swelling in face, hands, and legs
- Increased thirst
- High blood pressure
- Shortness of breath
- Heart failure

The ways to monitor sodium intake:

- Avoid processed foods
- Be attentive to serving sizes.
- Read food labels
- Utilize fresh meats instead of processed
- Choose fresh fruits and veggies.
- Compare brands, choosing the ones with the lowest sodium levels.
- Utilize spices that do not include salt
- Ensure the sodium content is less than 400 mg per meal and not more than 150 mg per snack
- Cook at home, not adding salt
- Foods to eat with lower sodium content:
- Fresh meats, dairy products, frozen veggies, and fruits
- Fresh herbs and seasonings like rosemary, oregano, dill, lime, cilantro, onion, lemon, and garlic
- Corn tortilla chips, pretzels, no salt added crackers, unsalted popcorn

POTASSIUM AND ITS ROLE IN THE BODY

The main function of potassium is keeping muscles working correctly and the heartbeat regular. This mineral is responsible for maintaining electrolyte and fluid balance in the bloodstream. The kidneys regulate the proper amount of potassium in the body, expelling excess amounts in the urine.

Monitoring potassium intake

- Limit high potassium food

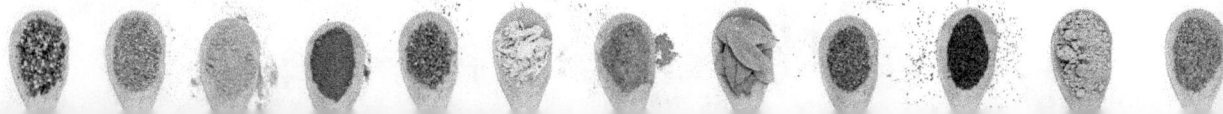

- Select only fresh fruits and veggies
- Limit dairy products and milk to 8 oz per day
- Avoid potassium chloride
- Read labels on packaged foods.
- Avoid seasonings and salt substitutes with potassium.

Foods to eat with lower potassium:

- Fruits: watermelon, tangerines, pineapple, plums, peaches, pears, papayas, mangoes, lemons and limes, honeydew, grapefruit/grapefruit juice, grapes/grape juice, clementine/satsuma, cranberry juice, berries, and apples/ applesauce, apple juice
- Veggies: summer squash (cooked), okra, mushrooms (fresh), lettuce, kale, green beans, eggplant, cucumber, corn, onions (raw), celery, cauliflower, carrots, cabbage, broccoli (fresh), bamboo shoots (canned), and bell peppers
- Plain Turkish delights, marshmallows and jellies, boiled fruit sweets, and peppermints
- Shortbread, ginger nut biscuits, plain digestives
- Plain flapjacks and cereal bars
- Plain sponge cakes like Madeira cake, lemon sponge, jam sponge
- Corn-based and wheat crisps
- Whole grain crispbreads and crackers
- Protein and other foods (bread (not whole grain), pasta, noodles, rice, eggs, canned tuna, turkey (white meat), and chicken (white meat)

PHOSPHORUS AND ITS ROLE IN THE BODY

This mineral is essential in bone development and maintenance. Phosphorus helps in the development of connective organs and tissue and assists in muscle movement. Extra phosphorus is possible to be removed by healthy kidneys. However, it is impossible with kidney dysfunction. High levels of phosphorus make bones weak by pulling calcium out of your bones. It might lead to dangerous calcium deposits in the heart, eyes, lungs, and blood vessels.

Monitoring phosphorus intake

- Pay attention to serving size
- Eat fresh fruits and veggies
- Eat smaller portions of foods that are rich in protein
- Avoid packaged foods
- Keep a food journal

Foods to eat with low phosphorus level:

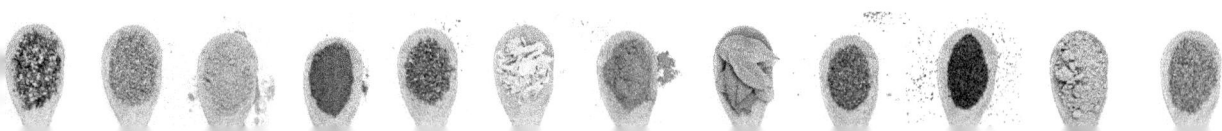

- grapes, apples
- lettuce, leeks
- Carbohydrates (white rice, corn, and rice Cereal, popcorn, pasta, crackers (not wheat), white bread)
- Meat (sausage, fresh meat)

PROTEIN

Damaged kidneys are unable to remove protein waste, so they accumulate in the blood. The amount of protein to consume differs depending on the stage of CKD. Protein is critical for tissue maintenance, and it is necessary to eat the proper amount of it according to the particular stage of kidneys disease.

Sources of protein for vegetarians:

- Vegans (allowing only plant-based foods): Wheat protein and whole grains, nut butter, soy protein, yogurt or soy milk, cooked no salt added canned and dried beans and peas, unsalted nuts.
- Lacto vegetarians (allowing dairy products, milk, and plant-based foods): reduced-sodium or low-sodium cottage cheese.
- Lacto-Ovo vegetarians (allowing eggs, dairy products, milk, and plant-based foods): eggs.

FOOD TO AVOID

Food with high sodium content:

- Onion salt, marinades, garlic salt, teriyaki sauce, and table salt
- Pepperoni, bacon, ham, lunch meat, hot dogs, sausage, processed meats
- Ramen noodles, canned produce, and canned soups
- Marinara sauce, gravy, salad dressings, soy sauce, BBQ sauce, and ketchup
- Chex Mix, salted nuts, Cheetos, crackers, and potato chips
- Fast food

Food with a high potassium level:

- Fruits: dried fruit, oranges/orange juice, prunes/prune juice, kiwi, nectarines, dates, cantaloupe, bananas, black currants, damsons, cherries, grapes, and apricots.
- Vegetables: tomatoes/tomato sauce/tomato juice, sweet potatoes, beans, lentils, split peas, spinach (cooked), pumpkin, potatoes, mushrooms (cooked), chile peppers, chard, Brussels sprouts (cooked), broccoli (cooked), baked beans, avocado, butternut squash, and acorn squash.

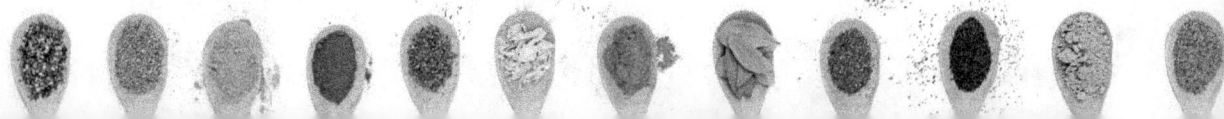

- Protein and other foods: peanut butter, molasses, granola, chocolate, bran, sardines, fish, bacon, ham, nuts and seeds, yogurt, milkshakes, and milk.
- Coconut-based snacks, nut-based snacks, fudge, and toffee
- Cakes containing marzipan.
- Potato crisps.

Foods with high phosphorus:

- Dairy products: pudding, ice cream, yogurt, cottage cheese, cheese, and milk
- Nuts and seeds: sunflower seeds, pumpkin seeds, pecans, peanut butter, pistachios, cashews, and almonds
- Dried beans and peas: soybeans, split peas, refried beans, pinto beans, lentils, kidney beans, garbanzo beans, black beans, and baked beans.
- Meat: veal, turkey, liver, lamb, beef, bacon, fish, and seafood.
- Carbohydrates: whole grain products, oatmeal, and bran cereals

RENAL DIET SHOPPING LIST

VEGETABLES:

- Arugula (raw)
- Alfalfa sprouts
- Bamboo shoots
- Asparagus
- Beans - pinto, wax, fava, green
- Bean sprouts
- Bitter melon (balsam pear)
- Beet greens (raw)
- Broccoli
- Broad beans (boiled, fresh)
- Cactus
- Cabbage - red, swamp, Napa/ Suey Choy, skunk
- Carrots
- Calabash
- Celery
- Cauliflower
- Chayote
- Celeriac (cooked)
- Collard greens

- Chicory
- Cucumber
- Corn
- Okra
- Onions
- Pepitas
- (Green) Peas
- Peppers
- Radish
- Radicchio
- Seaweed
- Rapini (raw)
- Shallots
- Spinach (raw)
- Snow peas
- Dandelion greens (raw)
- Daikon
- Plant Leaves
- Drumstick
- Endive

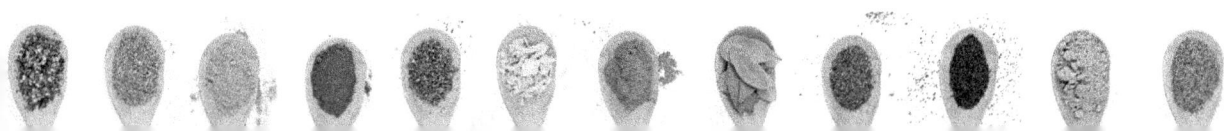

- Eggplant
- Fennel bulb
- Escarole
- Fiddlehead greens
- Ferns
- Hearts of Palm
- Irish moss
- Hominy
- Jicama, raw
- Leeks
- Kale(raw)
- Mushrooms (raw white)
- Lettuce (raw)

- Mustard greens
- Swiss chard (raw)
- Squash
- Turnip
- Tomatillos (raw)
- Watercress
- Turnip greens
- Wax beans
- Water chestnuts (canned)
- Winter melon
- Wax gourd
- Zucchini (raw)

FRUITS:

- Acerola Cherries
- Apple
- Blackberries
- Asian Pear
- Boysenberries
- Blueberries
- Cherries
- Casaba melon
- Clementine
- Chokeberries
- Crabapples
- Cloudberries
- Cranberries (fresh)
- Grapefruit
- Gooseberries
- Pomegranate
- Grapes
- Rambutan
- Quince
- Rhubarb
- Raspberries (fresh or frozen)
- Jujubes
- Golden Berry

- Kumquat
- Jackfruit
- Lingonberries
- Lemon
- Loganberries
- Lime
- Lychees
- Mango
- Mandarin orange
- Peach
- Pineapple
- Pear
- Plum
- Strawberries
- Rose-apple
- Tangerine
- Tangelo
- Watermelon

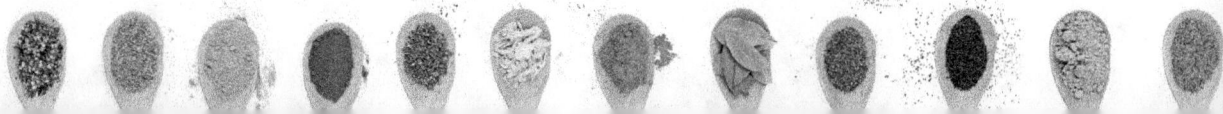

FRESH MEAT, SEAFOOD, AND POULTRY:

- Chicken
- Beef and Ground Beef
- Goat
- Duck
- Wild Game

- Pork
- Lamb
- Veal
- Turkey
- Fish

MILK, EGGS, AND DAIRY:

Milk:

- Milk (½-1 cup/day)

Non-Dairy Milk:

- Almond Fresh (Original, Unsweetened, Vanilla)
- Almond Breeze (Original, Vanilla, Vanilla Unsweetened, Original Unsweetened)
- Silk True Almond Beverage (Unsweetened Original, Original, Vanilla, Unsweetened Vanilla)
- Good Karma Flax Delight (Vanilla, Original, Unsweetened)
- Rice Dream Rice Drink (Vanilla Classic, Non-Enriched Original Classic)
- Silk Soy Beverage (Original, Vanilla, Unsweetened)
- Natura Organic Fortified Rice Beverage (Original, Vanilla)
- PC Organics Fortified Rice Beverage

Other Dairy Products:

- Non-Hydrogenated Margarine (Salt-Free or Regular)
- Butter (Unsalted or Regular)
- Whipping Cream
- Sour Cream
- Whipped Cream

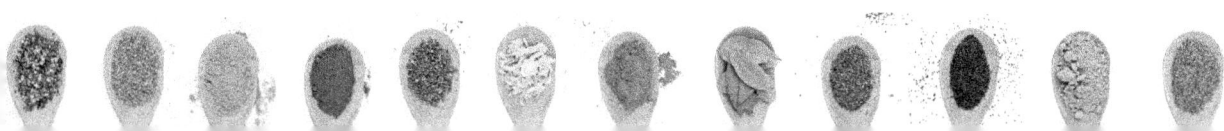

CHAPTER 9

JUICE AND BEVERAGES FOR THE RENAL DIET

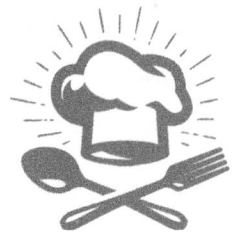

FRESH JUICES

There are plenty of delicious, thirst-quenching drinks available on the renal diet. It includes various teas and juices, both vegetable and fruit-based, to ensure you get the nutrients you need while helping your kidneys with the detoxification process. When choosing a juice, ensure that it's as natural as possible and freshly squeezed or pressed, if this option is available. Juices and smoothies can be squeezed, or prepared in a blender, though a freshly pressed juice is a best and easiest option.

POMEGRANATE JUICE

A tangy, delicious fruit, pomegranate is an excellent source of vitamin C and fiber. It's a great tasting snack on its own, sliced into quarters. The seeds have a variety of nutrients, including antioxidants. Juicing pomegranate is easily done with an electric juicer, or it can be pressed by hand. Before you discard the seeds after juicing, consider keeping them as a salad topping or a snack on their own. To prepare the pomegranate juice, take two large, ripe pomegranates and cut into quarters. Scrape the seeds and flesh from the peels and deposit into the juicer, and press. If you prefer to keep some of the seeds, remove them before adding the fruit to the press. Serve without any added sugar or salt and note that serving sizes may vary depending on the fruit's size and portion.

Pomegranate juice is a powerful support for the kidneys and especially effective while on dialysis. Studies support some benefits due to the high level of antioxidants, preventing the development of free radicals that contribute to infections and other complications such as inflammation, causing the overall condition to worsen if left untreated. It's a delicious juice that can easily fit into a daily

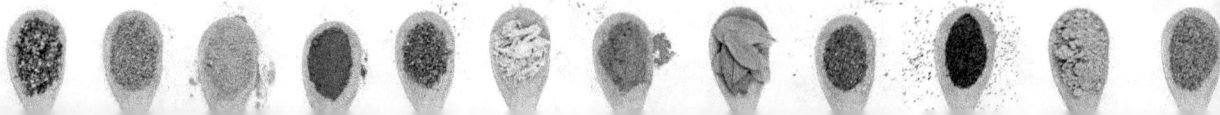

diet during any meal. Consuming pomegranate juice is also a good way to prevent kidney disease and high blood pressure while supporting overall immune health. (WebMD Health News, 2010)

APPLE CIDER VINEGAR

In recent years, apple cider vinegar has become a popular option for natural health remedies as a detoxifying agent and a way to support weight loss and overall health. While it's not considered a drink on its own, apple cider vinegar is often diluted to be consumed in water or juice, or taken in a capsule form, if not by spoon. One of the top benefits of regularly taking just one or two tablespoons each day is weight loss. Apple cider vinegar also improves hair and skin appearance and can help regulate insulin and decrease blood sugar. These benefits have the combined effect of supporting the kidneys and making their job a lot easier.

APPLE CIDER

A flavorful beverage hot or cold, apple cider is an excellent drink for kidney health. It's less intense than apple cider vinegar and often enjoyed as a warm beverage during the year's colder months. High in vitamin C, apple cider offers a good boost in antioxidants to the body, supporting the kidneys. It's a good alternative to hot chocolate and other hot drinks flavored with sugar and additives. To sweeten apple cider, add a dash of raw sugar, honey, or maple syrup.

CRANBERRY JUICE

Cranberry juice is an excellent diuretic and is often recommended to prevent and treat bladder infection and related difficulties. It acts as a diuretic because it helps the body flush out excess sodium while reducing water retention, much like water pills. It's a good source of vitamin C and fiber and can aid the kidneys in their function. Cranberry juice is naturally sweet and tangy, which makes it easy to enjoy. Cranberries also offer other benefits linked to kidney health, including fighting infection, improving urinary tract function, and improving digestion.

LEMON JUICE

Lemonade is often sweetened as the preferred lemon-based drink, though it's best to avoid sugary versions and add fresh lemon juice to various drinks or water to boost the vitamin C content. Adding one or two slices of lemon to a glass of iced or sparkling water is a good way to add a splash of flavor without sugar or artificial sweeteners.

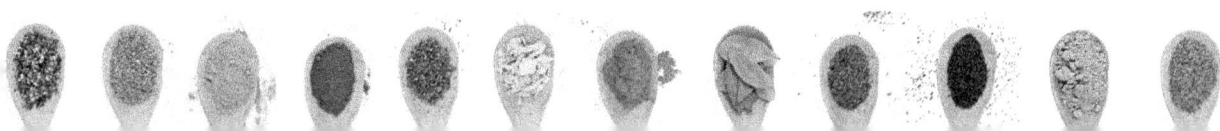

LIME JUICE

Like freshly squeezed lemon juice, lime can be used similarly as an added enhancement to water or another juice. Both limes and lemons are high in antioxidants and fiber, making them ideal for your overall health.

MINT AND LEMON WITH CRUSHED ICE

A thirst-quenching and refreshing drink, combining fresh mint leaves with squeezed lime and lemon juice, is a good way to satisfy your thirst and get many vitamins at once. Mint is easy to grow and harvest, or it can be found in fresh or dried varieties at your local market or grocery store. The leaves can be added whole, with ice cubes, sliced, and blended with lemon or lime juice and ice.

GRAPEFRUIT JUICE

Pink grapefruit is often chosen instead of the white variety due to its sweeter taste, though either option is excellent. Enjoyed as is or pressed into a juice, grapefruit can decrease the likelihood of kidney stone development while providing your body with vitamin C and fiber.

CARROT JUICE

The beta carotene in carrots is widely recognized as being good for your vision and eye health, but this is also the case when it comes to your renal function. Carrots offer a boost to the detoxification process, giving kidneys the added push, they need without causing any negative side effects. Carrots are also a delicious part of many meals, though the taste is stronger when consumed raw as a juice. For this reason, carrots are often juiced along with a few slices of apple or orange.

WINE

In moderation and small amounts, wine may offer some improvements in mild or moderate kidney disease cases. If you have a more advanced renal failure stage, you might want to avoid alcohol altogether or seek a medical opinion first. When selecting a wine, choose a dry, low-sugar option that will not increase glucose or blood sugar levels. Keep the drink size small and enjoy on occasion with a meal. Drink plenty of water after, like wine, like other alcoholic beverages, can deplete the body's water and require hydration. If you drink more than two glasses, be sure to increase your water intake and enjoy a small, healthy snack.

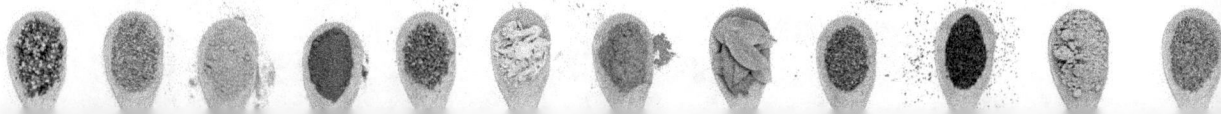

WATER

The best drink of all for any organs, including the kidneys, is water. Filtered and oxidized water options are often preferred in areas where there are high levels of contamination and concerns about toxicity, which, in large amounts, can harm the kidneys. If you are fortunate to have excellent quality water sources, make the most of it, and drink water often.

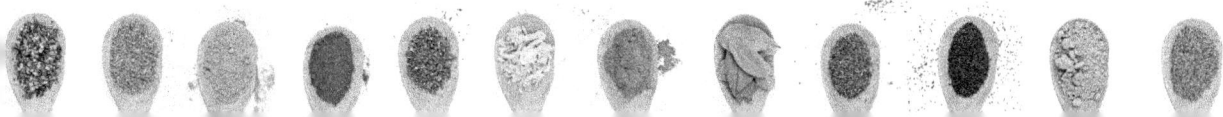

CHAPTER 10

BEST ADVICE TO AVOID DIALYSIS

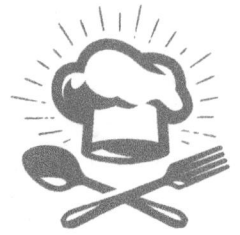

Even though it's frightening to be diagnosed with chronic kidney disease (CKD), if you discover in the beginning periods of the symptoms, there are steps you can take to keep away from dialysis. If you work intimately with your PCP, the odds are high you can, in any case, appreciate a refreshing personal satisfaction with kidney disease. Following excellent health practices and evading dialysis, remaining at work, and understanding social exercises are ways individuals can feel responsible for their condition. Notwithstanding doing everything physically and medicinally conceivable to maintain a strategic distance from dialysis, having an occupation with medical coverage gives security that pay, and medical advantages will be accessible. Here are portions of the means to take to maintain a strategic distance from the beginning of dialysis;

EAT RIGHT AND LOSE EXCESS WEIGHT

Consistently make sure to know about serving sizes. It's what you eat that includes calories, yet also how much. As you get in shape, make sure to follow a smart dieting plan that consists of an assortment of Nourishments.

EXERCISE CONSISTENTLY

Most dialysis patients accept they can't work out. In all certainty, most dialysis patients can work out. Numerous renal patients depict regular exercise as the principal action that made them feel "normal" again after beginning dialysis medications. Regardless of whether it is just for a brief timeframe every day, movement allows the patient with persistent kidney disease to feel good, more grounded, and more responsible for their health. Medicinal experts working in renal recovery have demonstrated that an ordinary exercise program, anyway restricted, not just upgrades an

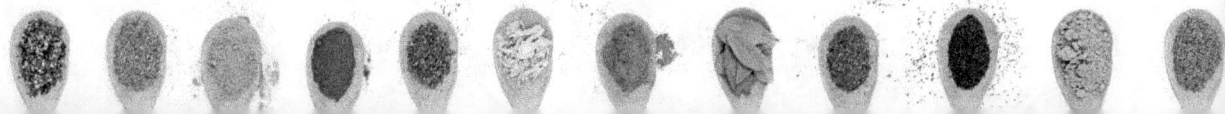

individual's potential for physical action, also improves the general personal satisfaction for individuals on dialysis. Exercise can also help the kidney symptoms patient recover the function to perform activities they were delighted in before being analyzed.

TRY NOT TO SMOKE

In case you smoke, there is, in all likelihood, no other choice you can make to help your health more than stopping. While an on-going examination found that smokers lose ten years of life expectancy at any rate than people who never smoked, in like manner found that people who halted by age 40 reduce their risk of smoking-related death by 90 rates.

BE CAUTIOUS OF YOUR GLUCOSE LEVELS

For good preventive health, cut back on soda pop, treats, and sugary baked goods, which can make glucose rise. If you have diabetes, this can hurt your heart, kidneys, eyes, and nerves after some time. Directing glucose is one of seven estimations for heart health, according to the American Heart Association. These equal estimations make it less slanted to be resolved to have malignancy.

FATTY INTAKE

the body needs calories for daily activities and looks after temperature, development, and sufficient body weight. Calories are provided mostly via starches and fats. The standard caloric necessity of CKD patients is 35 - 40 kcal/kg body weight every day. If caloric intake is insufficient, the body uses protein to get calories. This breakdown of protein can prompt severe impacts, for example, lack of healthy sustenance and a more prominent composition of waste items. It is along these lines basic to give a sufficient measure of calories to CKD patients. It is essential to ascertain the caloric necessity indicated by a patient's optimal body weight and not current weight.

STARCHES

These are the essential source of calories for the body. Starches are found in wheat, grains, rice, potatoes, organic products, sugar, nectar, treats, cakes, desserts, and beverages. People with diabetes and fat patients need to confine the measure of starches. It is ideal to use complex sugars from grains like entire wheat and unpolished rice, giving fiber. These should form a large segment of the sugars in the eating regimen. All other basic sugar-containing substances should form not over 20% of the total starch consumption, particularly in diabetic patients. Non-diabetic patients may exchange calories from protein with starches as natural products, pies, cakes, treats, jam, or nectar as long as sweets with chocolate, nuts, or bananas are restricted.

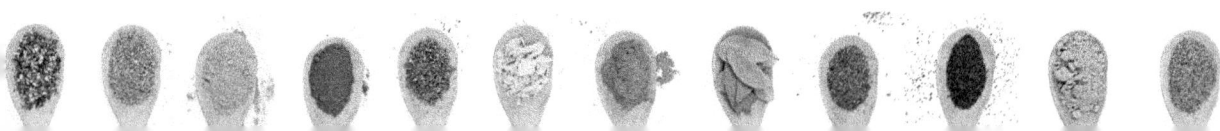

Unsaturated or great fats like olive oil, nut oil, canola oil, safflower oil, sunflower oil, fish, and nuts are superior to saturated or "terrible" fats, for example, red meat, poultry, whole milk, margarine, ghee, cheese, coconut, and grease. Patients with CKD ought to diminish their intake of immersed fats and cholesterol, as these can cause heart disease. Excessive omega-6 polyunsaturated fats (PUFA) and an extremely high omega-6/omega-3 proportion are unsafe, while low omega-6/omega-3 balance applies valuable impacts. Blends of vegetable oil, as opposed to single oil use, will accomplish this reason. Trans fat-containing substances like potato chips, doughnuts, financially arranged treats, and cakes are potentially hurtful and should be avoided.

LIMIT PROTEIN INTAKE

Protein is fundamental for the fix and upkeep of body tissues. It additionally helps in the mending of wounds and battling against disease. Protein confinement (< 0.8 gm/kg body weight/day) is prescribed for CKD patients not on dialysis to diminish the pace of decreased kidney function and defer the requirement for dialysis and kidney transplantation. Serious protein restriction should be kept away from anyway, given the danger of lack of healthy sustenance. Poor craving is normal in CKD patients. Poor hunger and severe protein restriction together can prompt poor sustenance, weight reduction, absence of vitality, and decrease in body opposition, which increment the danger of death. The consumption of protein enhancements and medications, like creatine utilized for muscle advancement, is best kept away from except if affirmed by a physician or dietician. Protein intake should be expanded to 1.0 – 1.2 gm./kg body weight/day to supplant the proteins lost during the methodology when a patient is on dialysis.

FLUID INTAKE

The kidneys play a significant role in maintaining the amount of water in the body by expelling excess fluid as urine. In patients with CKD, as the kidney function exacerbates, the volume of urine generally reduces. Decreased urine yield prompts fluid maintenance in the body, causing puffiness of the face, growing of the legs and hands, and hypertension. The gathering of fluid in the lungs (a condition called pneumonic blockage or edema) causes shortness of breath and trouble in relaxing. If this isn't controlled, it tends to be hazardous. Excess water in the body is called fluid over-burden. Leg growing (edema), ascites (aggregation of fluid in the stomach pit), the brevity of breath, and weight gain in a brief period are the pieces of information that suggest fluid over-burden.

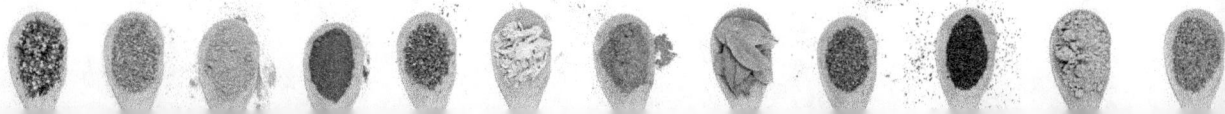

CHAPTER 11

30 DAY MEAL PLAN

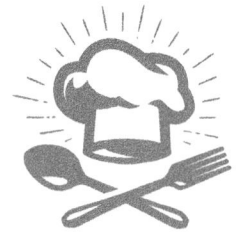

The right approach to a healthy diet is getting a balanced proportion of all necessary nutrients. Balanced diets are not meant for people with healthy kidneys alone. It is possible to get meals having all the vital body requirements even when you are on a specific nutrient restriction therapy. A balanced renal-healthy meal should have the right proportion of calories, proteins, vegetables, fruits, and water. As you know, they have their specific roles in ensuring that the kidneys remain healthy.

Meal planning involves including these in a single serving of food. The point of emphasis is that food should be enjoyed, even when you may have to let go of some things. There are essentials to successful meal planning. The following are some generally useful tips:

- Have an objective. Why are you planning your meals? In this case, the goal is to have healthier kidneys. Your overall aim may be broken down into measurable aims to assess how you are doing.
- A handy knowledge of what you need. Equip yourself with the pros and cons of the renal diet so that there are no blurred lines.
- Although you may not need to make regular visits to a dietician at this stage, it will be good to have one look over the meal plan. There may need to make additions or subtractions. Emphasis is on individuality in this plan. Therefore, your dietician may need to go over the plan to be sure it is tailored to meet your specific needs. If you don't have one, consult your doctor.
- Be open-minded. There may be restrictions that make you unhappy but bear in mind that this is not for nothing. The little inconvenience can't be compared with the healthy results.

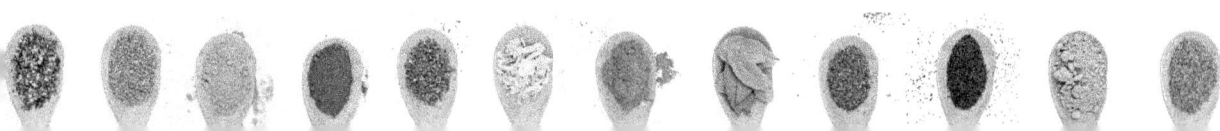

- Be flexible with your plans. It is good to have interchangeable alternatives when planning meals.
- Work with your budget. What is the essence of organizing what you will eat if you end up stressing yourself over the money? Work on a diet based on your financial capability.

Meal planning is not without its benefits.

- It helps to maximize time, resources, and money.

With meal planning, you can reason thoroughly on the menu, putting whatever is available into good use, and minimizing wastage. There is no rush, and you are relaxed. You also end up saving yourself some energy because everything is organized.

- Planning your meals puts a personal touch on it.

It gives you gratification and a sense of belonging. It does feel good to do something meaningful for oneself, especially when the news of chronic kidney disease is taking its toll on your emotions.

- Helps in creating colorful, delicious, and appealing meals.

Eating goes beyond just having to put something in the stomach. It should come with a satisfaction that is more than just killing your hunger.

- It helps in adherence.

Dieting needs discipline. When you think about the food or edibles you need to do without, you may get tempted to ditch everything and throw caution to the wind.

- It takes care of the craving.

You may feel the urge to binge on some forbidden foods at times. However, with a handy meal menu from adequate planning, it becomes easier to curb it and go with what you have. Sometimes, excessive hunger is what leads to bingeing. When you feel hungry, and there is nothing to satisfy it, your body changes, secreting hormones that heighten the sense of hunger so much that you will eat the available food if there is no control.

- Meal planning curbs extravagant spending during shopping.

You know what you need. Therefore, your trip to the grocery yields only the essentials and unnecessary stuff, something most people find difficult to do.

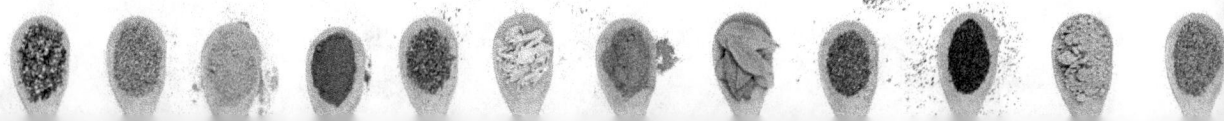

DAYS	BREAKFAST	LUNCH	DINNER
1	Apple Cherry Breakfast Risotto	Lettuce Wraps with Chicken	Cilantro-Lime Flounder
2	Creamy Keto Cucumber Salad	Peanut Butter and Jelly Grilled Sandwich	Minced Beef Samosa
3	Tasty Beef and Liver Burger	Crispy Lemon Chicken	Green Tuna Salad
4	Shredded Chicken Chili	Grilled Corn on the Cob	Meatloaf Sandwiches
5	Hot Fruit Salad	Cucumber Sandwich	Roasted Chicken and Vegetables
6	Bacon and Cheese Quiche	Ciabatta Rolls with Chicken Pesto	Salmon and Green Beans
7	Egg and Broccoli Casserole	Mexican Steak Tacos	Mango Cheesecake Smoothie
8	Berries and Cream Breakfast Cake	Marinated Shrimp Pasta Salad	Cucumber and Dill Cold Soup
9	Spinach Goat Cheese & Chorizo Omelet	Pizza Pitas	Herb-Crusted Baked Haddock
10	Rice Milk	Beer Pork Ribs	Pizza Pitas
11	Mexican Style Burritos	Grilled Shrimp with Cucumber Lime Salsa	Baked Macaroni & Cheese
12	Blueberry Muffins	Eggplant Casserole	Beef Enchiladas
13	Berry Chia with Yogurt	Turkey Pinwheels	Eggplant Casserole
14	Cheesy Scrambled Egg with Fresh Herbs	Asparagus Fried Rice	Chicken Stew
15	Egg and Veggie Muffins	Shrimp Scampi Linguine	Simple Cabbage Soup
16	Turkey and Spinach Scramble	Vegetable Minestrone	Cilantro and Chili Infused Swordfish

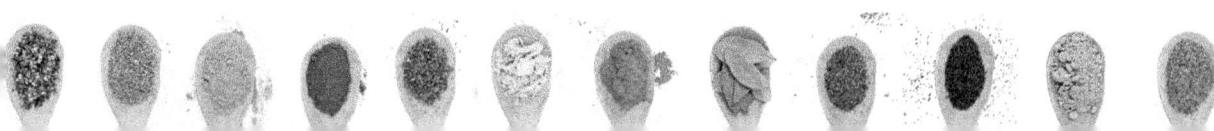

17	Bucket wheat and Grapefruit Porridge	Thai Fish Soup	Feta Bean Salad
18	Apple Pie	Chicken Tacos	Chicken and Savory Rice
19	Eggplant Chicken Sandwich	Curried Carrot and Beet Soup	Chicken and Broccoli Casserole
20	Panzanella Salad	Chicken and Broccoli Casserole	Couscous with Veggies
21	Chorizo Bowl with Corn	Vegetable Biryani	Pork Souvlaki
22	Eggs in Tomato Rings	Simple Chicken and Rice Soup	Cauliflower Rice
23	Arugula Eggs with Chili Peppers	Tuna Twist	Meatball Soup
24	Hot Cocoa	Mexican Chorizo Sausage	Sunny Pineapple Smoothie
25	Bulgur, Couscous and Bucket wheat Cereal	Pesto Pasta Salad	Mexican Chorizo Sausage
26	Poached Asparagus and Egg	Tuna Twist	Creamy Shells with Peas and Bacon
27	Spinach and Ham Frittata	Grilled Onion and Pepper Jack Grilled Cheese Sandwich	Double-Boiled Stewed Potatoes
28	Blueberry Smoothie	Shrimp Quesadilla	Barley Blueberry Avocado Salad
29	Egg Drop Soup	Spicy Mushroom Stir-Fry	Taco Soup
30	Hot Fruit Salad	Pizza with Chicken and Pesto	Spicy Mushroom Stir-Fry

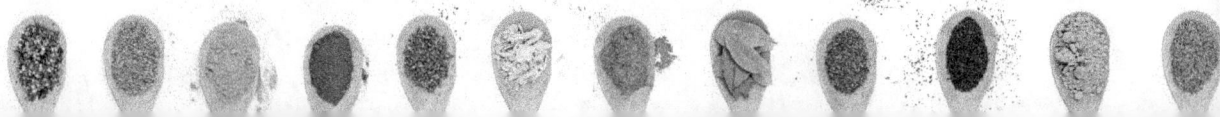

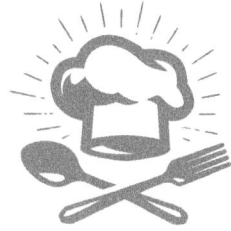

CHAPTER 12

BREAKFAST RECIPES

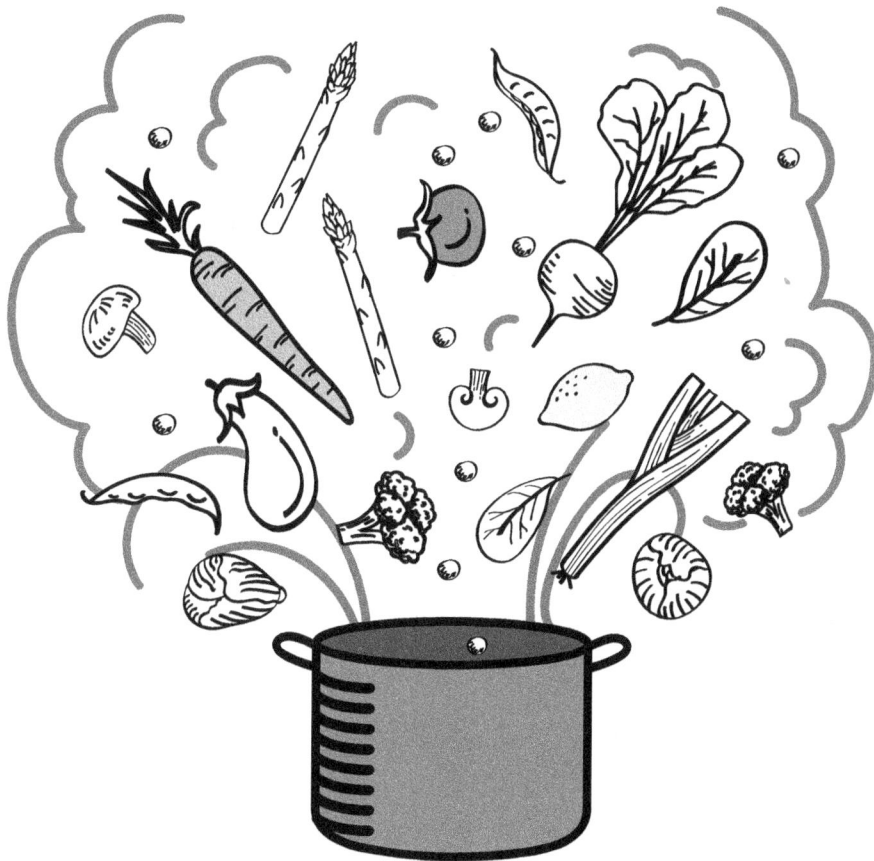

1 TASTY BEEF AND LIVER BURGER

Preparation Time: 5 minutes

Cooking Time: 5 minutes

Servings: 4

INGREDIENTS:

- ½ medium red onion, peeled
- 1 tsp sea salt
- 1 tsp poultry seasoning
- ¼ pound chicken livers
- pounds beef
- 1 ½ tsp coriander
- 1 tsp ground black pepper

DIRECTIONS:

1. Add the onion and chicken liver to a food processor and process until blended.
2. Put in the ground beef and all the ingredients.
3. Blend for about 1 minute until the ingredients combined thoroughly.
4. Mold the mixture into four-inch wide patties.
5. Broil patties until it is done to your desired taste.
6. Serve on a lettuce wrap or hamburger and enjoy it.

NUTRITION:

Calories: 220
Fat: 4g
Protein: 23g
Sodium: 78mg
Potassium: 344.7mg
Phosphorus: 461mg

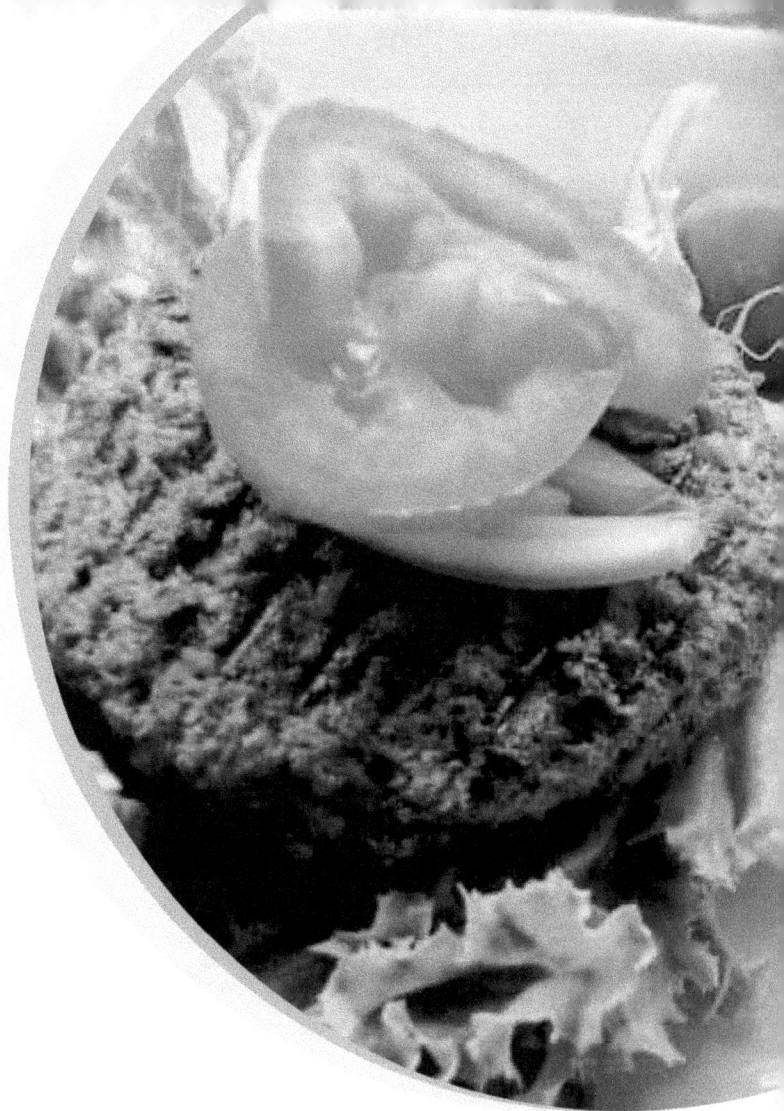

2 CREAMY KETO CUCUMBER SALAD

Preparation Time: 5 minutes

Cooking Time: 5 minutes

Servings: 1

INGREDIENTS:

- 2 tbsp of mayo
- Freshly ground pepper
- 2 tbsp lemon juice
- 1 cucumber about 220grams, sliced

DIRECTIONS:

1. Combine the mayo, lemon juice, and cucumber strips in a medium bowl
2. Put salt and pepper to taste.
3. Serve and enjoy.

NUTRITION:

Calories: 77
Fat: 5g
Carbs: 6g
Protein: 1g
Sodium: 150mg
Potassium: 99mg
Phosphorus: 17mg

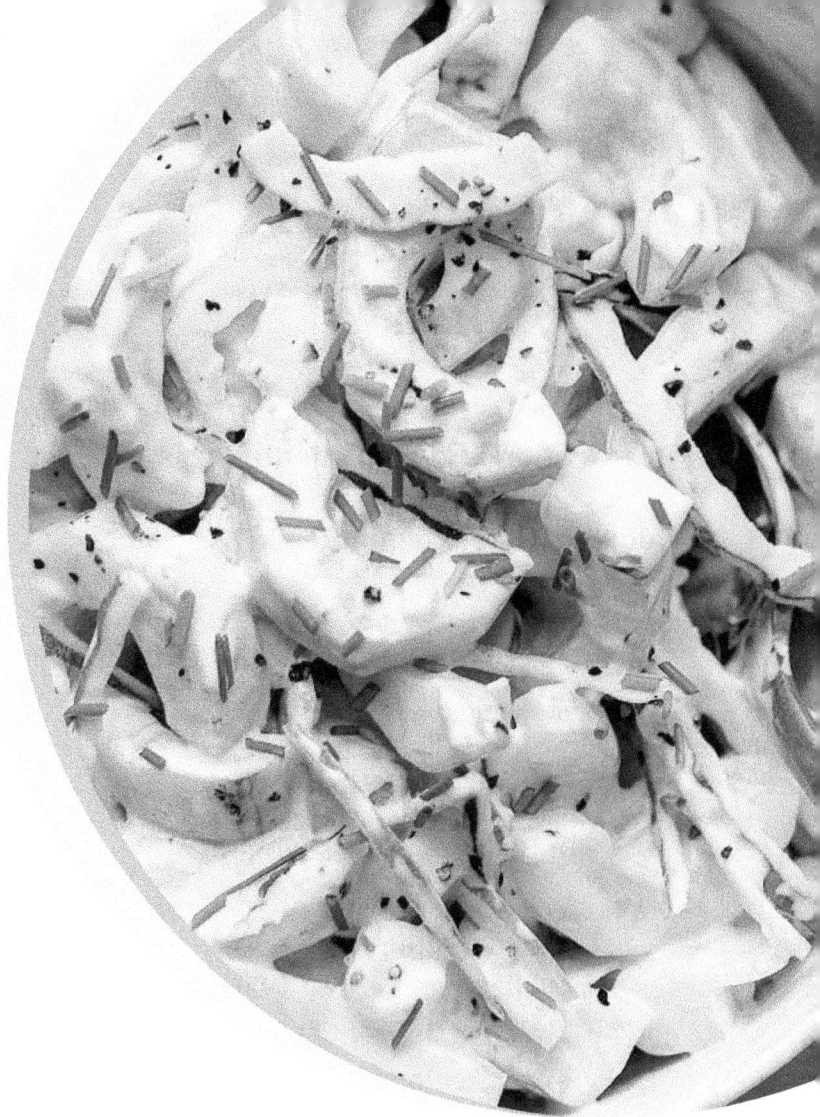

3 SHREDDED CHICKEN CHILI

Preparation Time: 10 minutes

Cooking Time: 25 minutes

Servings: 1

INGREDIENTS:

- 1 tbsp butter
- 1 jalapeno pepper, diced
- 2 oz tomato paste
- ½ tbsp garlic powder
- 10 oz diced tomatoes canned
- Salt and pepper to taste
- 4 chicken breasts, shredded
- 1 tbsp chili powder
- 2 cups chicken broth
- 4 oz cream cheese
- ½ onion, diced
- 1 tbsp cumin

DIRECTIONS:

1. Add chicken breast and water to a sizable pot and bring to a boil for 10 to 12 minutes.
2. Once well cooked, take out of the heat and crumble with two forks.
3. Add butter to a large pot and melt over medium to high heat.
4. Add onion and sauté until tender.
5. Add the chicken broth, chili powder, shredded chicken, garlic powder, cumin, and jalapeno to the pot and stir well until evenly blended.
6. Cook over medium to low heat and cover with lid for 10 minutes.
7. Chop cream cheese into 1-inch small strips.

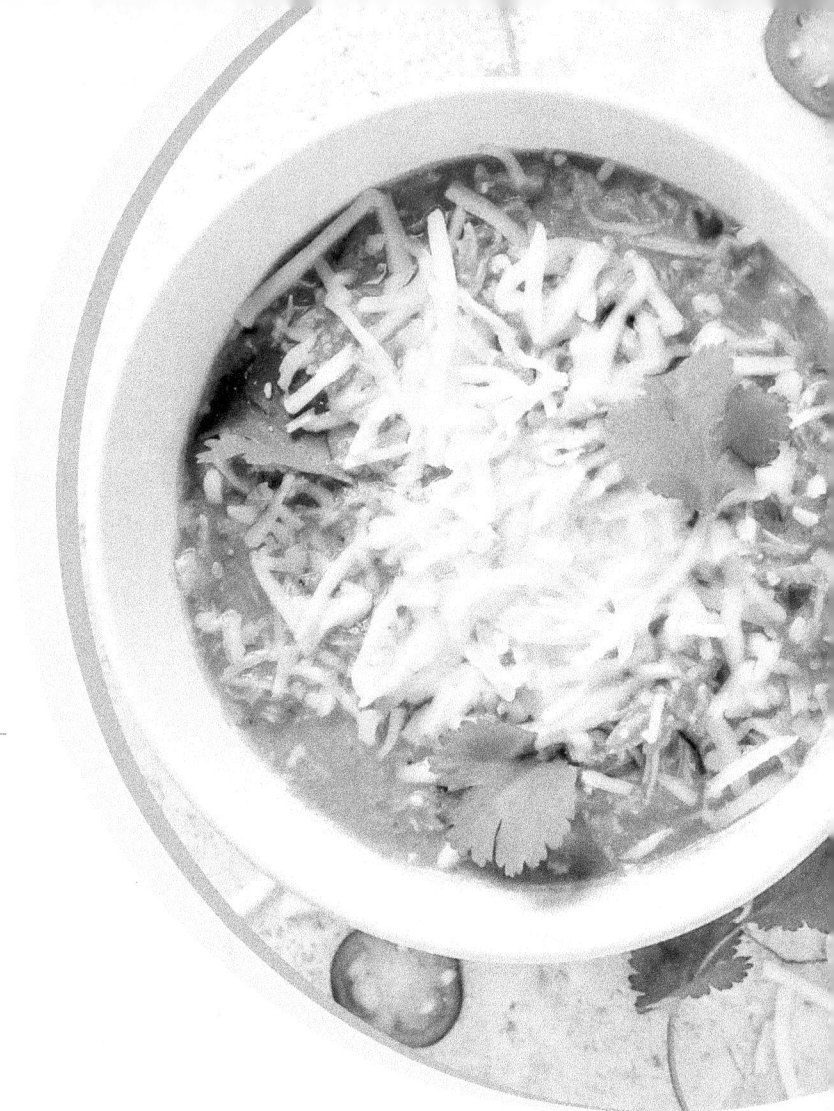

8. Remove the cover and whisk in the cream cheese. Increase the heat to medium-high and keep on whisking until the cream cheese combined thoroughly.

9. Take out of the heat and add salt and pepper to taste. Serve and sprinkle with any desired toppings and enjoy.

NUTRITION:

Calories: 330
Fat: 2.8g
Carbs: 38g
Protein: 38g
Sodium: 716mg
Potassium: 970.7mg
Phosphorus: 421mg

4 SPINACH, GOAT CHEESE & CHORIZO OMELET

Preparation Time: 5 minutes

Cooking Time: 10 minutes

Servings: 1

INGREDIENTS:

- 4 eggs
- 4 ounces chorizo sausage
- ½ tbsp butter
- 1/4 cup salsa Verde (optional)
- 1 tbsp water
- 2 cups baby spinach leaves
-
  2 ounces shredded fresh goat cheese
- Avocado, diced

DIRECTIONS:

1. In a medium-sized frying pan, take out chorizo from the casing and sauté until thoroughly cooked.
2. Meanwhile, add water to a small bowl and beat in the eggs.
3. Remove the chorizo from the skillet with a spoon and keep aside. Clean off the skillet of the remaining oil with a paper towel.
4. Over a moderate flame, melt the butter in the same skillet.
5. Put the cracked eggs in the skillet, and then add the spinach, chorizo, and shredded goat cheese to half of the mixture of the eggs.
6. Heat on low flame for about 3 minutes until a bit dense, then add in the filling and fold over.

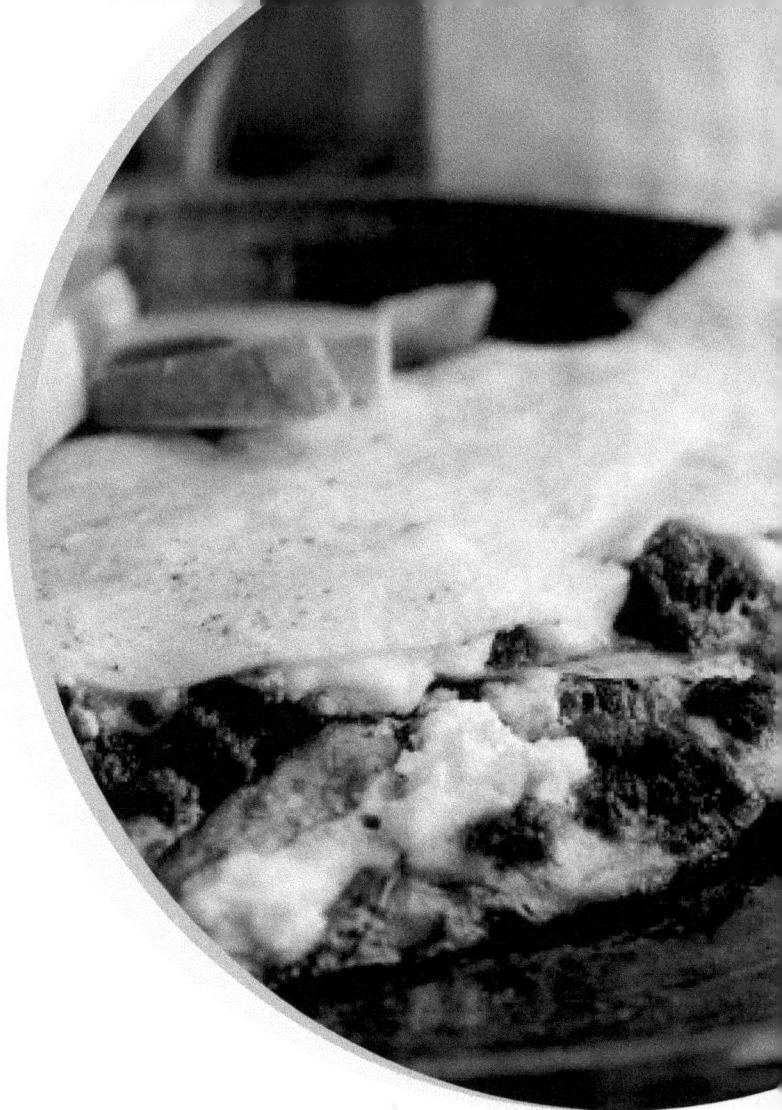

7. Cover the skillet with a pot cover and cook on a moderate flame for few minutes until the eggs are evenly cooked.

8. Turn off the stove and allow skillet cover for about 8 minutes while it gets cooked with the extra heat. Serve with slices of avocado and salsa.

NUTRITION:

Calories: 324
Fat: 15.5g
Carbs: 26g
Protein: 21g
Sodium: 389mg
Potassium: 501.3mg
Phosphorus: 238mg

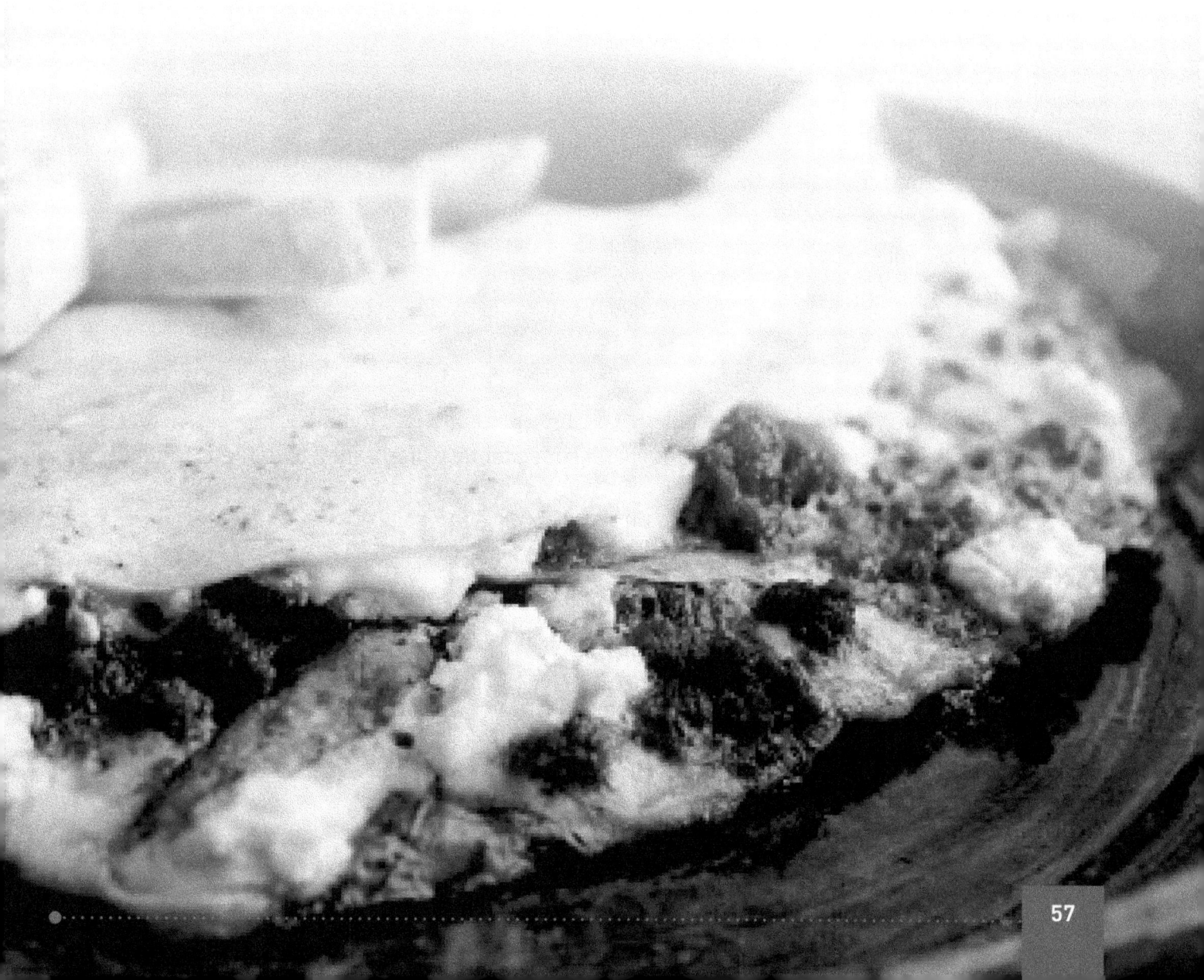

5 APPLE CHERRY BREAKFAST RISOTTO

Preparation Time: 10 minutes

Cooking Time: 15 minutes

Servings: 1

INGREDIENTS:

- 2 large apples, cored and chopped
- 1 ½ cups arborio rice
- ½ cup dried cherries
- 1 ½ tsp cinnamon
- 2 tbsp butter
- ¼ tsp salt
- 1 cup apple juice
- 3 cups of milk

DIRECTIONS:

1. Add butter to the pressure-cooking pot and heat for 2 to 3 minutes.
2. Whisk in the rice, continue heating, and consistently whisk until rice darkens for about 3 to 4 minutes.
3. Put the spices, brown sugar, and apples.
4. Whisk in the juice and milk.
5. Set pressure cooker to high pressure and select 6 minutes cook time and heat.
6. Once the timer beeps, unplug the cooker and use a fast pressure release to release the pressure.
7. Gently remove the lid of the pressure cooker and whisk in dried cherries.
8. Serve hot, and garnish with extra sliced almonds, brown sugar, and milk.

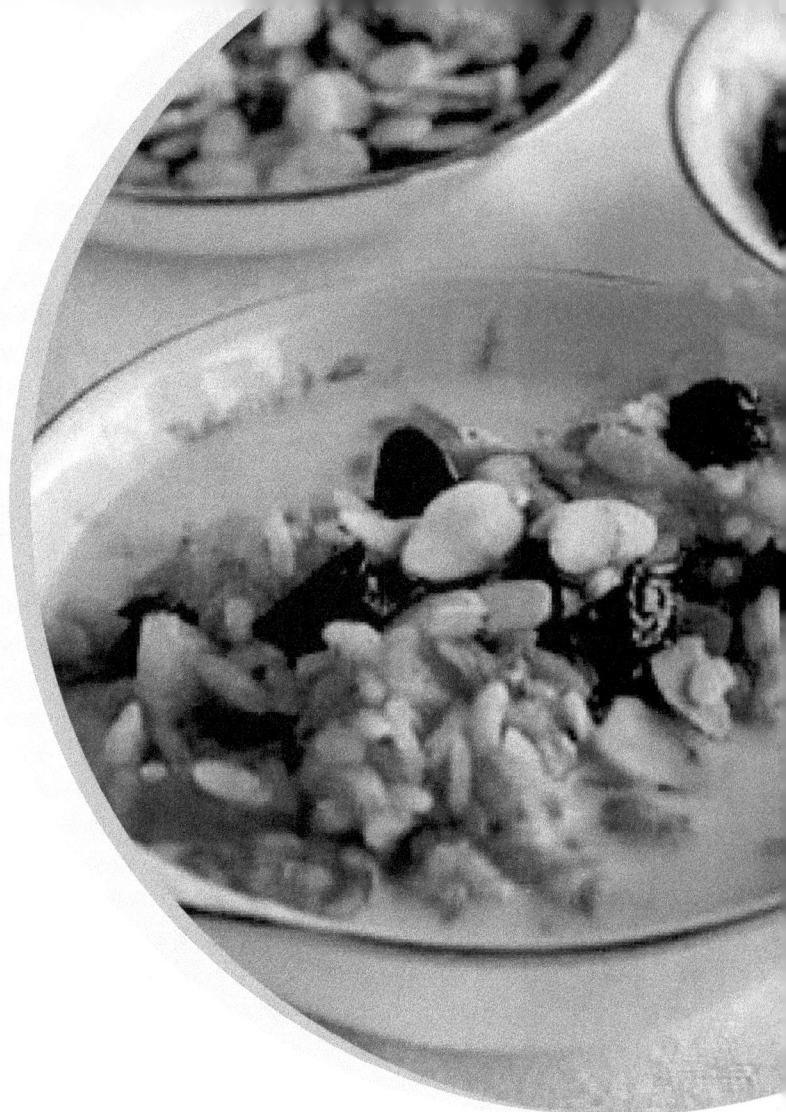

Calories: 258
Fat: 3g
Carbs: 50g
Protein: 10g
Sodium: 227mg
Potassium: 580mg
Phosphorus: 150mg

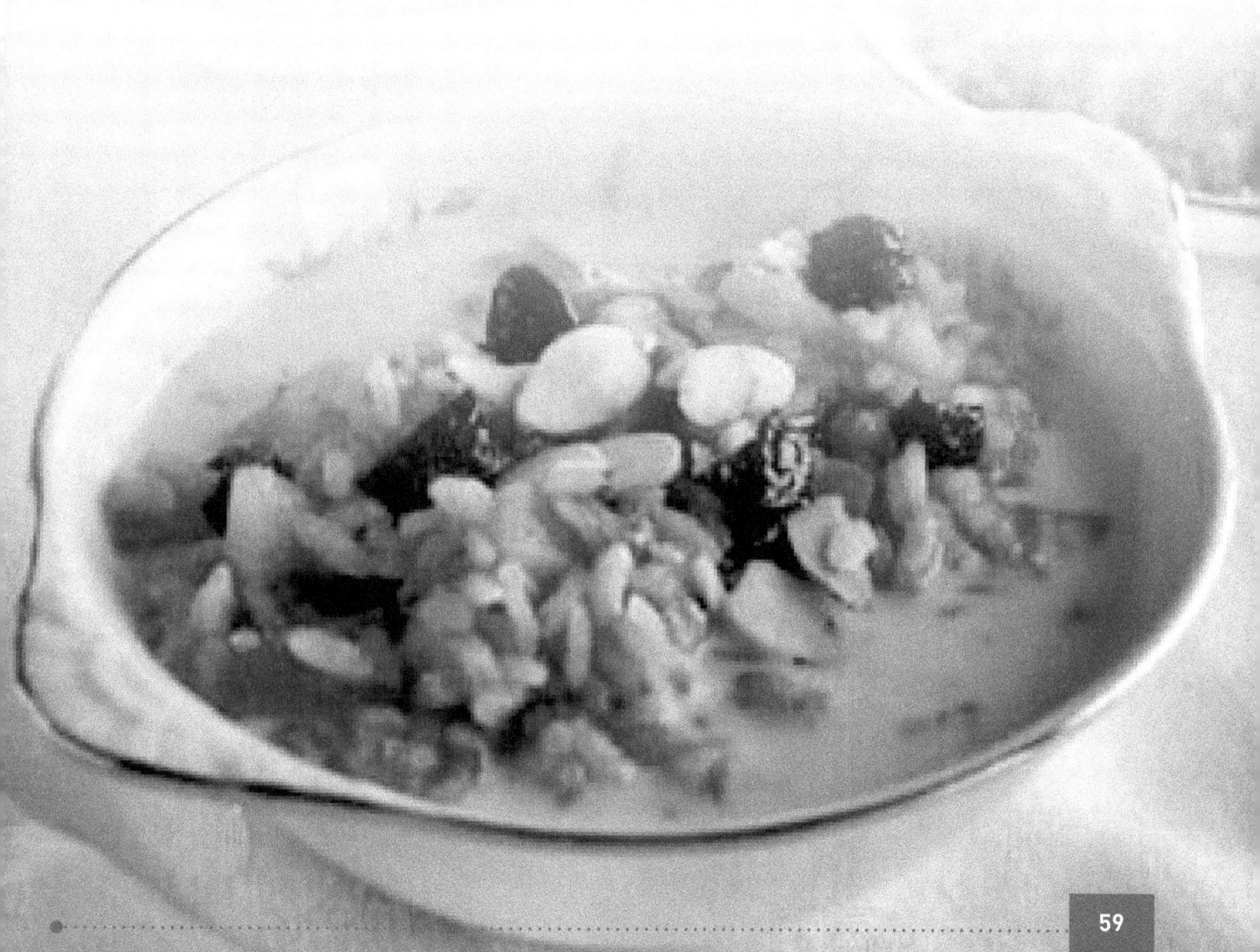

6 BERRIES AND CREAM BREAKFAST CAKE

Preparation Time: 15 minutes

Cooking Time: 35 minutes

Servings: 1

INGREDIENTS:

- 5 eggs
- ¼ cup of sugar
- 2 tbsp butter, melted
- ¾ cup ricotta cheese
- Sweet yogurt glaze
- Berry Compote
- 2 tsp vanilla extract
- ½ tsp salt
- 1 cup of whole white wheat flour or wheat pastry flour
- 2 tsp baking powder
- ½ cup berry compote

For the sweet yogurt glaze

- ½ tsp vanilla extract
- ¼ cup yogurt
- 1 to 2 tbsp powdered sugar
- 1 tsp milk

DIRECTIONS:

1. First, make ready the berry compote to chill and become thick.
2. For the cake, thoroughly oil a pan with a non-stick cooking spray.
3. Mix the eggs and sugar until blended.

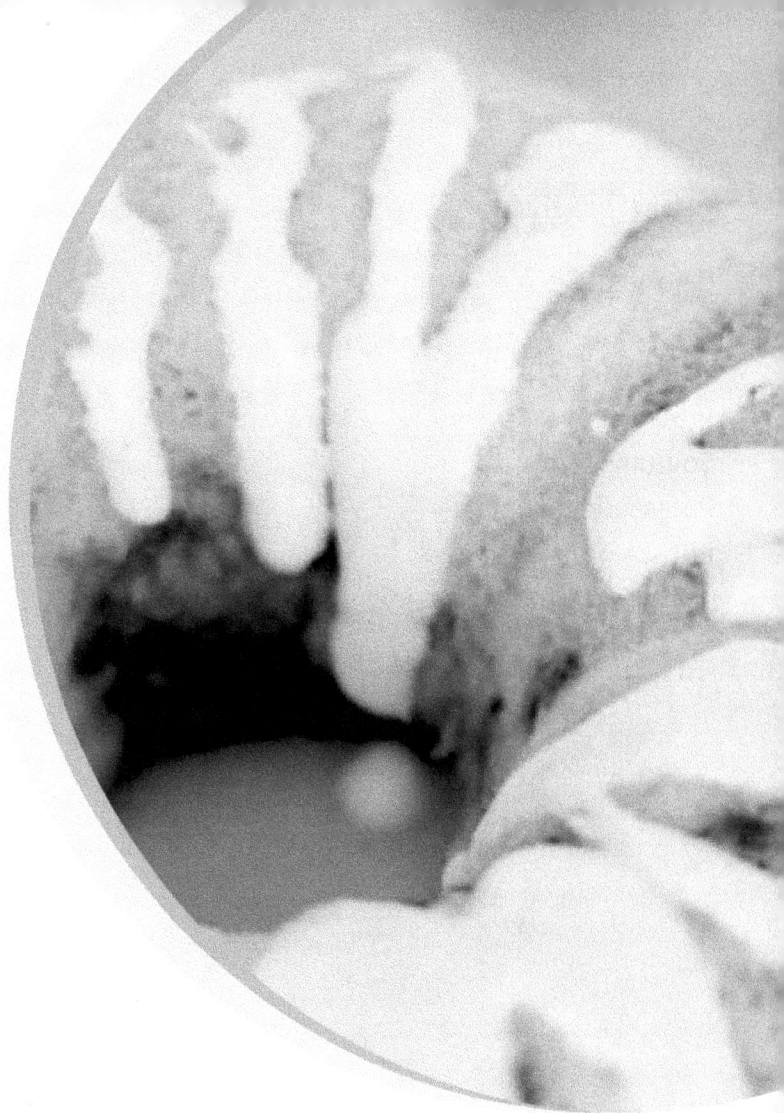

4. Add the ricotta cheese, butter, vanilla, yogurt, and stir until blended.
5. Mix salt, baking powder, and the flour in a separate bowl.
6. Add to the egg mixture. Turn into the prepared pan.
7. With a tablespoon, drop 1/2 cup of berry compote on top of the batter and whisk with a knife.
8. Turn 1 cup of water in the pressure cooker pot and set in the steamer basket. Gently position the pan on the steamer basket.
9. Set the pressure to high. Heat for about 25 minutes.
10. While cooking the cake, prepare the sweet yogurt glaze by mixing the vanilla, yogurt, powdered sugar, and milk.
11. Keep aside. Once cooking is completed, use a normal release to vent pressure for 10 minutes and then release any further pressure.
12. Take out the pan from the pressure cooker. Allow chilling a bit. Loosen the edges of the cake off the pan and lightly pour on a plate.
13. Sprinkle with sweet yogurt glaze and serve hot.

NUTRITION:

Calories: 275
Fat: 13g
Carbs: 36g
Protein: 5g
Sodium: 110.8mg
Potassium: 175.6mg
Phosphorus: 78mg

EGG AND BROCCOLI CASSEROLE

Preparation Time: 15 minutes

Cooking Time: 3 hours

Servings: 1

INGREDIENTS:

- ½ tsp salt
- 3 cups frozen, sliced broccoli, thawed and drained
- 6 eggs
- 3 tbsp thinly sliced onion
- 2 cups crumbled cheddar cheese
- ¼ cup butter softened
- 3 cups of cottage cheese
- Extra crumbled cheddar cheese, optional
- 1/3 cup all-purpose flour

DIRECTIONS:

1. Combine all the ingredients in a sizable bowl. Turn into a greased instant pot.
2. Set in the lid and cook on high for 1 hour, then whisk.
3. Lower the heat, place in the lid and cook for an additional 2 hours 30 minutes to 3 hours until a thermometer shows 160 degrees.
4. Unplug the cooker, take out your meal and spread in cheese, and enjoy.

NUTRITION:

Calories: 260
Fat: 13g
Carbs: 10g
Protein: 23g

Sodium: 335mg
Potassium: 161.6mg
Phosphorus: 82.8mg

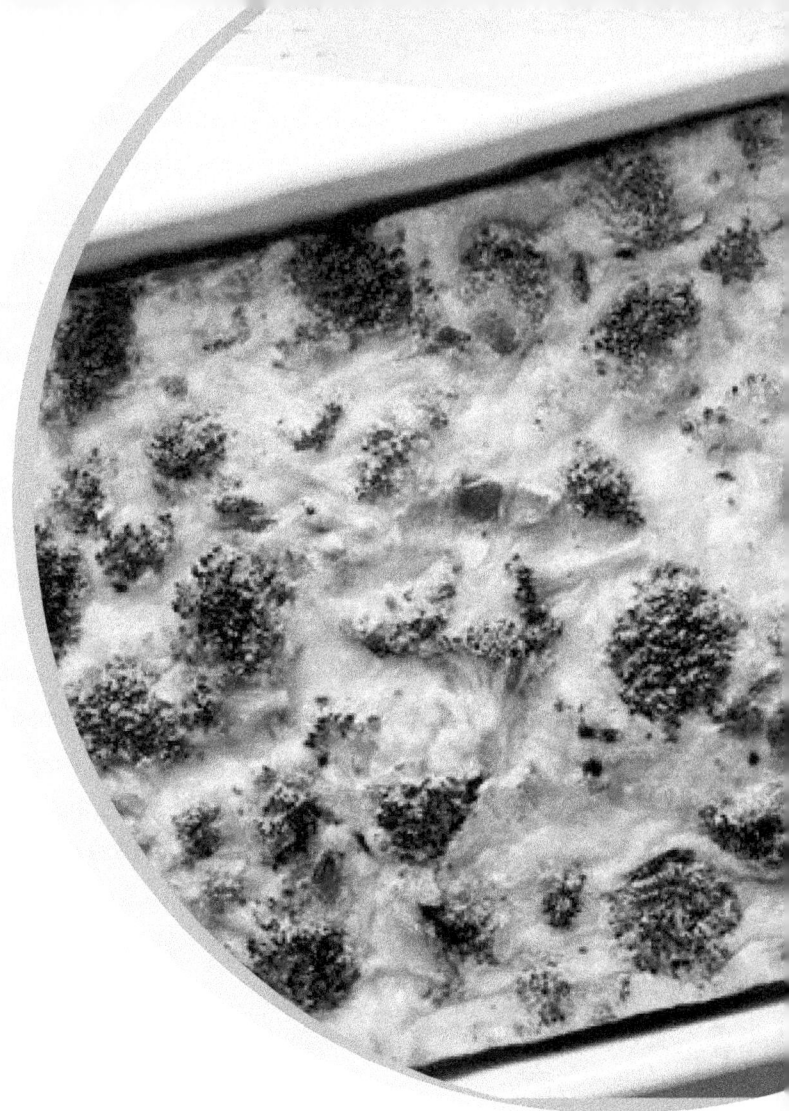

8 SPINACH AND HAM FRITTATA

Preparation Time: 15 minutes

Cooking Time: 2 – 3 hours

Servings: 1

INGREDIENTS:

- 1 tsp coconut oil
- 8 eggs, whisked
- ½ tsp pepper
- 1 small onion, sliced
- 1 tsp sea salt
- 2 cloves garlic
- 2 cups spinach, diced
- 1 cup ham, sliced
- ½ cup of canned coconut milk

DIRECTIONS:

1. Melt coconut oil in a medium pan.
2. Put onion and garlic and cook until softened.
3. Pour the mixture of the garlic and onion in the instant pot.
4. Add in the ham and spinach.
5. Whisk ingredients until well blended.
6. In a separate bowl, combine coconut milk, whisked egg mixture, salt, pepper, and whisked with a stirrer until well blended.
7. Turn the mixture into the cooking pot and stir well.
8. Set the cooker to low and cook for 4 to 6 hours until the egg is set. You can as well set to high and cook for 2 to 3 hours.
9. Once done, serve warm and enjoy.

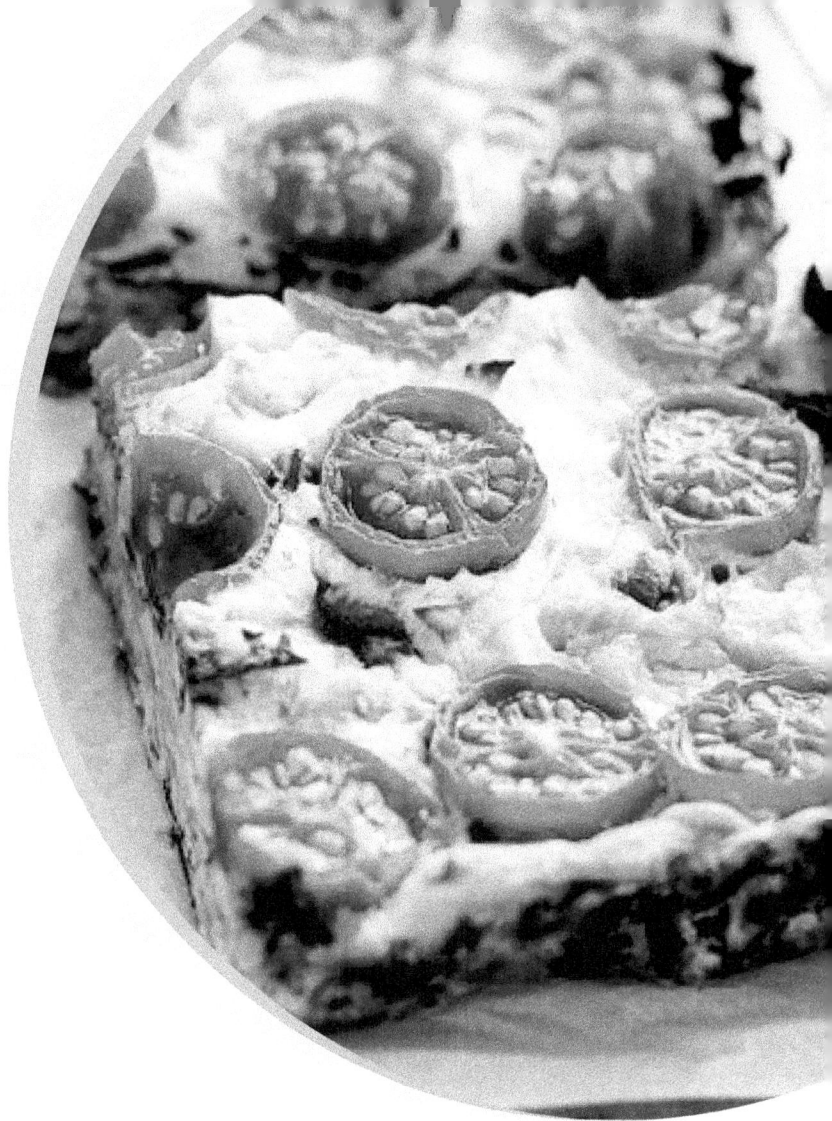

Calories: 390
Fat: 24g
Carbs: 6g
Protein: 35g
Sodium: 847mg
Potassium: 145.9mg
Phosphorus: 41mg

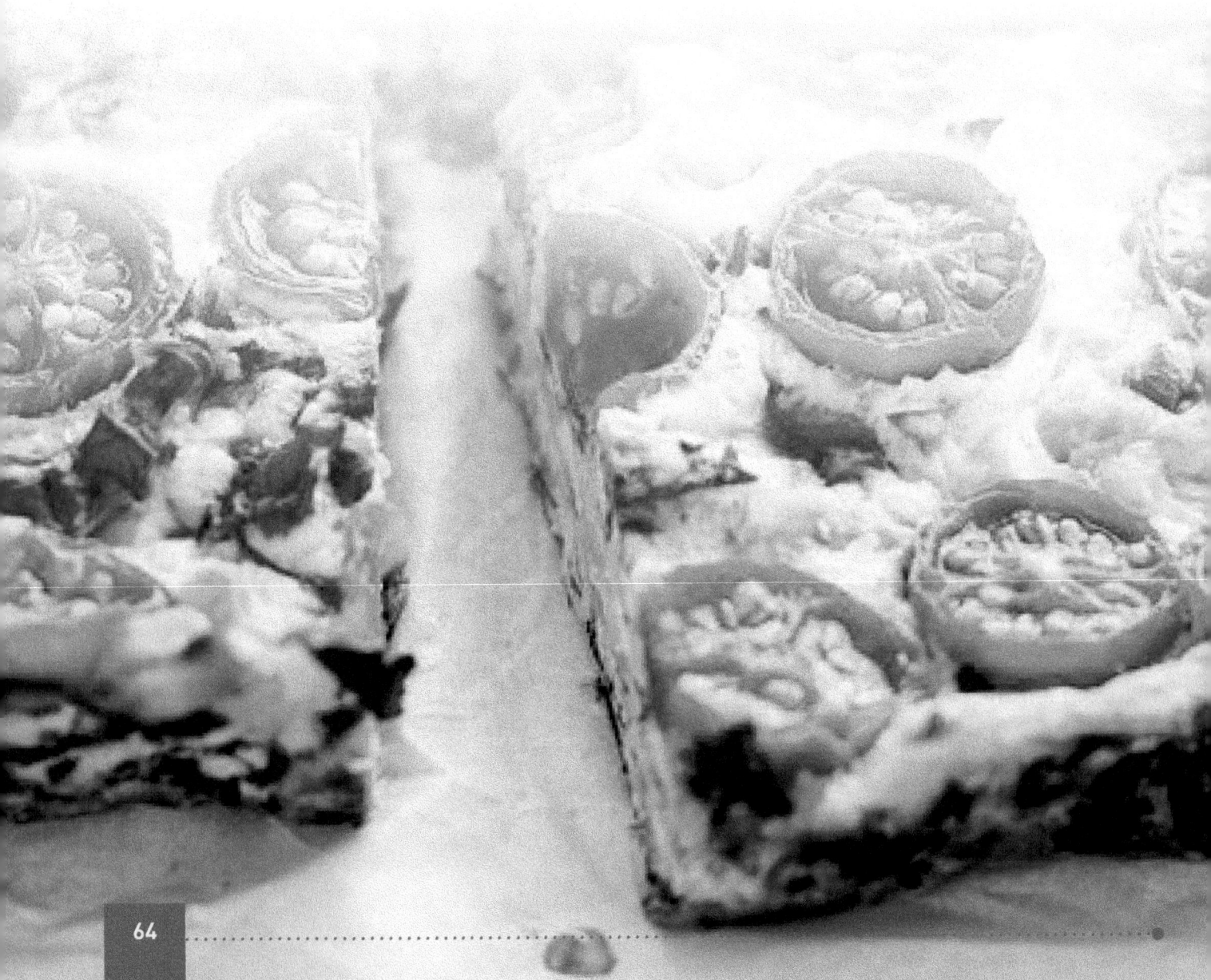

9 HOT FRUIT SALAD

Preparation Time: 10 minutes

Cooking Time: 2 – 3 hours

Servings: 1

INGREDIENTS:

- ¾ cups of sugar
- ¼ tsp ground nutmeg
- ¼ cup dried cranberries
- ½ cup butter, melted
- ¼ tsp ground cinnamon
- 1/8 tsp salt
- ½ cup dried apricots, sliced
- 2 (15 1/4-ounce) cans of chopped peaches, drained
- 2 (15 1/4-ounce) cans of diced pears, not drained
- One 23-ounce jar of chunky applesauce

DIRECTIONS:

1. Mix the butter, sugar, nutmeg, cinnamon, and salt in the instant pot.
2. Turn in the rest ingredients.
3. Place in the lid and cook on high until evenly cooked.
4. Allow cooling and then serve.

NUTRITION:

Calories: 152
Fat: 0.1g
Carbs: 39g
Protein: 0.7g
Sodium: 15mg
Potassium: 220.6mg
Phosphorus: 21mg

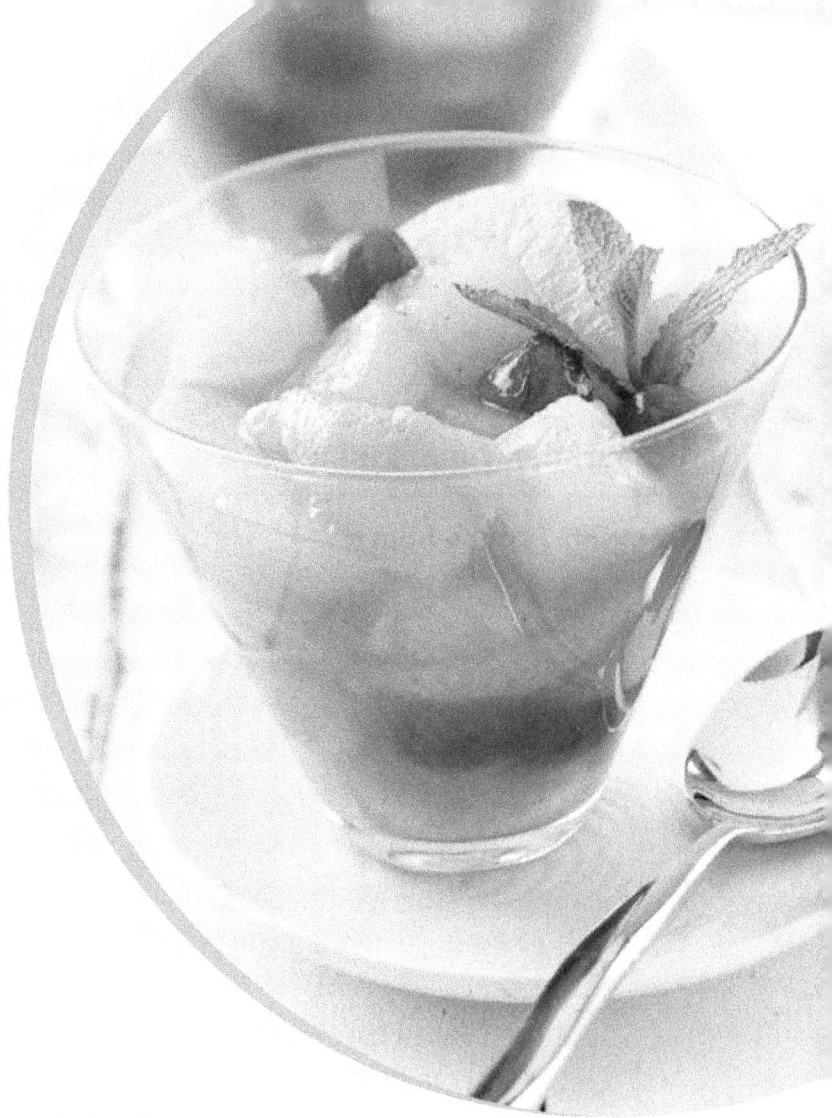

10 BACON AND CHEESE QUICHE

Preparation Time: 5 minutes

Cooking Time: 4 hours

Servings: 1

INGREDIENTS:

- 1 cup milk
- ¼ tsp salt
- ¼ tsp freshly ground pepper
- 1 box refrigerated pie crusts
- 6 eggs
- 1 cup cooked bacon
- 2 cups crumbled Monterrey jack cheese

DIRECTIONS:

1. Grease 5 to 6-quart slow oval cooker with a cooking spray.
2. Press halves of pie crust 2 inches up the side and halve in the bottom in the cooker, to extend over seams by 1/4 inch.
3. Heat for 1 hour 30 minutes on high.
4. Turn in stirred eggs and bacon over the mixture.
5. Garnish with cheese and seasonings.
6. Heat on low for 2 hours 30 minutes

NUTRITION:

Calories: 524
Fat: 34g
Carbs: 22g
Protein: 25g

Sodium: 826mg
Potassium: 174.8mg
Phosphorus: 287.1mg

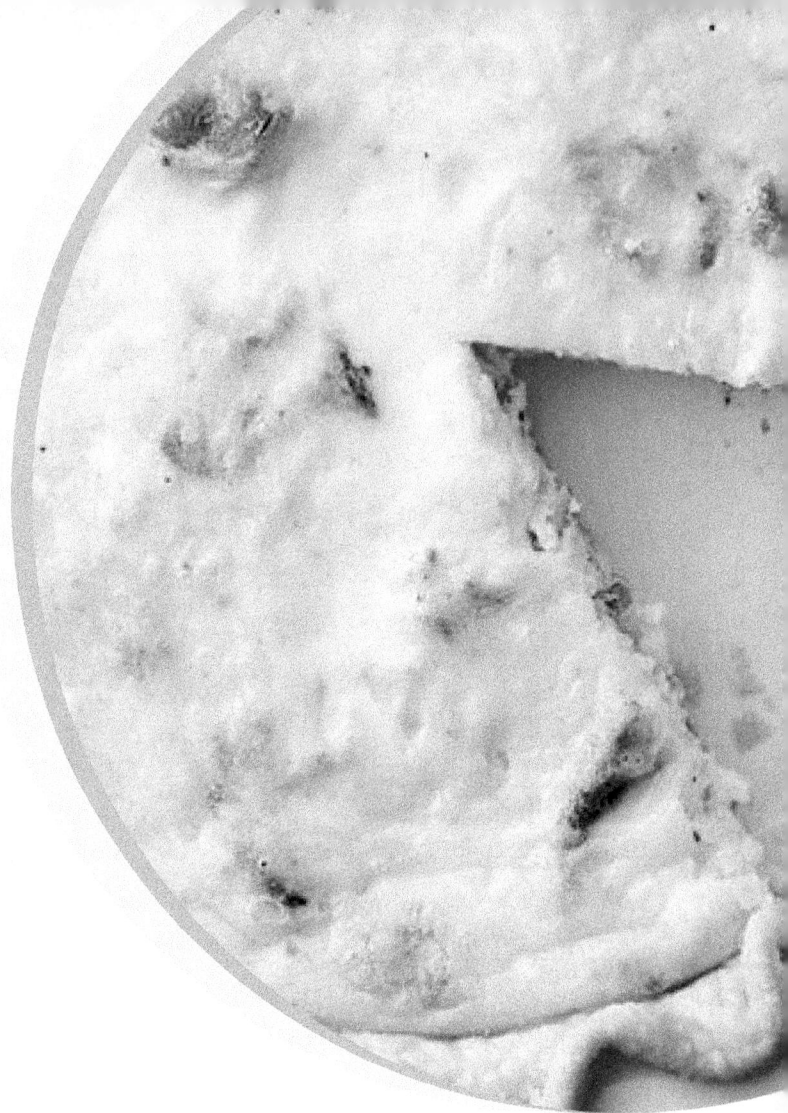

11 TURKEY AND SPINACH SCRAMBLE ON MELBA TOAST

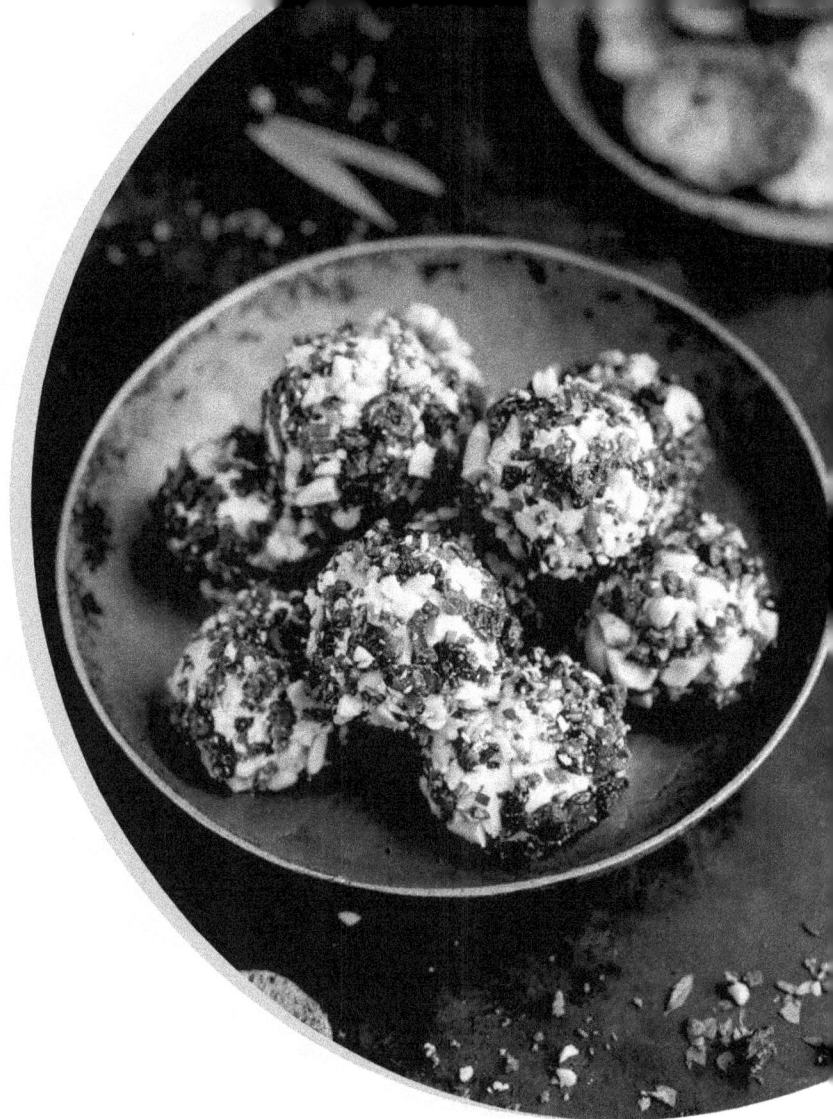

Preparation Time: 5 minutes

Cooking Time: 15 minutes

Servings: 2

INGREDIENTS:

- 1 tsp. Extra virgin olive oil
- 1 cup Raw spinach
- ½ clove, minced Garlic
- 1 tsp. grated Nutmeg
-
  1 cup Cooked and diced turkey breast
- 4 slices Melba toast
- 1 tsp. Balsamic vinegar

DIRECTIONS:

1. Heat a skillet over medium heat and add oil.
2. Add turkey and heat through for 6 to 8 minutes.
3. Add spinach, garlic, and nutmeg and stir-fry for 6 minutes more.
4. Plate up the Melba toast and top with spinach and turkey scramble.
5. Drizzle with balsamic vinegar and serve.

NUTRITION:

Calories: 301

Fat: 19g

Carb: 12g

Protein: 19g

Sodium: 360mg

Potassium: 269mg

Phosphorus: 215mg

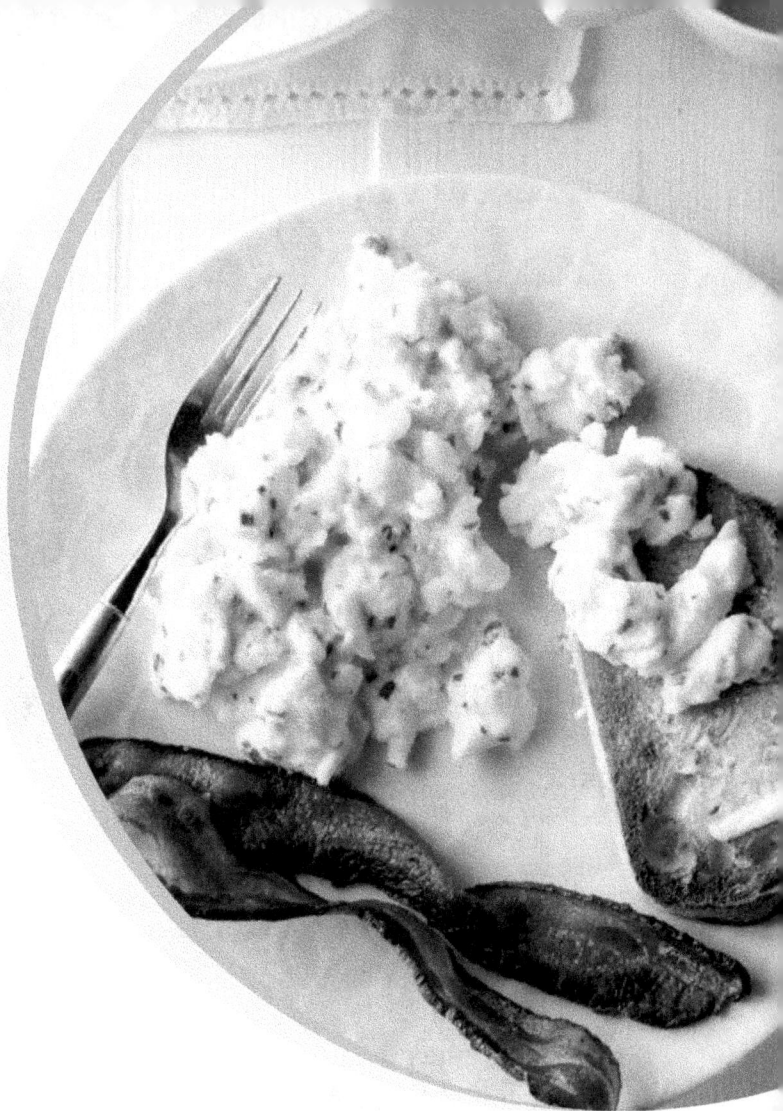

12 CHEESY SCRAMBLED EGGS WITH FRESH HERBS

Preparation Time: 15 minutes

Cooking Time: 10 minutes

Servings: 4

INGREDIENTS:

- 3 Eggs
- 2 Egg whites
- ½ cup Cream cheese
- ¼ cup Unsweetened rice milk
-
    1 tbsp. green part only Chopped scallion
- 1 tbsp. Chopped fresh tarragon
- 2 tbsps. Unsalted butter
- Ground black pepper to taste

DIRECTIONS:

1. Whisk the eggs, egg whites, cream cheese, rice milk, scallions, and tarragon. Mix until smooth.
2. Melt the butter in a skillet.
3. Put egg mixture and cook for 5 minutes or until the eggs are thick and curds creamy.
4. Season with pepper and serve.

NUTRITION:

Calories: 221

Fat: 19g

Carb: 3g

Protein: 8g

Sodium: 193mg

Potassium: 140mg

Phosphorus: 119mg

13 MEXICAN STYLE BURRITOS

Preparation Time: 5 minutes

Cooking Time: 15 minutes

Servings: 2

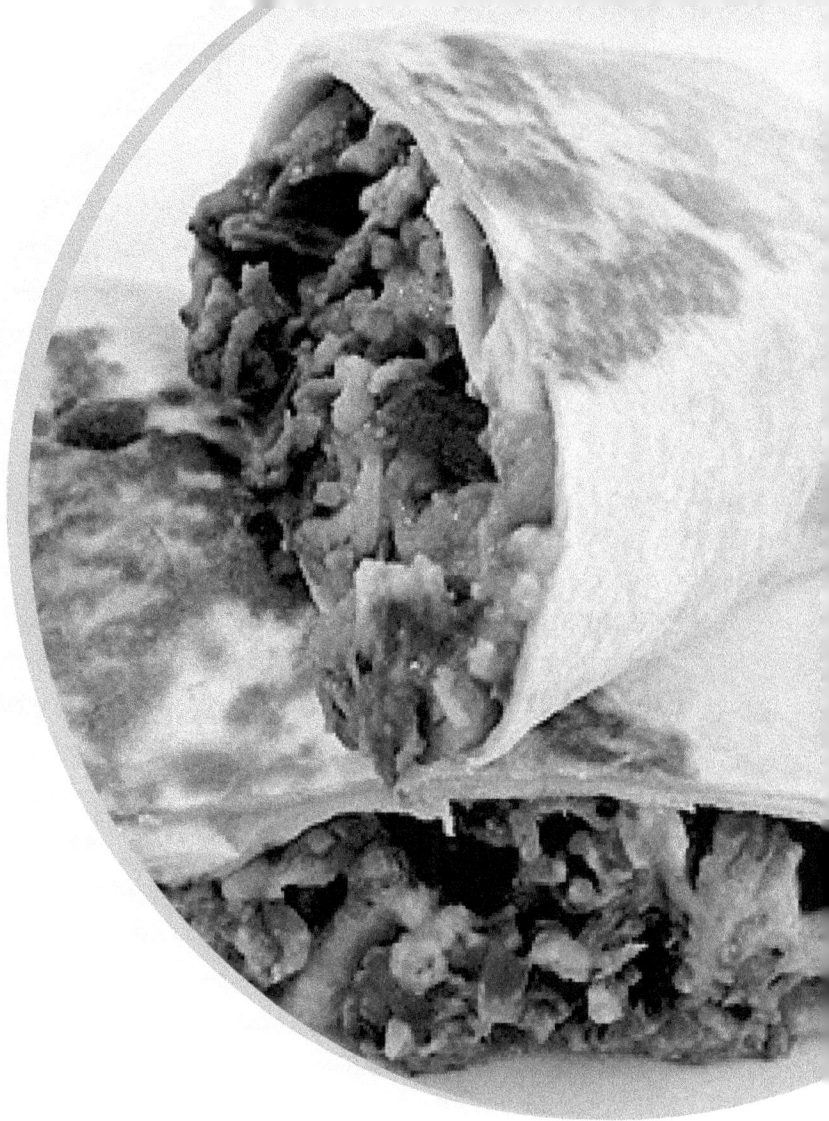

INGREDIENTS:

- 1 tbsp. Olive oil
- 2 Corn tortillas
- ¼ cup chopped Red onion
- ¼ cup chopped Red bell peppers
- ½, deseeded and chopped red chili
- 2 Eggs
- 1 lime juice
- 1 tbsp. chopped Cilantro

DIRECTIONS:

1. Place the tortillas in medium heat for 1 to 2 minutes on each side or until lightly toasted.
2. Remove and keep the broiler on.
3. Heat the oil in a skillet and sauté onion, chili, and bell peppers for 5 to 6 minutes or until soft.
4. Crack the eggs over the top of the onions and peppers.
5. Place skillet under the broiler for 5 to 6 minutes or until the eggs are cooked.
6. Serve half the eggs and vegetables on top of each tortilla and sprinkle with cilantro and lime juice to serve.

NUTRITION:

Calories: 202

Fat: 13g

Carb: 19g

Protein: 9g

Sodium: 77mg

Potassium: 233mg

Phosphorus: 184mg

14 | BULGUR, COUSCOUS, AND BUCKWHEAT CEREAL

Preparation Time: 10 minutes

Cooking Time: 25 minutes

Servings: 4

INGREDIENTS:

2 ¼ cups Water
1 ¼ cups Vanilla rice milk
6 Tbsps. Uncooked bulgur
2 Tbsps. Uncooked whole buckwheat
1 cup Sliced apple
6 Tbsps. Plain uncooked couscous
½ tsp. Ground cinnamon

DIRECTIONS:

1. Heat the water and milk in the saucepan over medium heat. Let it boil.
2. Put the bulgur, buckwheat, and apple.
3. Reduce the heat to low and simmer, occasionally stirring until the bulgur is tender, about 20 to 25 minutes.
4. Remove the saucepan and stir in the couscous and cinnamon—cover for 10 minutes.
5. Put the cereal before serving.

NUTRITION:

Calories: 159
Fat: 1g
Carb: 34g
Protein: 4g

Sodium: 33mg
Potassium: 116m
Phosphorus: 130mg

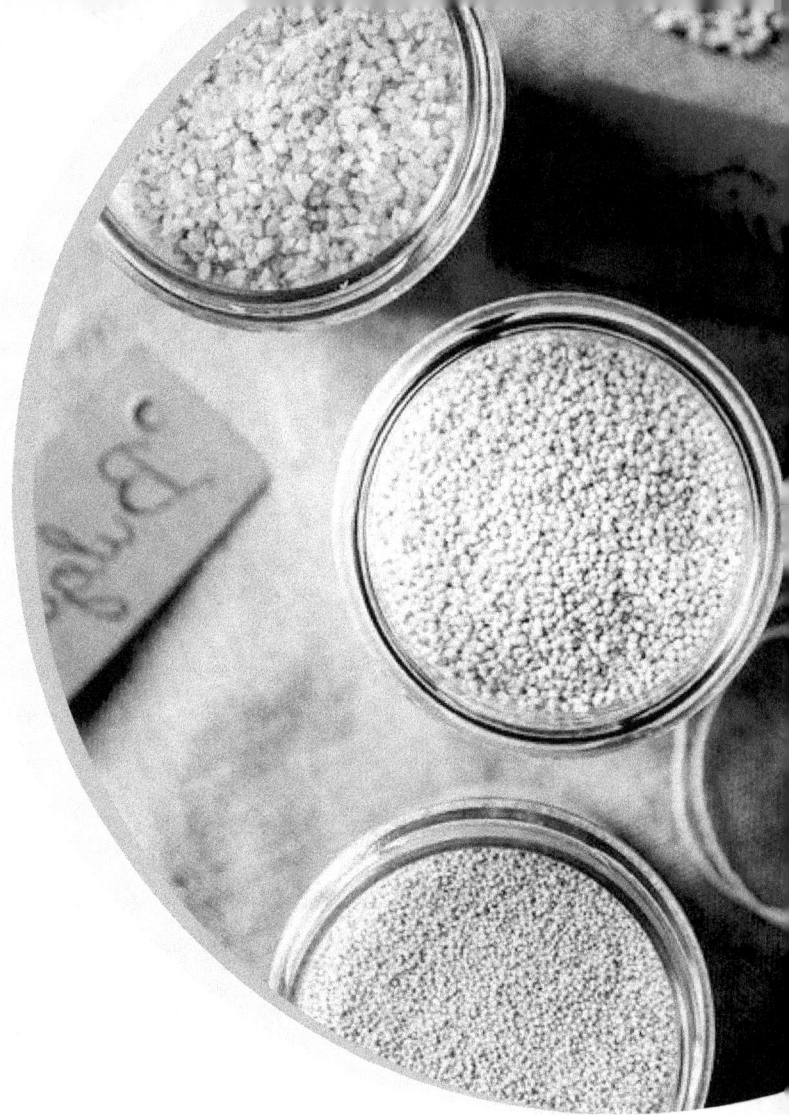

15 BLUEBERRY MUFFINS

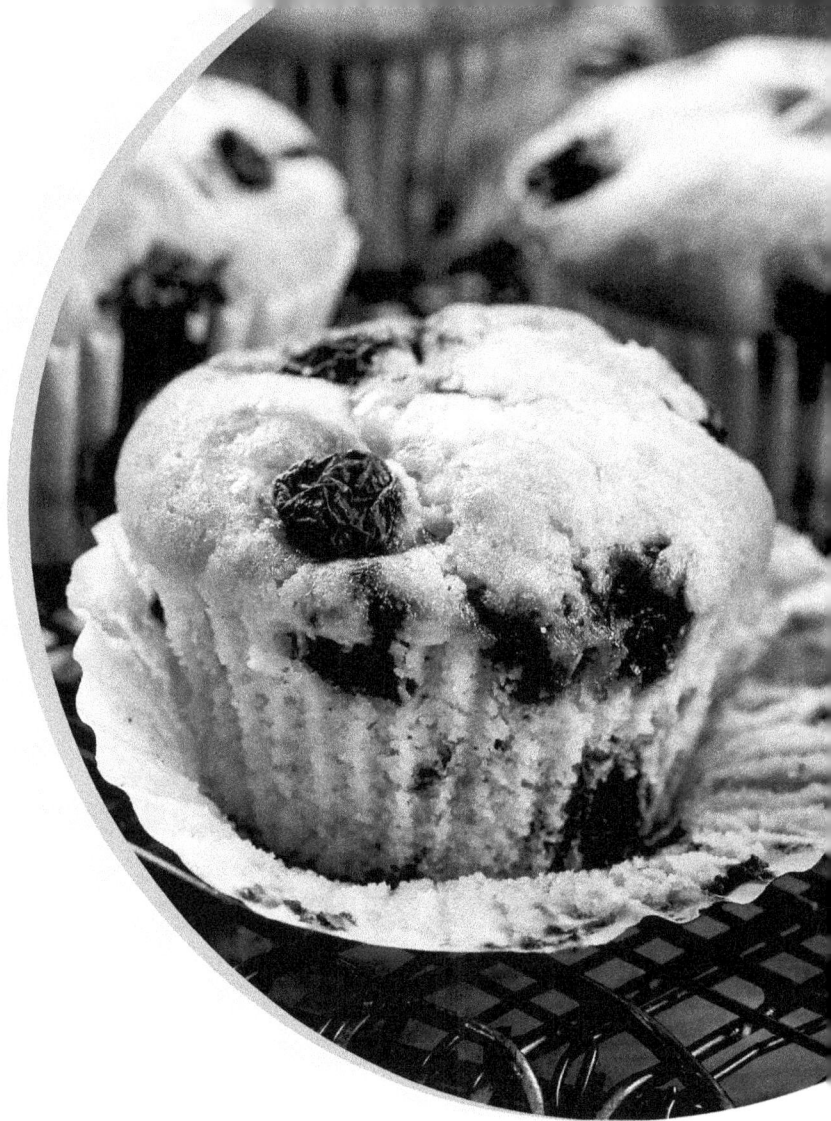

Preparation Time: 15 minutes

Cooking Time: 30 minutes

Servings: 12

INGREDIENTS:

- 2 cups Unsweetened rice milk
- 1 Tbsp. Apple cider vinegar
- 3 ½ cups All-purpose flour
- 1 cup Granulated sugar
- 1 Tbsp. Baking soda substitute
- 1 tsp. Ground cinnamon
- ½ tsp. Ground nutmeg
- Pinch ground ginger
- ½ cup Canola oil
- 2 Tbsps. Pure vanilla extract
- 2 ½ cups Fresh blueberries

DIRECTIONS:

1. Preheat the oven to 375F.
2. Prepare a muffin pan and set aside.
3. Stir together the rice milk and vinegar in a small bowl. Set aside for 10 minutes.
4. In a large bowl, stir together the sugar, flour, baking soda, cinnamon, nutmeg, and ginger until well mixed.
5. Add oil and vanilla to the milk and mix.
6. Put milk mixture to dry ingredients and stir well to combine.
7. Put the blueberries and spoon the muffin batter evenly into the cups.
8. Bake the muffins for 25 to 30 minutes or until golden and a toothpick inserted comes out clean.
9. Cool for 15 minutes and serve.

Calories: 331
Fat: 11g
Carb: 52g
Protein: 6g
Sodium: 35mg
Potassium: 89mg
Phosphorus: 90mg

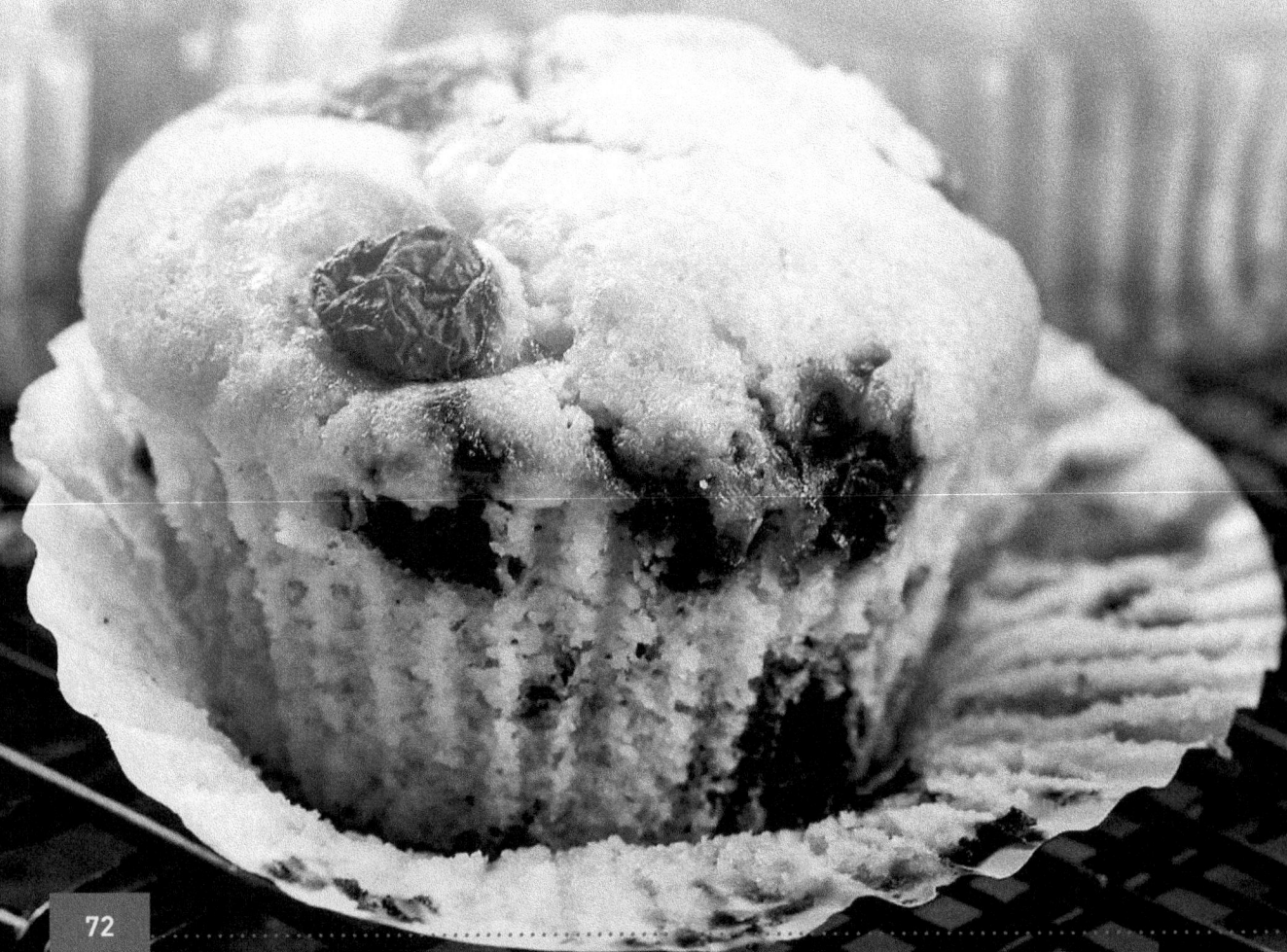

16 BUCKWHEAT AND GRAPEFRUIT PORRIDGE

Preparation Time: 5 minutes

Cooking Time: 20 minutes

Servings: 2

INGREDIENTS:

- ½ cup Buckwheat
- ¼ chopped Grapefruit
- 1 Tbsp. Honey
- 1 ½ cups Almond milk
- 2 cups Water

DIRECTIONS:

1. Let the water boil on the stove. Add the buckwheat and place the lid on the pan.
2. Lower heat slightly and simmer for 7 to 10 minutes, checking to ensure water does not dry out.
3. When most of the water is absorbed, remove, and set aside for 5 minutes.
4. Drain any excess water from the pan and stir in almond milk, heating through for 5 minutes.
5. Add the honey and grapefruit.
6. Serve.

NUTRITION:

Calories: 231
Fat: 4g
Carb: 43g
Protein: 13g
Sodium: 135mg
Potassium: 370mg
Phosphorus: 165mg

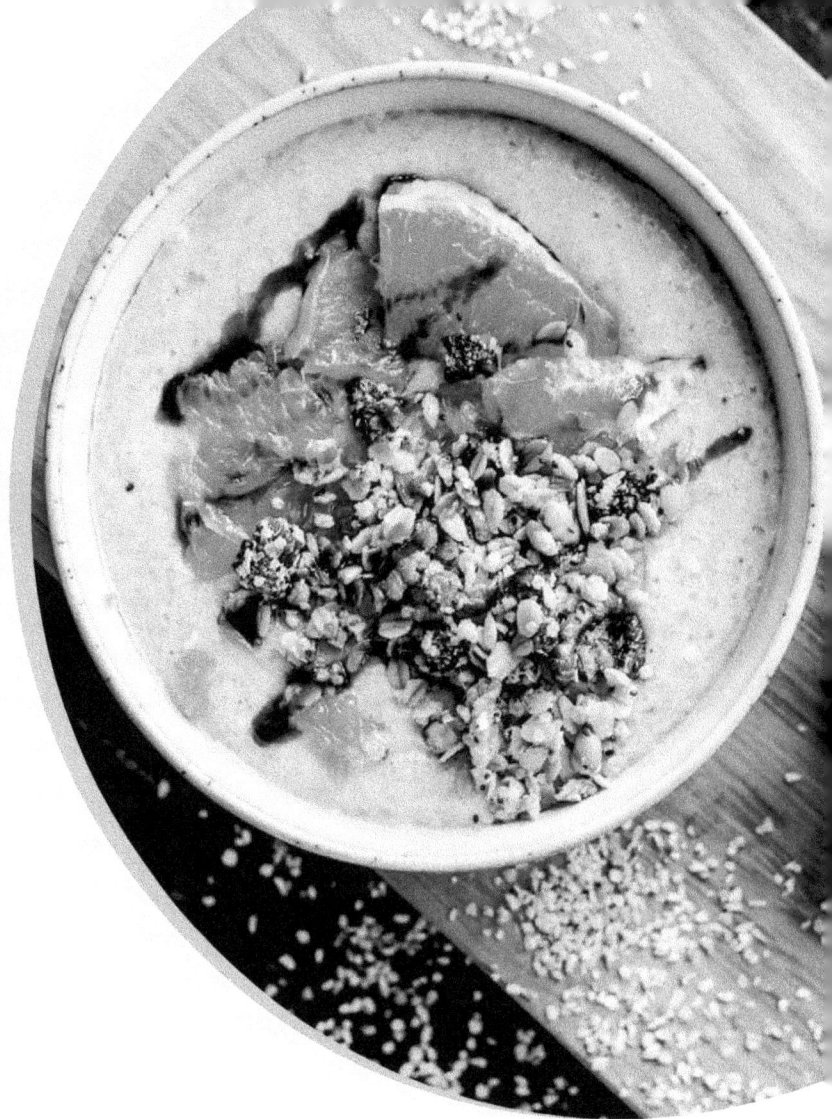

17 EGG AND VEGGIE MUFFINS

Preparation Time: 15 minutes

Cooking Time: 20 minutes

Servings: 4

INGREDIENTS:

- 4 Eggs
- 2 Tbsp. Unsweetened rice milk
- ½ chopped Sweet onion
- ½ chopped Red bell pepper
- Pinch red pepper flakes
- Pinch ground black pepper

DIRECTIONS:

1. Preheat the oven to 350F.
2. Spray 4 muffin pans with cooking spray. Set aside.
3. Whisk the milk, eggs, onion, red pepper, parsley, red pepper flakes, and black pepper until mixed.
4. Pour the egg mixture into prepared muffin pans.
5. Bake until the muffins are puffed and golden, about 18 to 20 minutes. Serve.

NUTRITION:

Calories: 84
Fat: 5g
Carb: 3g
Protein: 7g
Sodium: 75mg
Potassium: 117mg
Phosphorus: 110mg

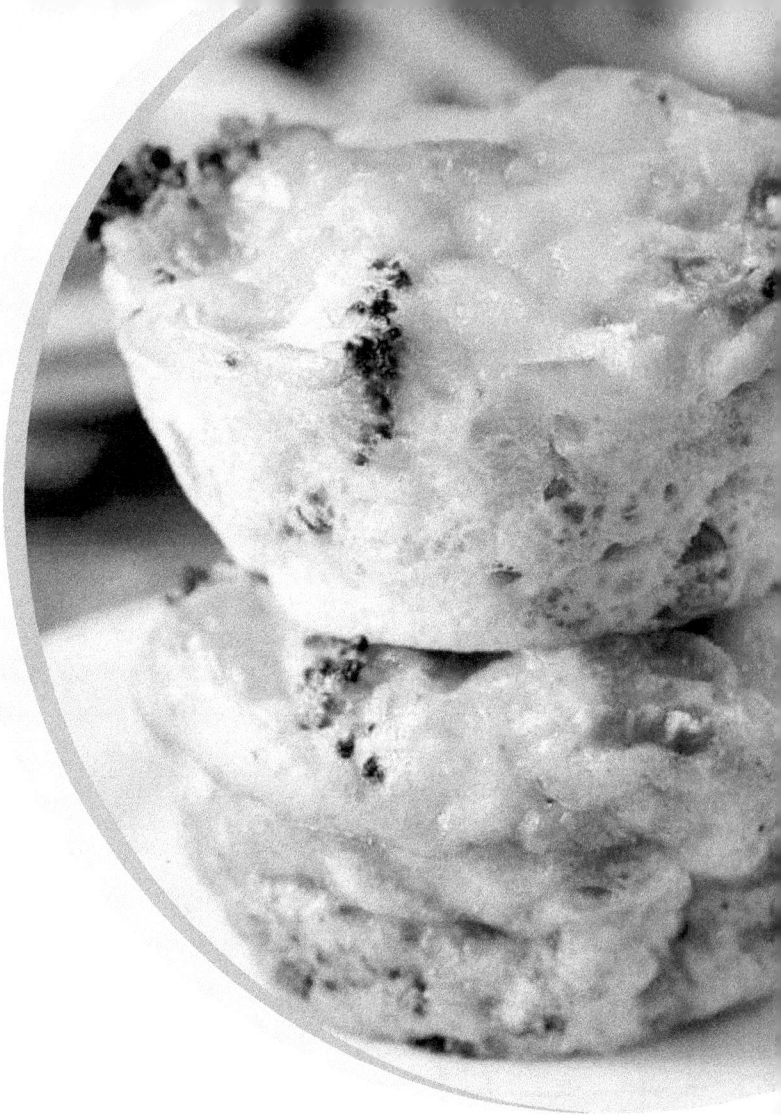

18 BERRY CHIA WITH YOGURT

Preparation Time: 35 minutes

Cooking Time: 5 minutes

Servings:4

INGREDIENTS:

- ½ cup chia seeds, dried
- 2 cup Plain yogurt
- 1/3 cup strawberries, chopped
- ¼ cup blackberries
- ¼ cup raspberries
- 4 teaspoons Splenda

DIRECTIONS:

1. Mix up together Plain yogurt with Splenda, and chia seeds.
2. Transfer the mixture into the serving ramekins (jars) and leave for 35 minutes.
3. After this, add blackberries, raspberries, and strawberries. Mix up the meal well.
4. Serve it immediately or store it in the fridge for up to 2 days.

NUTRITION:

Calories: 150
Fat: 5g
Carbs: 19g
Protein: 6.8g
Sodium: 65mg
Potassium: 226mg
Phosphorus: 75mg

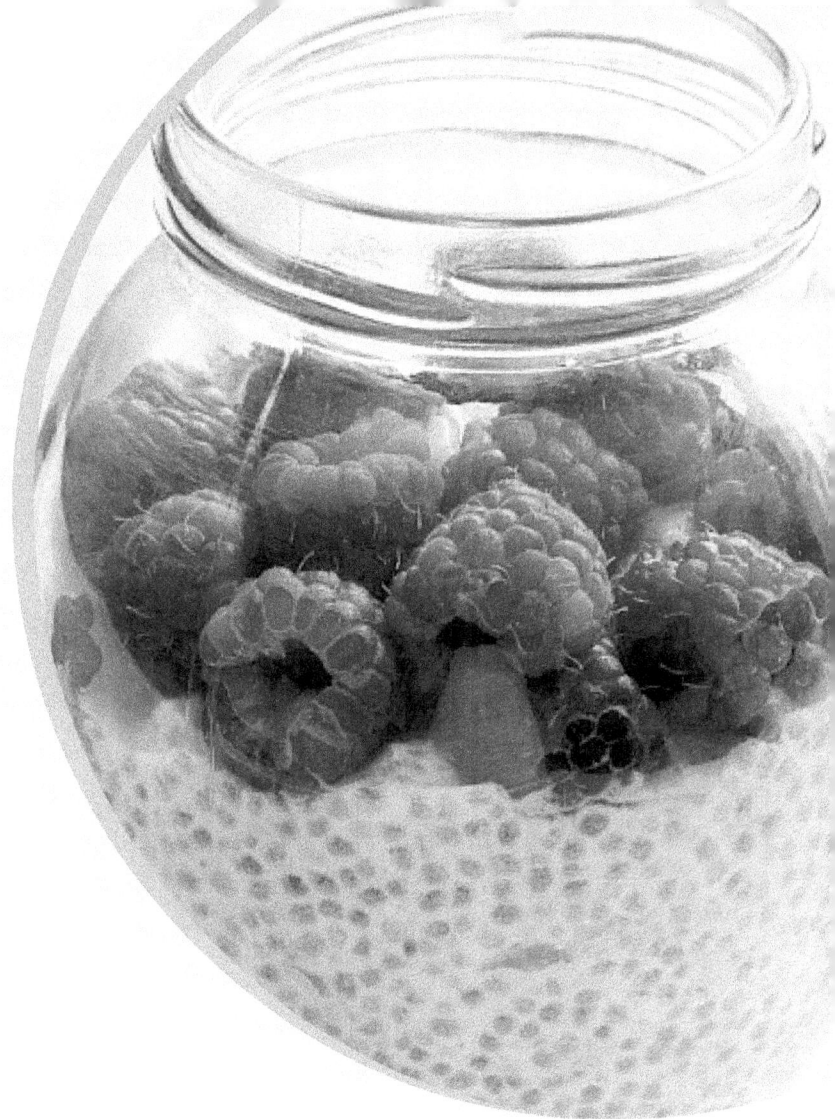

19 ARUGULA EGGS WITH CHILI PEPPERS

Preparation Time: 7 minutes

Cooking Time: 10 minutes

Servings: 4

INGREDIENTS:

- 2 cups arugula, chopped
- 3 eggs, beaten
- ½ chili pepper, chopped
- 1 tablespoon butter
- 1 oz Parmesan, grated

DIRECTIONS:

1. Toss butter in the skillet and melt it.
2. Add arugula and sauté it over medium heat for 5 minutes. Stir it from time to time.
3. Meanwhile, mix up together Parmesan, chili pepper, and eggs.
4. Pour the egg mixture over the arugula and scramble well.
5. Cook for 5 minutes more over medium heat.

NUTRITION:

Calories: 218
Fat: 15g
Carbs: 2.8g
Protein: 17g
Sodium: 656mg
Potassium: 243mg
Phosphorus: 310mg

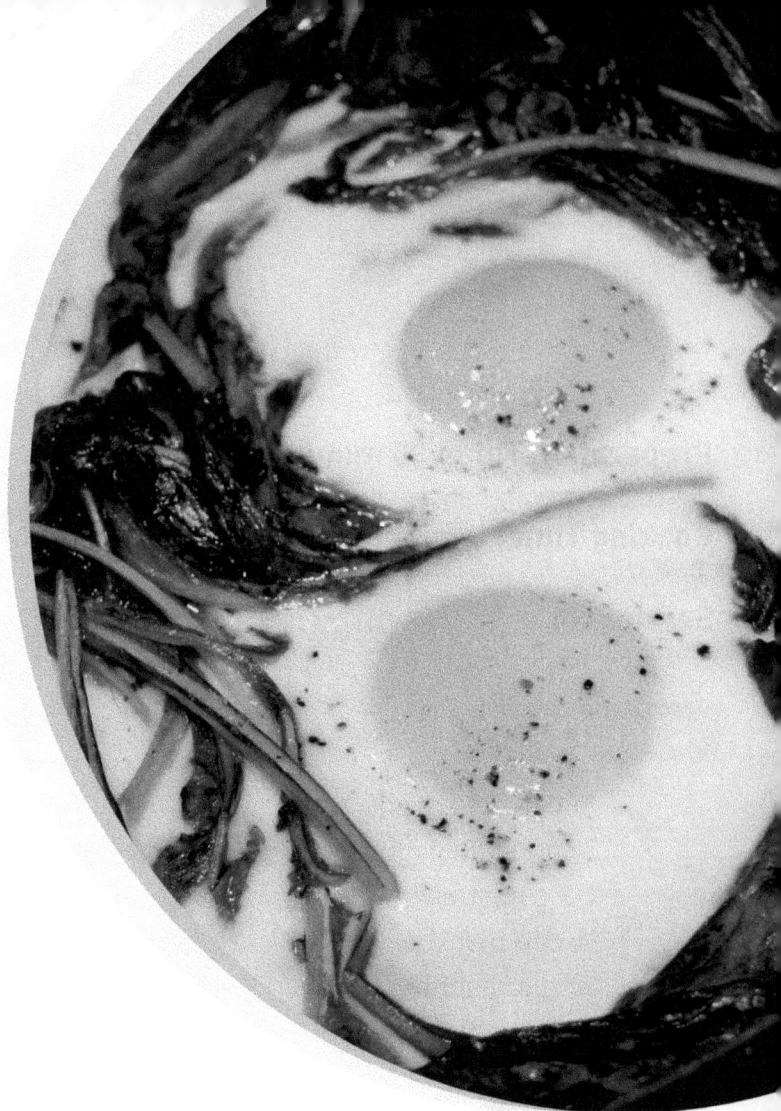

20 EGGPLANT CHICKEN SANDWICH

Preparation Time: 10 minutes

Cooking Time: 15 minutes

Servings: 2

INGREDIENTS:

- 1 eggplant, trimmed
- 10 oz chicken fillet
- 1 teaspoon Plain yogurt
- ½ teaspoon minced garlic
- 1 tablespoon fresh cilantro, chopped
- 2 lettuce leaves
- 1 teaspoon olive oil
- ½ teaspoon salt
- ½ teaspoon chili pepper
- 1 teaspoon butter

DIRECTIONS:

1. Slice the eggplant lengthwise into 4 slices.
2. Rub the eggplant slices with minced garlic and brush with olive oil.
3. Grill the eggplant slices on the preheated to 375F grill for 3 minutes from each side.
4. Meanwhile, rub the chicken fillet with salt and chili pepper.
5. Place it in the skillet and add butter.
6. Roast the chicken for 6 minutes from each side over medium-high heat.
7. Cool the cooked eggplants gently and spread one side of them with Plain yogurt.
8. Add lettuce leaves and chopped fresh cilantro.
9. After this, slice the cooked chicken fillet and add over the lettuce.
10. Cover it with the remaining sliced eggplant to get the sandwich shape. Pin the sandwich with the toothpick if needed.

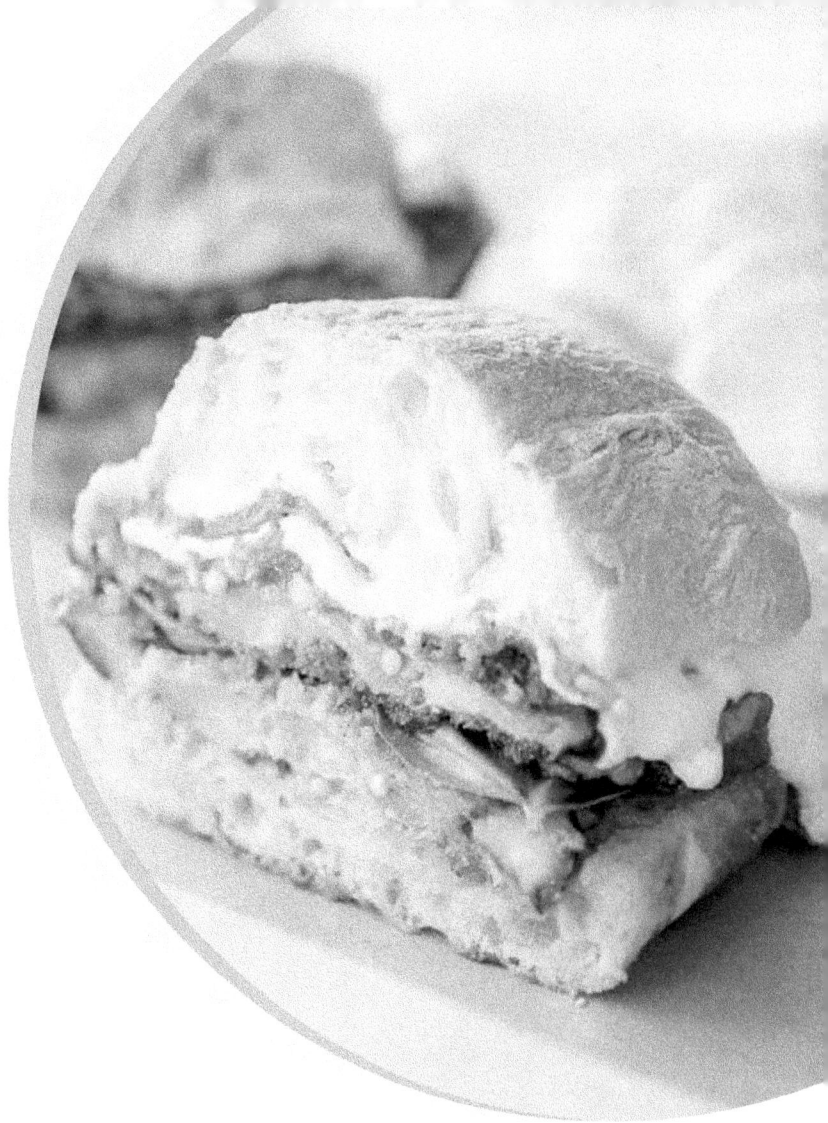

NUTRITION:

Calories: 276
Fat: 11g
Carbs: 41g
Protein: 13.8g
Sodium: 775mg
Potassium: 532mg
Phosphorus: 187mg

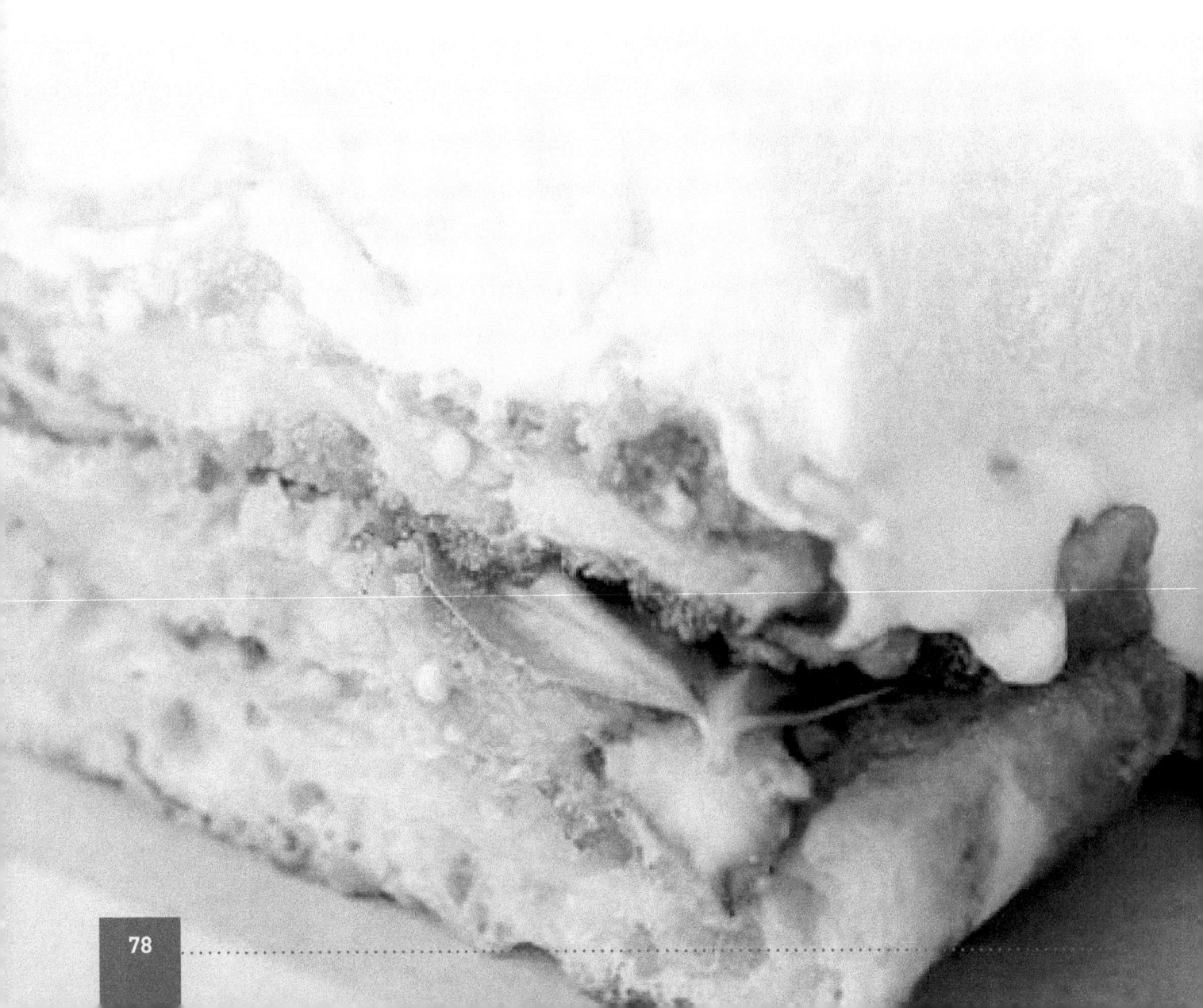

21 EGGS IN TOMATO RINGS

Preparation Time: 8 minutes

Cooking Time: 5 minutes

Servings: 2

INGREDIENTS:

- 1 tomato
- 2 eggs
- ¼ teaspoon chili flakes
- ¾ teaspoon salt
- ½ teaspoon butter

DIRECTIONS:

1. Trim the tomato and slice it into 2 rings.
2. Remove the tomato flesh.
3. Toss butter in the skillet and melt it.
4. Then arrange the tomato rings.
5. Crack the eggs in the tomato rings. Sprinkle them with salt and chili flakes.
6. Cook the eggs for 4 minutes over medium heat with the closed lid.
7. Transfer the cooked eggs into the serving plates with the help of the spatula.

NUTRITION:

Calories: 237
Fat: 16g
Carbs: 7g
Protein: 16g
Sodium: 427mg
Potassium: 391.5mg
Phosphorus: 291mg

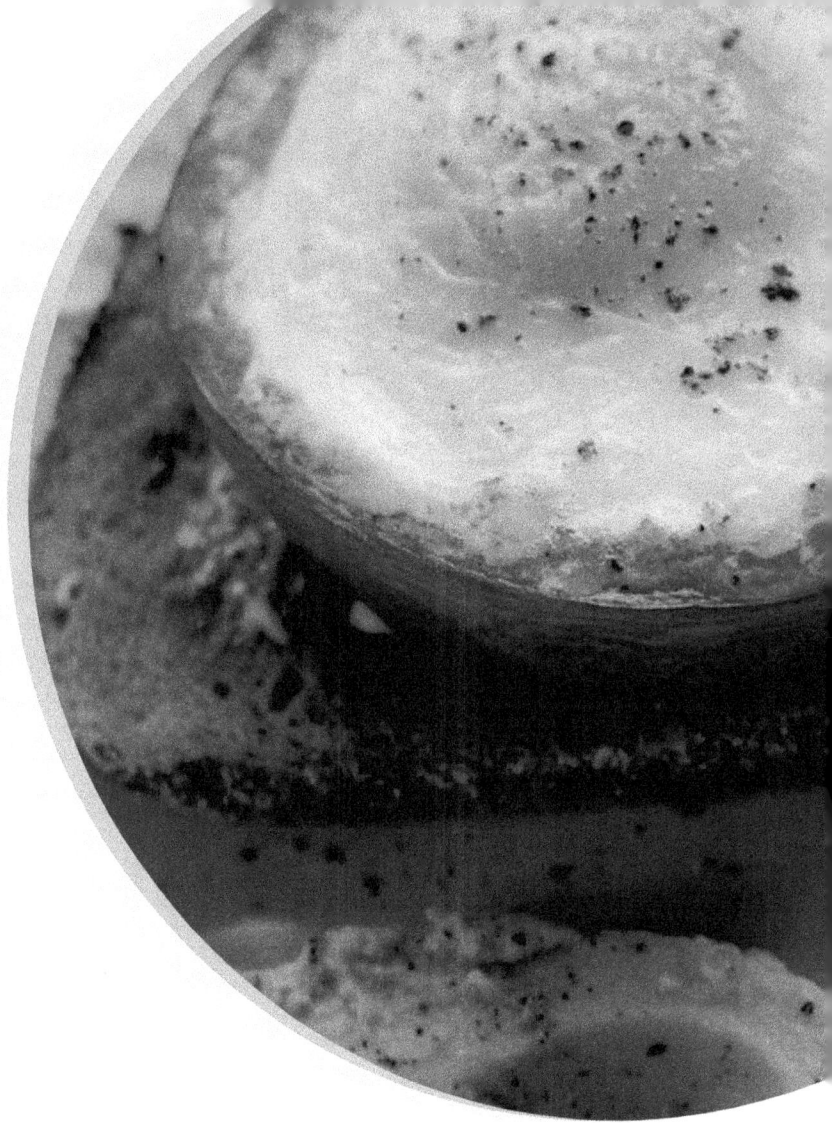

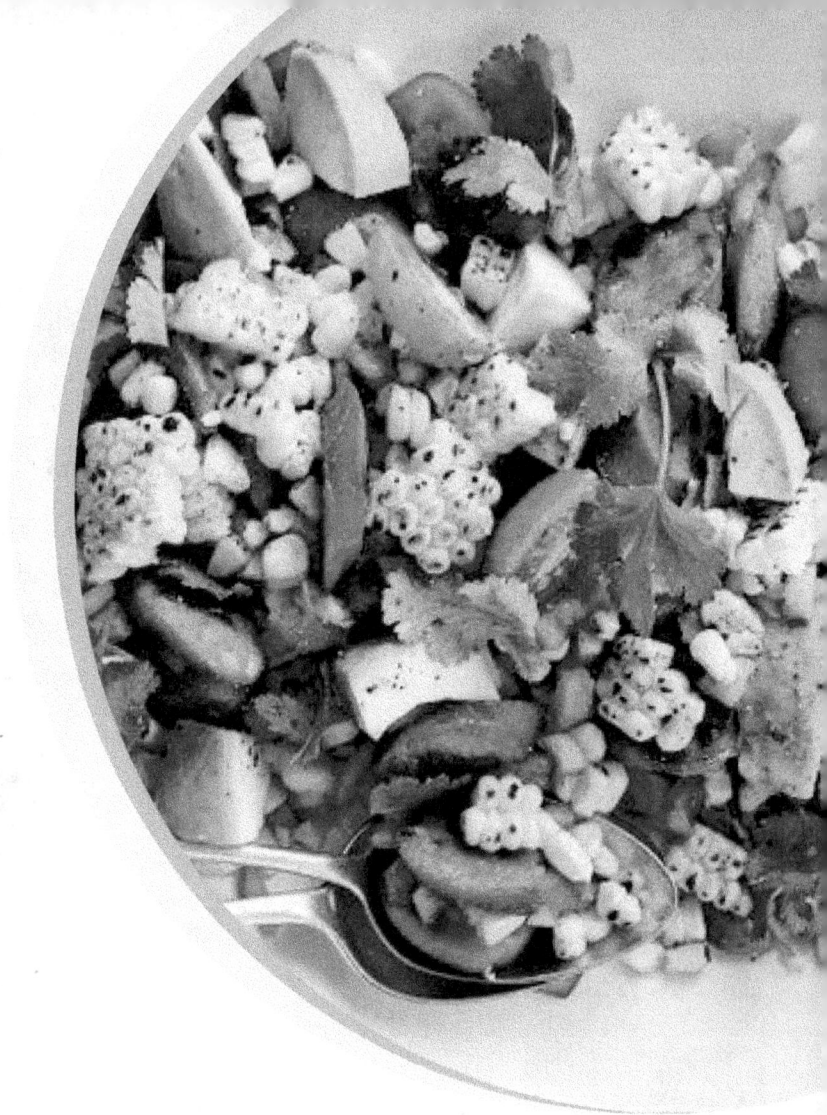

22 CHORIZO BOWL WITH CORN

Preparation Time: 10 minutes

Cooking Time: 15 minutes

Servings: 4

INGREDIENTS:

- 9 oz chorizo
- 1 tablespoon almond butter
- ½ cup corn kernels
- 1 tomato, chopped
- ¾ cup heavy cream
- 1 teaspoon butter
- ¼ teaspoon chili pepper
- 1 tablespoon dill, chopped

DIRECTIONS:

1. Chop the chorizo and place it in the skillet.
2. Add almond butter and chili pepper.
3. Roast the chorizo for 3 minutes.
4. After this, add tomato and corn kernels.
5. Add butter and chopped the dill. Mix up the mixture well—Cook for 2 minutes.
6. Close the lid and simmer for 10 minutes over low heat.
7. Transfer the cooked meal into the serving bowls.

NUTRITION:

Calories: 286
Fat: 15g
Carbs: 26g
Protein: 13g

Sodium: 228mg
Potassium: 255mg
Phosphorus: 293mg

23 PANZANELLA SALAD

Preparation Time: 10 minutes

Cooking Time: 5 minutes

Servings: 4

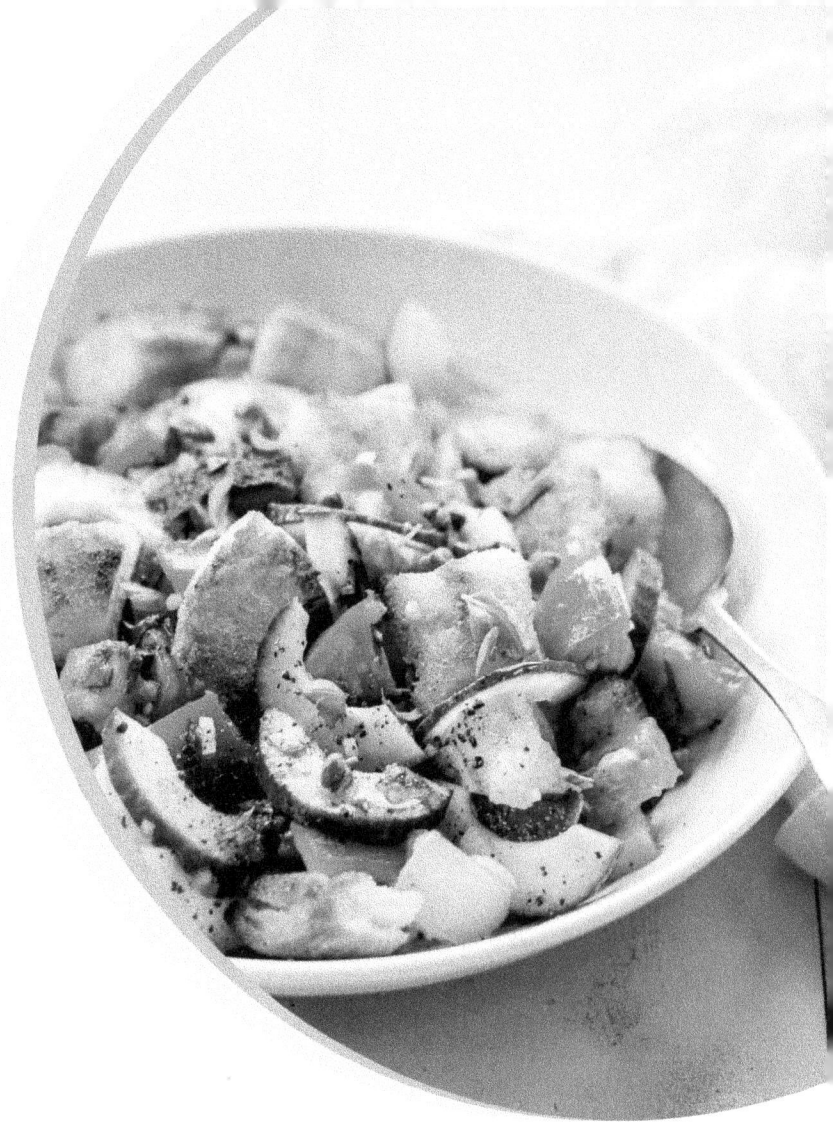

INGREDIENTS:

- 3 tomatoes, chopped
- 2 cucumbers, chopped
- 1 red onion, sliced
- 2 red bell peppers, chopped
- ¼ cup fresh cilantro, chopped
- 1 tablespoon capers
- 1 oz whole-grain bread, chopped
- 1 tablespoon canola oil
- ½ teaspoon minced garlic
- 1 tablespoon Dijon mustard
- 1 teaspoon olive oil
- 1 teaspoon lime juice

DIRECTIONS:

1. Pour canola oil into the skillet and bring it to boil.
2. Add chopped bread and roast it until crunchy (3-5 minutes).
3. Meanwhile, in the salad bowl, combine sliced red onion, cucumbers, tomatoes, bell peppers, cilantro, capers, and mix up gently.
4. Make the dressing: mix up together lime juice, olive oil, Dijon mustard, and minced garlic.
5. Put the dressing over the salad and stir it directly before serving.

NUTRITION:

Calories: 224.3
Fat: 10g
Carbs: 26g

Protein: 6.6g
Sodium: 401mg

Potassium: 324.9mg
Phosphorus: 84mg

24 POACHED ASPARAGUS AND EGG

Preparation time: 3 minutes

Cooking Time: 15 minutes

Servings: 1

INGREDIENTS:

- 1 egg
- 4 spears asparagus
- Water

DIRECTIONS:

1. Half-fill a deep saucepan with water set over high heat. Let the water come to a boil.
2. Dip asparagus spears in water. Cook until they turn a shade brighter, about 3 minutes. Remove from saucepan and drain on paper towels. Keep warm—lightly season before serving.
3. Use a slotted spoon to lower the egg into boiling water gently.
4. Cook for only 4 minutes. Remove from pan immediately. Place on egg holder.
5. Slice off the top. The egg should still be fluid inside.
6. Place asparagus spears on a small plate and serve egg on the side.
7. Dip asparagus into the egg and eat while warm.

NUTRITION:

Calories: 178
Fat: 13g
Carbs: 1g
Protein: 7.72g

Calories 178
Sodium: 71mg
Potassium: 203mg
Phosphorus: 124mg

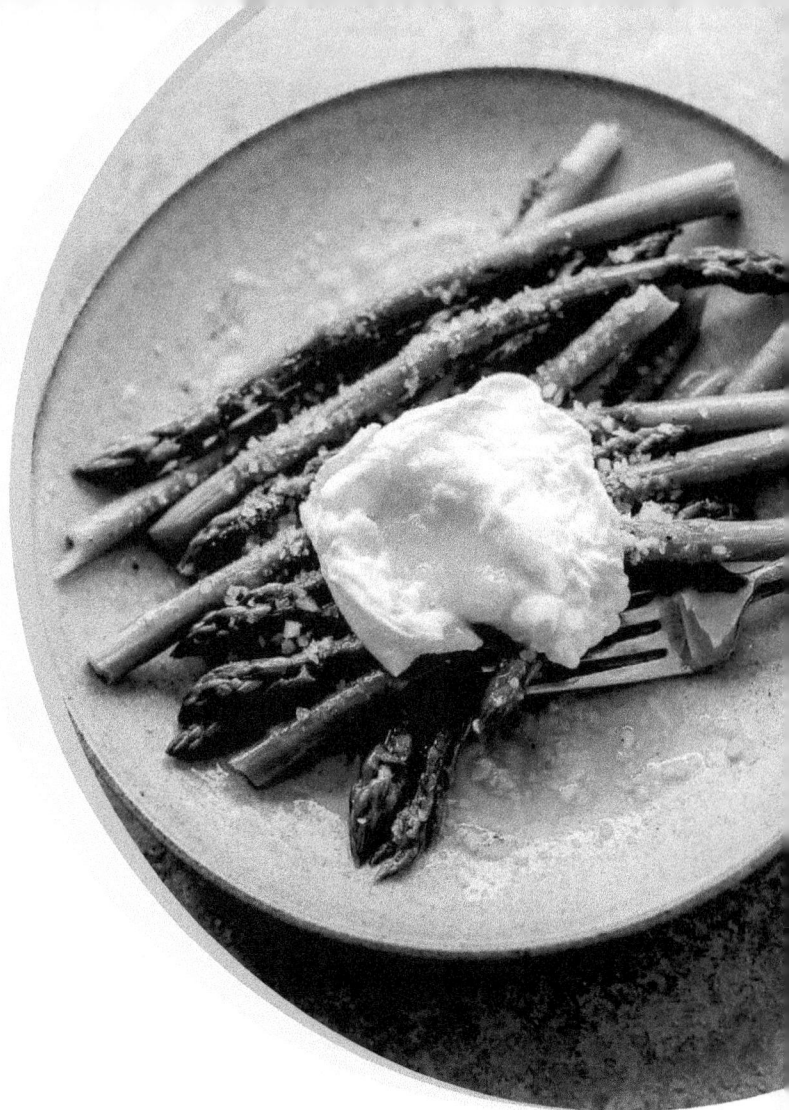

25 EGG DROP SOUP

Preparation Time: 5 minutes

Cooking Time: 10 minutes

Servings:4

INGREDIENTS:

- ¼ cup minced fresh chives
- 4 cups unsalted vegetable stock
- 4 whisked eggs

DIRECTIONS:

1. Pour unsalted vegetable stock into the oven set over high heat. Bring to a boil. Lower heat.
2. Pour in the eggs. Stir until ribbons form into the soup.
3. Turn off the heat immediately. The residual heat will cook eggs through.
4. Cool slightly before ladling the desired amount into individual bowls. Garnish with a pinch of parsley, if using.
5. Serve immediately.

NUTRITION:

Calories: 73
Fat: 3g
Carbs: 1g
Protein: 7g
Sodium: 891mg
Potassium: 53mg
Phosphorus: 36mg

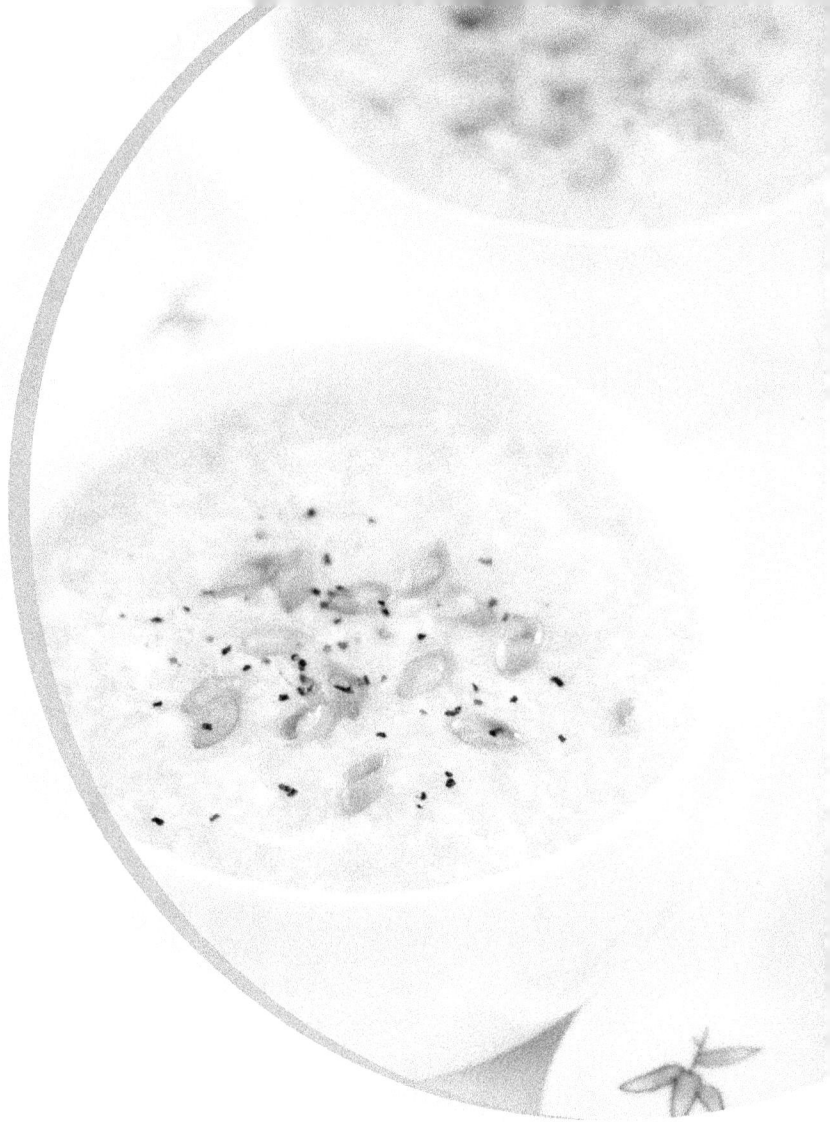

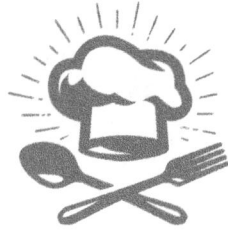

CHAPTER 13

LUNCH RECIPES

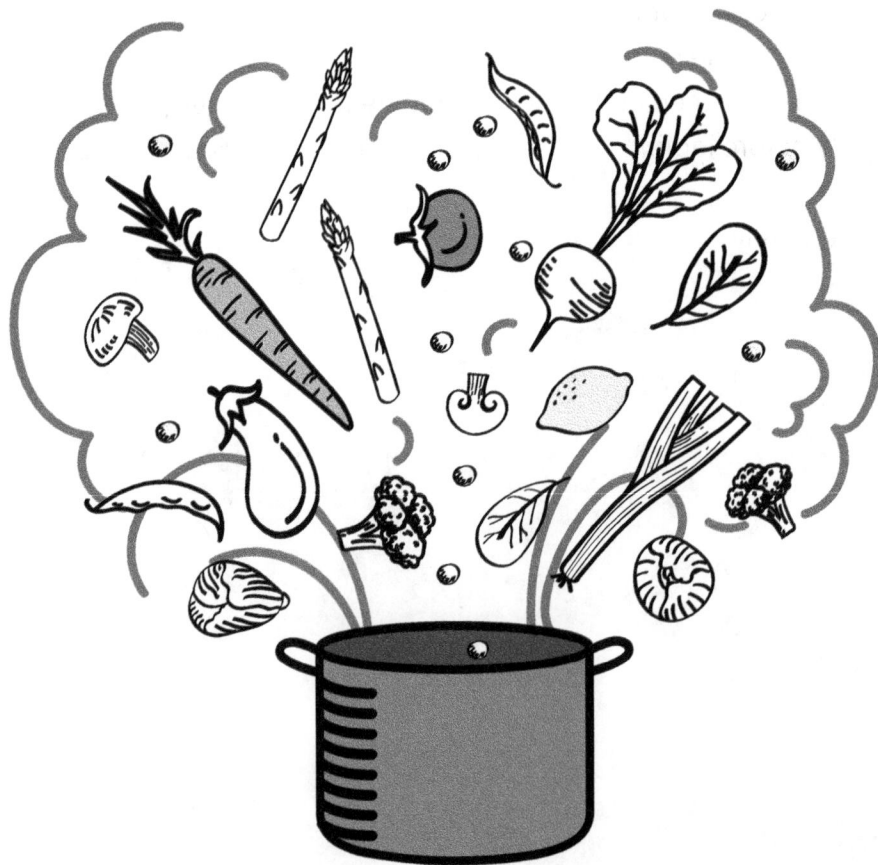

26 CUCUMBER SANDWICH

Preparation Time: 1 hour

Cooking Time: 5 minutes

Servings: 2

INGREDIENTS:

- 6 tsp. of cream cheese
- 1 pinch of dried dill weed
- 3 tsp. of mayonnaise
- .25 tsp. dry Italian dressing mix
- 4 slices of white bread
- .5 of a cucumber

DIRECTIONS:

1. Prepare the cucumber and cut it into slices.
2. Mix cream cheese, mayonnaise, and Italian dressing. Chill for one hour.
3. Distribute the mixture onto the white bread slices.
4. Place cucumber slices on top and sprinkle with the dill weed.
5. Cut in halves and serve.

NUTRITION:

Calories: 143

Fat: 6g

Carbs: 16.7g

Protein: 4g

Sodium: 255mg

Potassium: 127mg

Phosphorus: 64mg

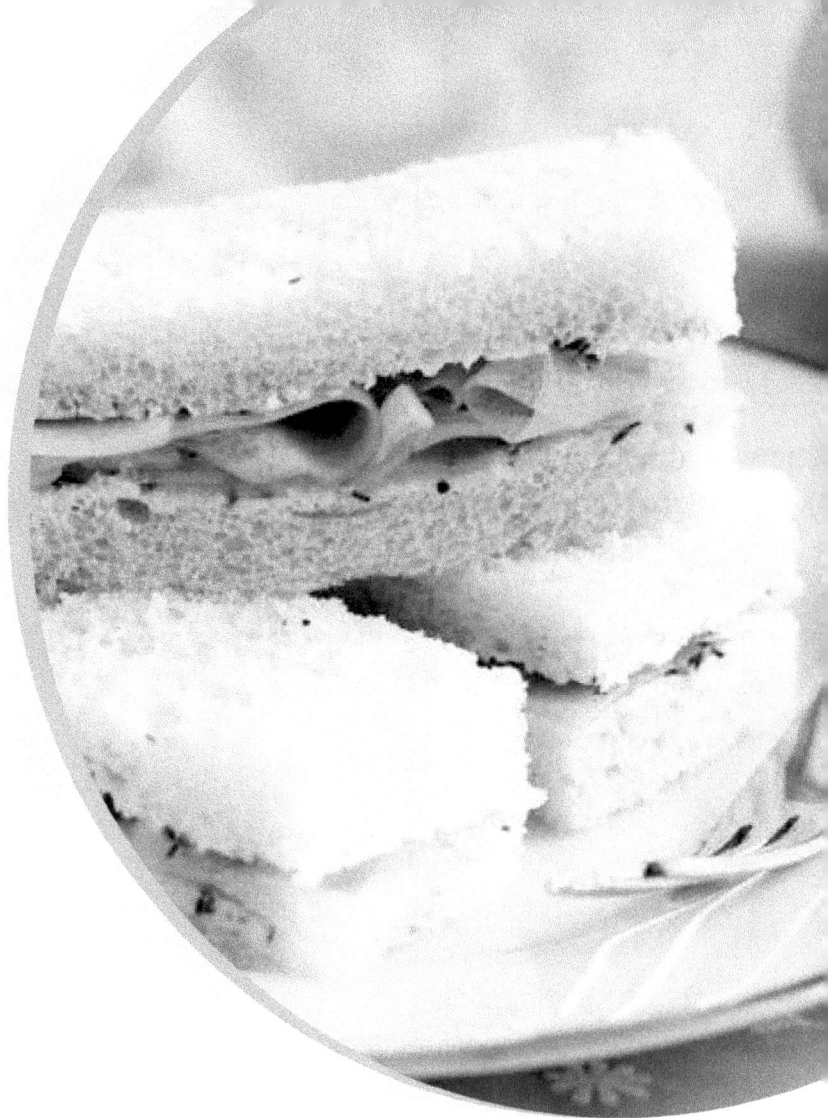

27 PIZZA PITAS

Preparation Time: 10 minutes

Cooking Time: 10 minutes

Servings: 1

INGREDIENTS:

- .33 cup of mozzarella cheese
- 2 pieces of pita bread, 6 inches in size
- 6 tsp. of chunky tomato sauce
- 2 cloves of garlic (minced)
- .25 cups of onion, chopped small
- .25 tsp. of red pepper flakes
- .25 cup of bell pepper, chopped small
- 2 ounces of ground pork, lean
- No-stick oil spray
- .5 tsp. of fennel seeds

DIRECTIONS:

1. Preheat oven to 400.
2. Put the garlic, ground meat, pepper flakes, onion, and bell pepper in a pan. Sauté until cooked.
3. Grease a flat baking pan and put pitas on it. Use the mixture to spread on the pita bread.
4. Spread one tablespoon of the tomato sauce and top with cheese.
5. Bake for five to eight minutes, until the cheese is bubbling.

NUTRITION:

Calories: 284
Fat: 10g
Carbs: 34g
Protein: 16g

Sodium: 795mg
Potassium: 706mg
Phosphorus: 416mg

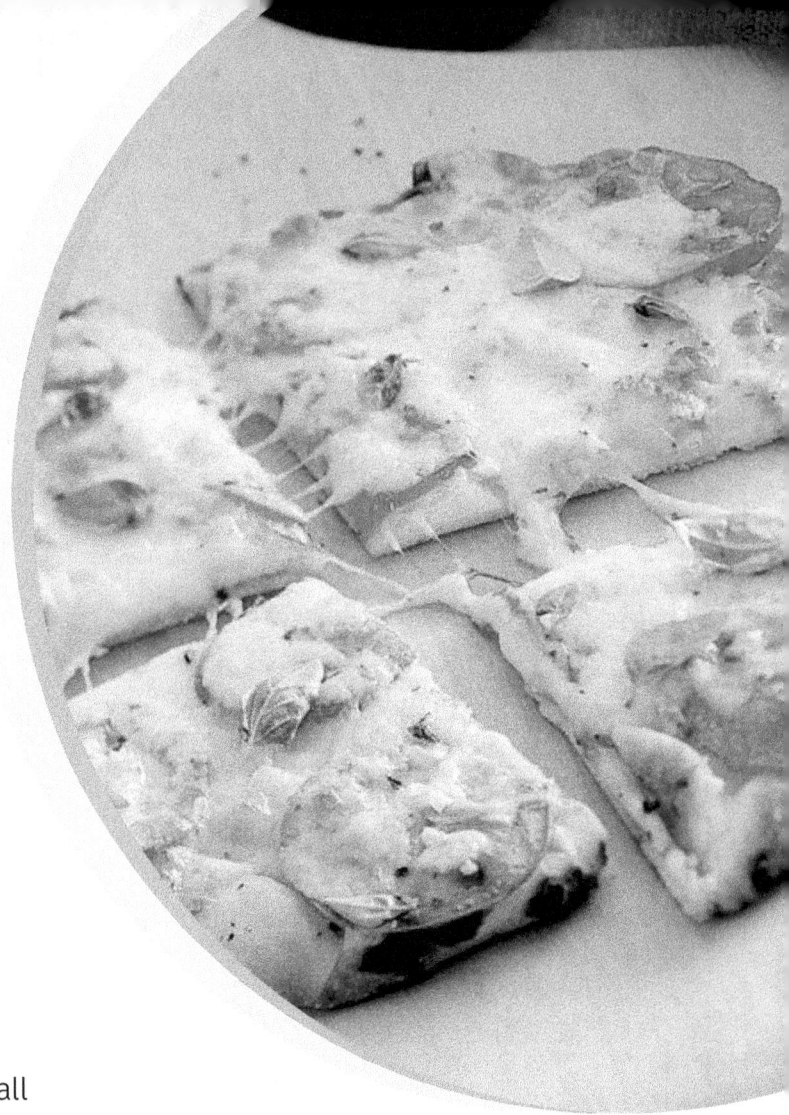

28 LETTUCE WRAPS WITH CHICKEN

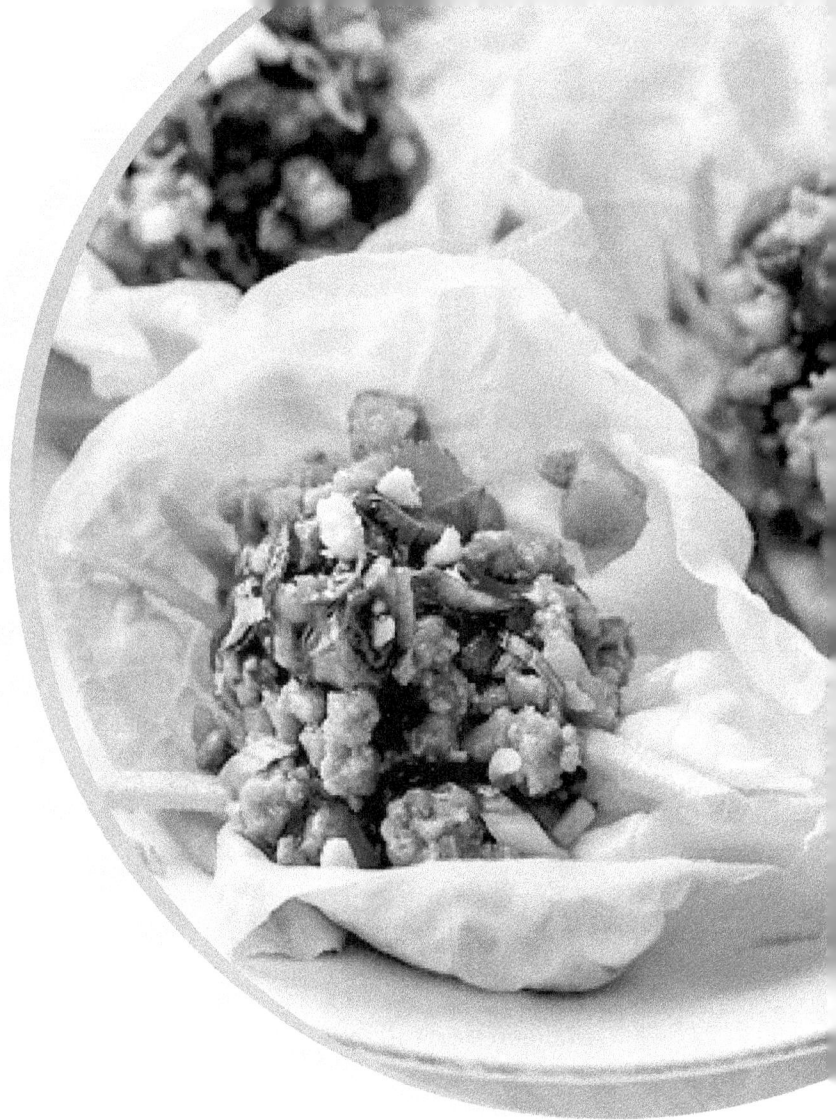

Preparation Time: 10 minutes

Cooking Time: 15 minutes

Servings: 4

INGREDIENTS:

- 8 lettuce leaves
- .25 cups of fresh cilantro
- .25 cups of mushroom
- 1 tsp. of five spices seasoning
- .25 cups of onion
- 6 tsp. of rice vinegar
- 2 tsp. of hoisin
- 6 tsp. of oil (canola)
- 3 tsp. of oil (sesame)
- 2 tsp. of garlic
- 2 scallions
- 8 ounces of cooked chicken breast

DIRECTIONS:

1. Mince together the cooked chicken and the garlic. Chop up the onions, cilantro, mushrooms, and scallions.
2. Use a skillet overheat, combine chicken to all remaining ingredients, minus the lettuce leaves. Cook for fifteen minutes, stirring occasionally.
3. Place .25 cups of the mixture into each leaf of lettuce.
4. Wrap the lettuce around like a burrito and eat.

NUTRITION:

Calories: 84

Fat: 4g

Carbs: 9g

Protein: 5.9g

Sodium: 618mg

Potassium: 258mg

Phosphorus: 64mg

29 TURKEY PINWHEELS

Preparation Time: 10 minutes

Cooking Time: 15 minutes

Servings: 6

INGREDIENTS:

- 6 toothpicks
- 8 oz of spring mix salad greens
- 1 ten-inch tortilla
- 2 ounces of thinly sliced deli turkey
- 9 tsp. of whipped cream cheese
- 1 roasted red bell pepper

DIRECTIONS:

1. Cut the red bell pepper into ten strips about a quarter-inch thick.
2. Spread the whipped cream cheese on the tortilla evenly.
3. Add the salad greens to create a base layer and then lay the turkey on top of it.
4. Space out the red bell pepper strips on top of the turkey.
5. Tuck the end and begin rolling the tortilla inward.
6. Use the toothpicks to hold the roll into place and cut it into six pieces.
7. Serve with the swirl facing upward.

NUTRITION:

Calories: 206
Fat: 9g
Carbs: 21g
Protein: 9g

Sodium: 533mg
Potassium: 145mg
Phosphorus: 47mg

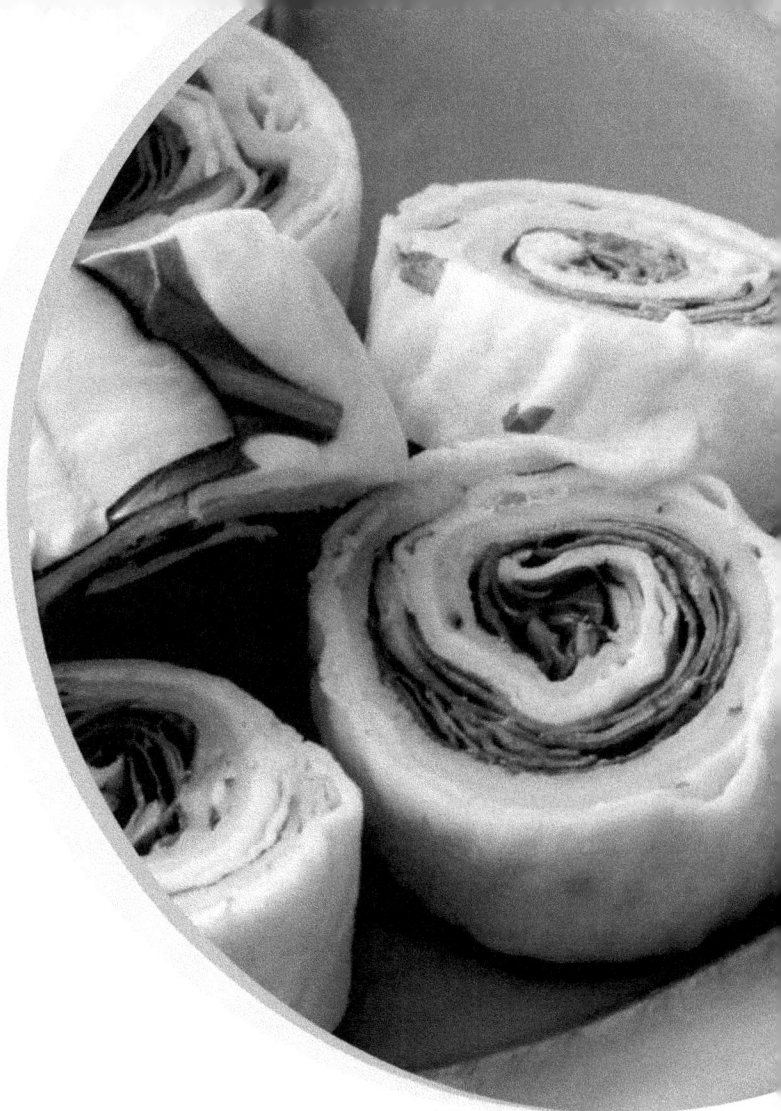

30 | CHICKEN TACOS

Preparation Time: 5 minutes

Cooking Time: 20 minutes

Servings: 4

INGREDIENTS:

- 8 corn tortillas
- 1.5 tsp. of Sodium-free taco seasoning
- 1 juiced lime
- .5 cups of cilantro
- 2 green onions, chopped
- 8 oz of iceberg or romaine lettuce, shredded or chopped
- .25 cup of sour cream
- 1 pound of boneless and skinless chicken breast

DIRECTIONS:

1. Cook chicken, by boiling, for twenty minutes. Shred or chop cooked chicken into fine bite-sized pieces.
2. Mix the seasoning and lime juice with the chicken.
3. Put chicken mixture and lettuce in tortillas.
4. Top with the green onions, cilantro, sour cream.

NUTRITION:

Calories: 260
Fat: 3g
Carbs: 36g
Protein: 23g

Sodium: 922mg
Potassium: 445mg
Phosphorus: 357mg

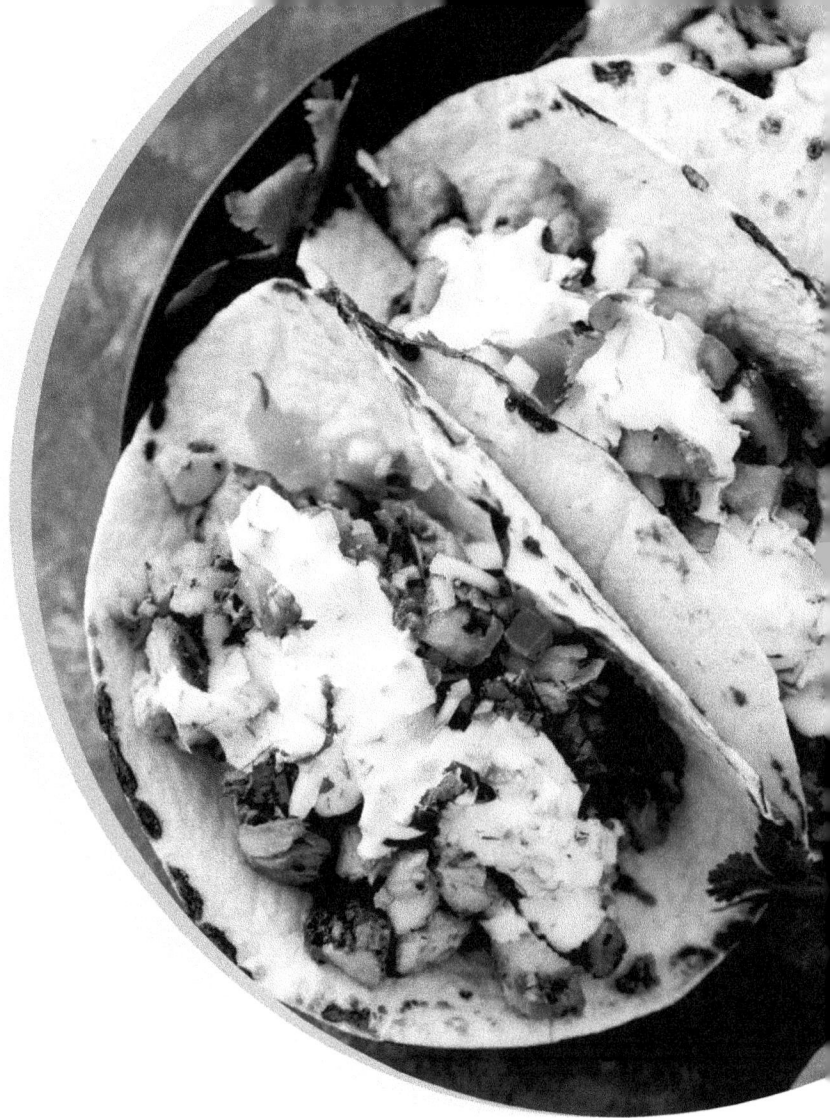

31 | TUNA TWIST

Preparation Time: 10 minutes

Cooking Time: 30 minutes

Servings: 4

INGREDIENTS:

- 1 can of unsalted or water packaged tuna, drained
- 6 tsp. of vinegar
- .5 cup of cooked peas
- .5 cup celery (chopped)
- 3 tsp. of dried dill weed
- 12 oz cooked macaroni
- .75 cup of mayonnaise

DIRECTIONS:

1. Stir together the macaroni, vinegar, and mayonnaise together until blended and smooth.
2. Stir in remaining ingredients.
3. Chill before serving.

NUTRITION:

Calories: 290
Fat: 10g
Carbs: 32g
Protein: 16g
Sodium: 307mg
Potassium: 175mg
Phosphorus: 111mg

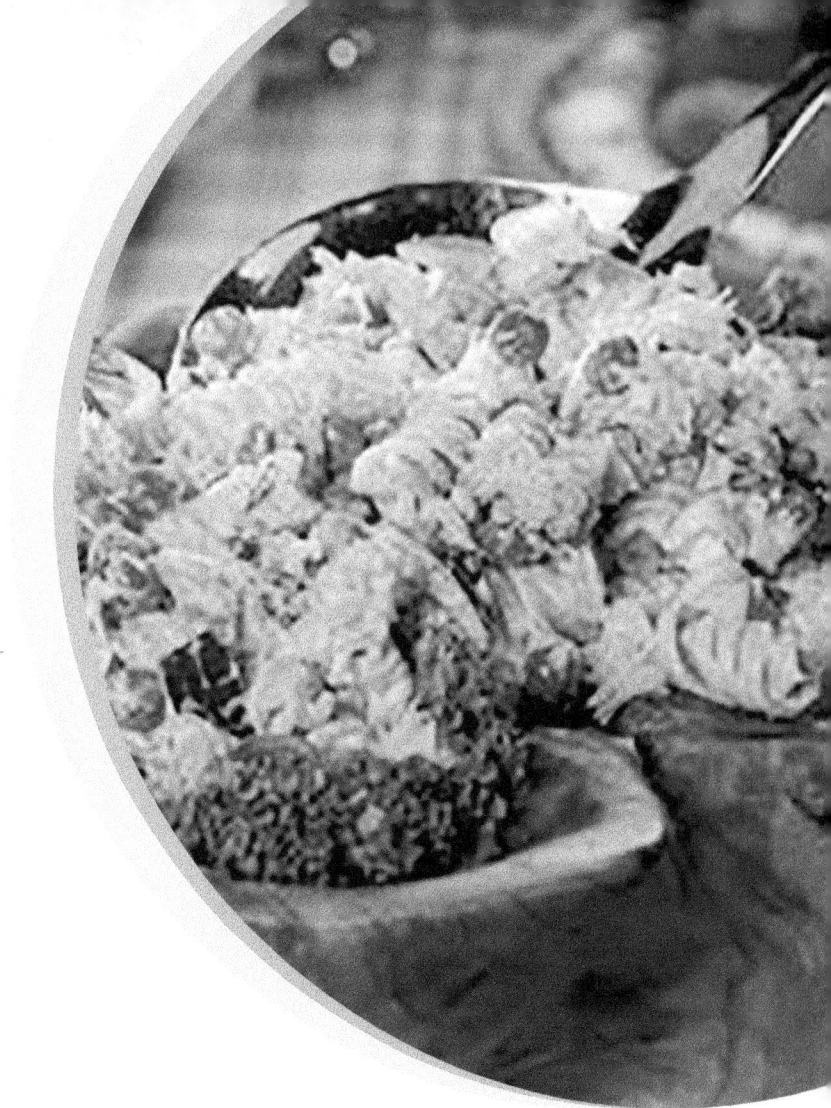

32 CIABATTA ROLLS WITH CHICKEN PESTO

Preparation Time: 10 minutes

Cooking Time: 20 minutes

Servings: 2

INGREDIENTS:

- 6 tsp. of Greek yogurt
- 6 tsp. of pesto
- 2 small ciabatta rolls
- 8 oz of a shredded iceberg or romaine lettuce
- 8 oz of cooked boneless and skinless chicken breast, shredded
- .125 tsp. of pepper

DIRECTIONS:

1. Combine the shredded chicken, pesto, pepper, and Greek yogurt in a medium-sized bowl.
2. Slice and toast the ciabatta rolls.
3. Divide the shredded chicken and pesto mixture in half and make sandwiches with the ciabatta rolls.
4. Top with shredded lettuce if desired.

NUTRITION:

Calories: 374
Fat: 10g
Carbs: 40g
Protein: 30g
Sodium: 522mg

Potassium: 360mg
Phosphorus: 84mg

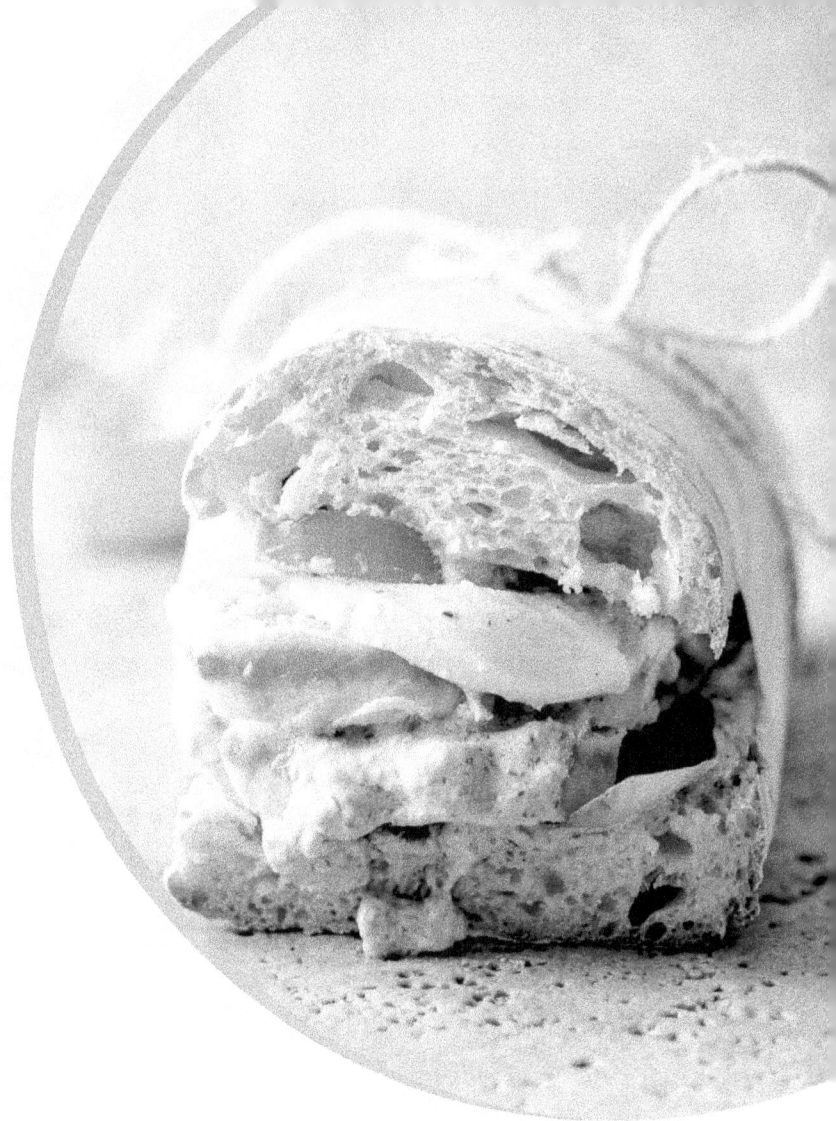

33 MARINATED SHRIMP PASTA SALAD

Preparation Time: 15 minutes

Cooking Time: 5 hours

Servings: 1

INGREDIENTS:

- 1/4 cup of honey
- 1/4 cup of balsamic vinegar
- 1/2 of an English cucumber, cubed
- 1/2 pound of fully cooked shrimp
- 15 baby carrots
- 1.5 cups of dime-sized cut cauliflower
- 4 stalks of celery, diced
- 1/2 large yellow bell pepper (diced)
- 1/2 red onion (diced)
- 1/2 large red bell pepper (diced)
- 12 ounces of uncooked tri-color pasta (cooked)
- 3/4 cup of olive oil
- 3 tsp. of mustard (Dijon)
- 1/2 tsp. of garlic (powder)
- 1/2 tsp. pepper

DIRECTIONS:

1. Cut vegetables and put them in a bowl with the shrimp.
2. Whisk together the honey, balsamic vinegar, garlic powder, pepper, and Dijon mustard in a small bowl. While still whisking, slowly add the oil and whisk it all together.
3. Add the cooled pasta to the bowl with the shrimp and vegetables and mix it.

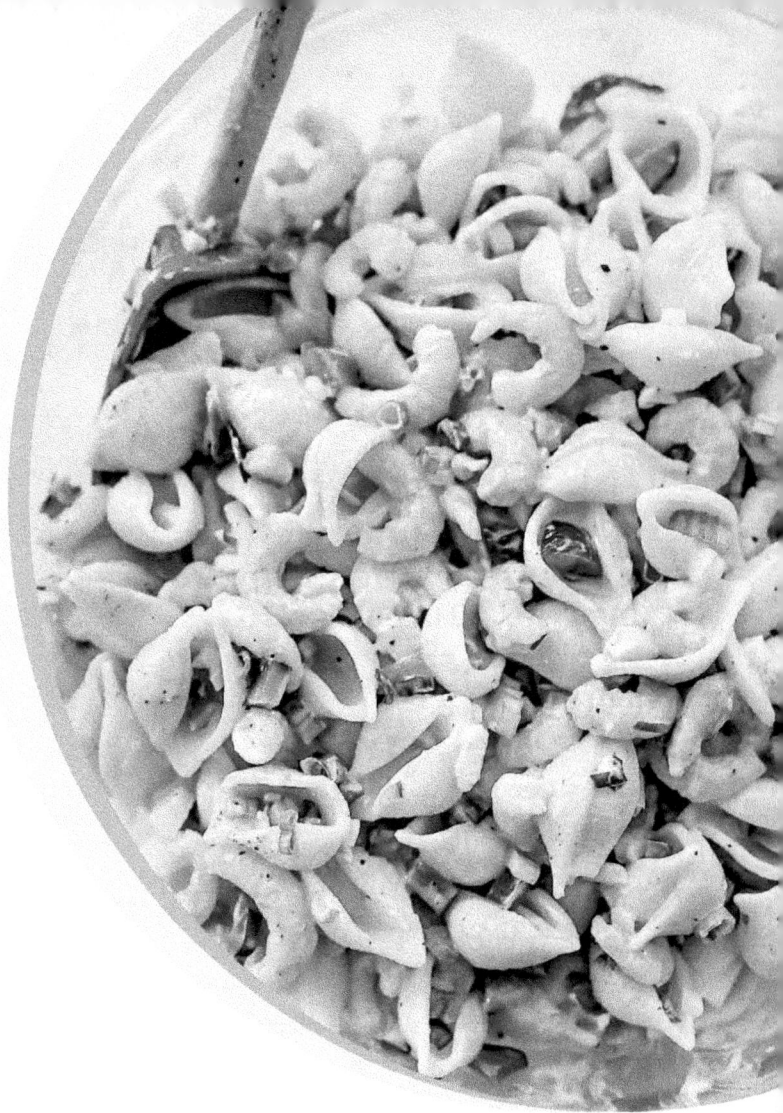

4. Toss the sauce to coat the pasta, shrimp, and vegetables evenly.
5. Cover and chill for a minimum of five hours before serving. Stir and serve while chilled.

NUTRITION:

Calories: 205
Fat: 13g
Carbs: 10g
Protein: 12g
Sodium: 363mg
Potassium: 156mg
Phosphorus: 109mg

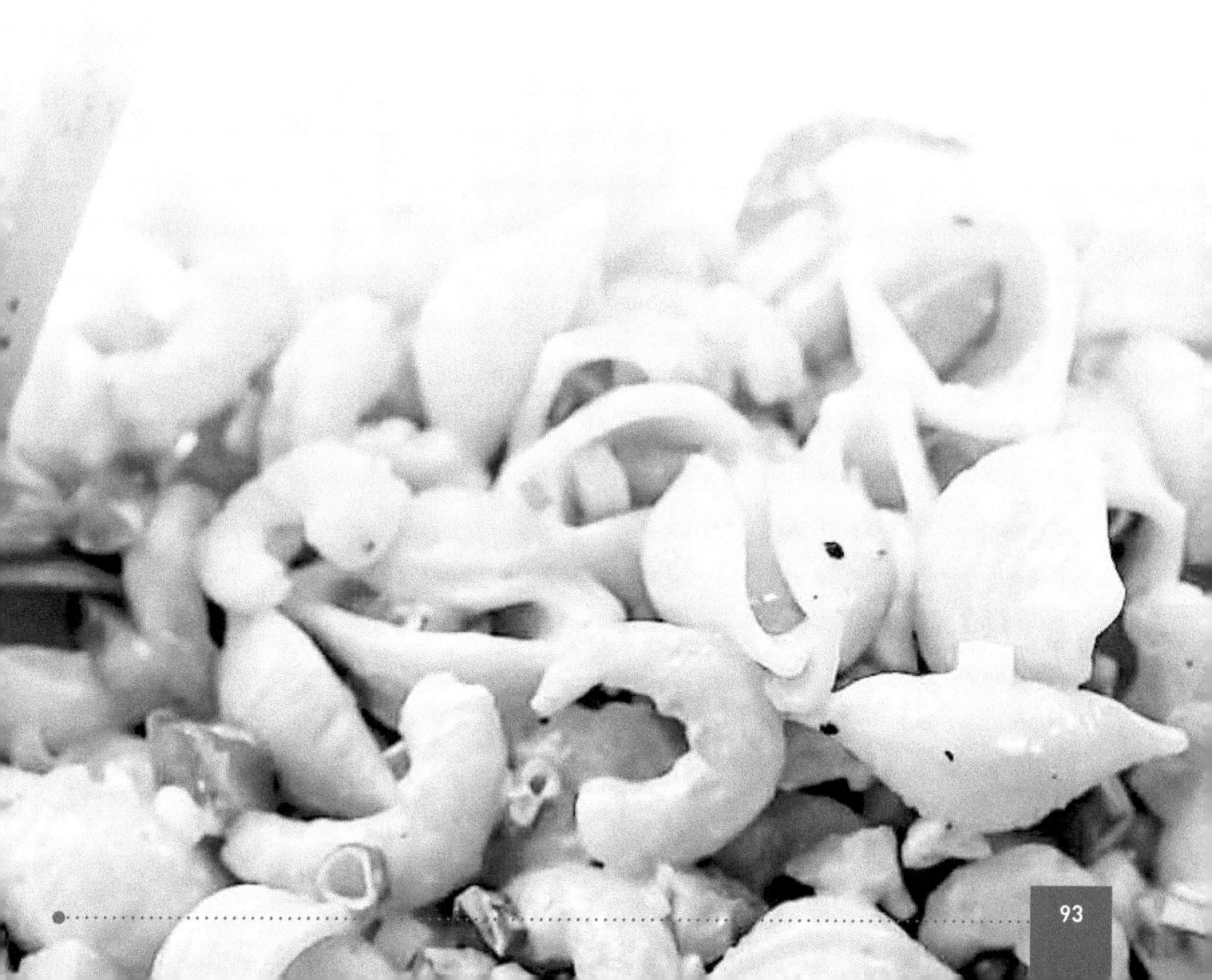

34 PEANUT BUTTER AND JELLY GRILLED SANDWICH

Preparation Time: 5 minutes

Cooking Time: 5 minutes

Servings: 1

INGREDIENTS:

- 2 tsp. butter (unsalted)
- 6 tsp. butter (peanut)
- 3 tsp. of flavored jelly
- 2 pieces of bread

DIRECTIONS:

1. Put the peanut butter evenly on one bread. Add the layer of jelly.
2. Butter the outside of the pieces of bread.
3. Add the sandwich to a frying pan and toast both sides.

NUTRITION:

Calories: 300
Fat: 7g
Carbs: 49g
Protein: 8g
Sodium: 460mg
Potassium: 222mg
Phosphorus: 80mg

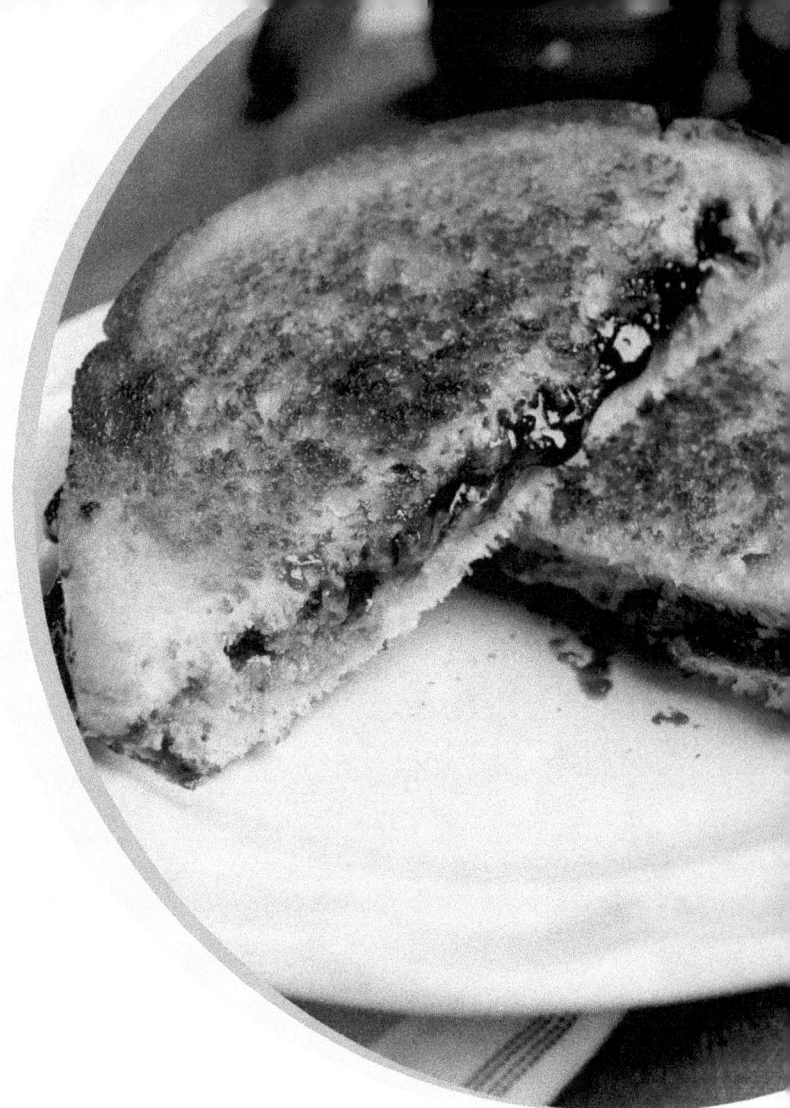

35 | GRILLED ONION AND PEPPER JACK GRILLED CHEESE SANDWICH

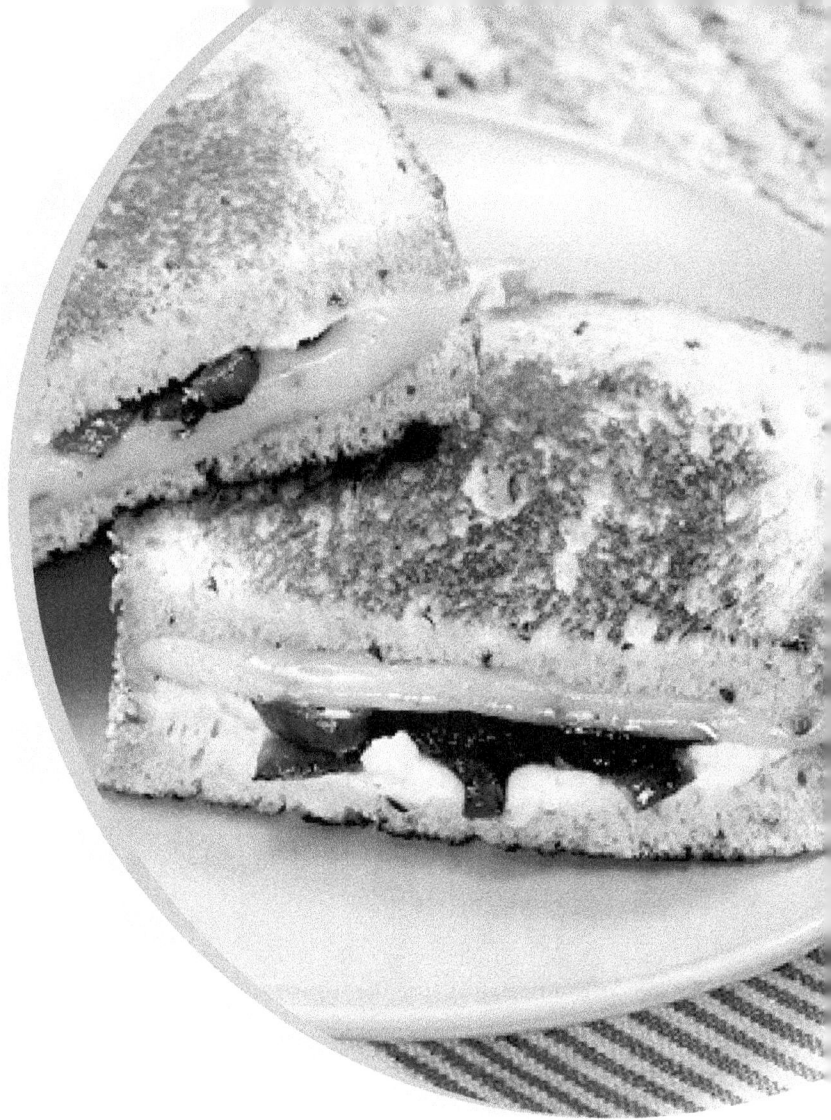

Preparation Time: 5 minutes

Cooking Time: 5 minutes

Servings: 2

INGREDIENTS:

- 1 tsp. of oil (olive)
- 6 tsp. of whipped cream cheese
- 1/2 of a medium onion
- 2 ounces of pepper jack cheese
- 4 slices of rye bread
- 2 tsp. of unsalted butter

DIRECTIONS:

1. Set out the butter so that it becomes soft. Slice up the onion into thin slices.
2. Sauté onion slices. Continue to stir until cooked. Remove and put it to the side.
3. Spread one tablespoon of the whipped cream cheese on two of the slices of bread.
4. Then add grilled onions and cheese to each slice. Then top using the other two bread slices.
5. Spread the softened butter on the outside of the slices of bread.
6. Use the skillet to toast the sandwiches until lightly brown and the cheese is melted.

NUTRITION:

Calories: 350
Fat: 18g
Carbs: 34g
Protein: 13g

Sodium: 589mg
Potassium: 184mg
Phosphorus: 226mg

36 CRISPY LEMON CHICKEN

Preparation Time: 10 minutes

Cooking Time: 10 minutes

Servings: 6

INGREDIENTS:

- 1 lb. boneless and skinless chicken breast
- ½ cup of all-purpose flour
- 1 large egg
- ½ cup of lemon juice
- 2 tbsp of water
- ¼ tsp salt
- ¼ tsp lemon pepper
- 1 tsp of mixed herb seasoning
- 2 tbsp of olive oil
- A few lemon slices for garnishing
- 1 tbsp of chopped parsley (for garnishing)
- 2 cups of cooked plain white rice

DIRECTIONS:

1. Slice the chicken breast into thin and season with the herb, salt, and pepper.
2. In a small bowl, whisk together the egg with the water.
3. Keep the flour in a separate bowl.
4. Dip the chicken slices in the egg bath and then into the flour.
5. Heat your oil in a medium frying pan.
6. Shallow fry the chicken in the pan until golden brown.
7. Add the lemon juice and cook for another couple of minutes.
8. Taken the chicken out of the pan and transfer on a wide dish with absorbing paper to absorb any excess oil.

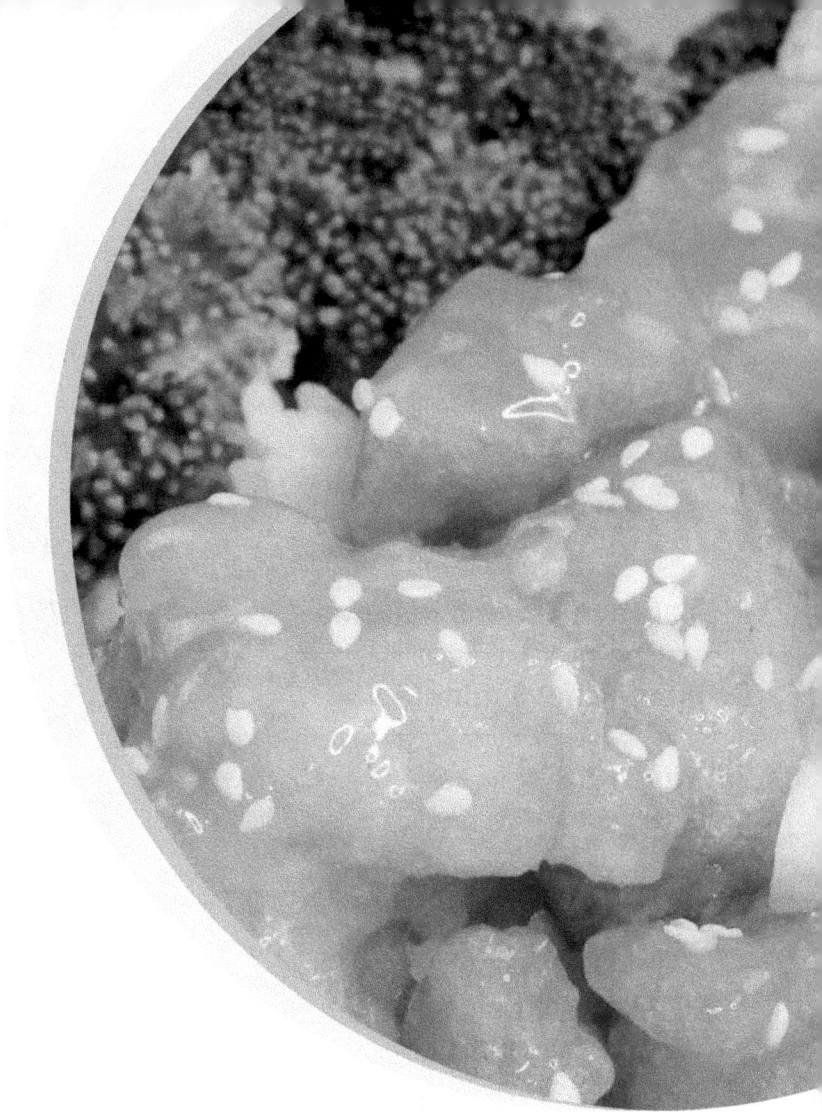

9. Garnish with some chopped parsley and lemon wedges on top.
10. Serve with rice.

NUTRITION:

Calories: 232
Carbohydrate: 24g
Protein: 18g
Fat: 8g
Sodium: 100g
Potassium: 234mg
Phosphorus: 217mg

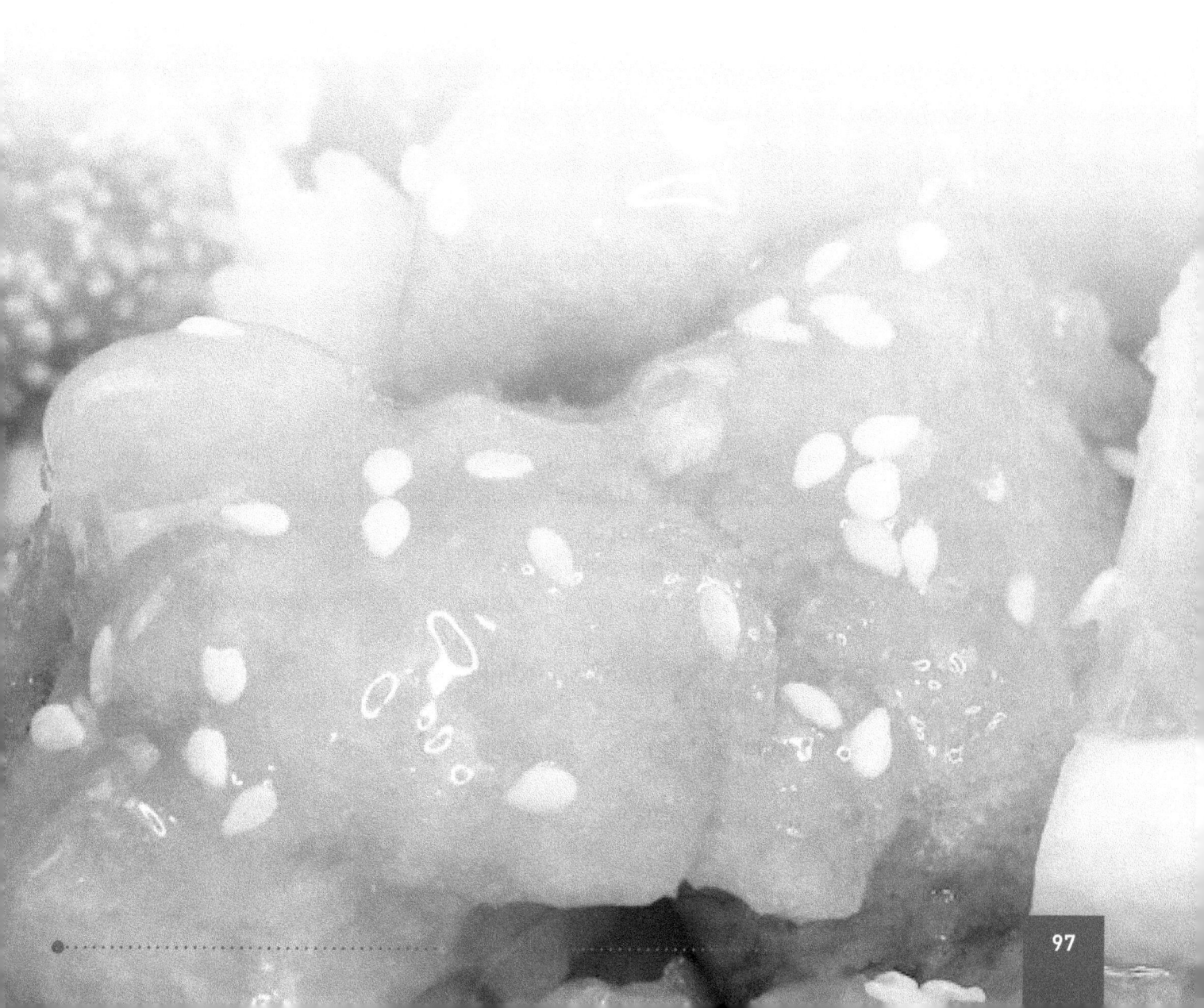

37 MEXICAN STEAK TACOS

Preparation Time: 10 minutes

Cooking Time: 15 minutes

Servings: 8

INGREDIENTS:

- 1 pound of flank or skirt steak
- ¼ cup of fresh cilantro, chopped
- ¼ cup white onion, chopped
- 3 limes, juiced
- 3 cloves of garlic, minced
- 2 tsp of garlic powder
- 2 tbsp of olive oil
- ½ cup of Mexican or mozzarella cheese, grated
- 1 tsp of Mexican seasoning
- 8 medium-sized (6") corn flour tortillas

DIRECTIONS:

1. Combine the juice from two limes, Mexican seasoning, and garlic powder in a dish or bowl and marinate the steak with it for at least half an hour in the fridge.
2. In a separate bowl, combine the chopped cilantro, garlic, onion, and juice from one lime to make your salsa. Cover and keep in the fridge.
3. Slice steak into thin strips and cook for approximately 3 minutes on each side.
4. Preheat your oven to 350F/180C.
5. Distribute evenly the steak strips in each tortilla. Top with a tablespoon of the grated cheese on top.
6. Wrap each taco in aluminum foil and bake in the oven for 7-8 minutes or until cheese is melted.
7. Serve warm with your cilantro salsa.

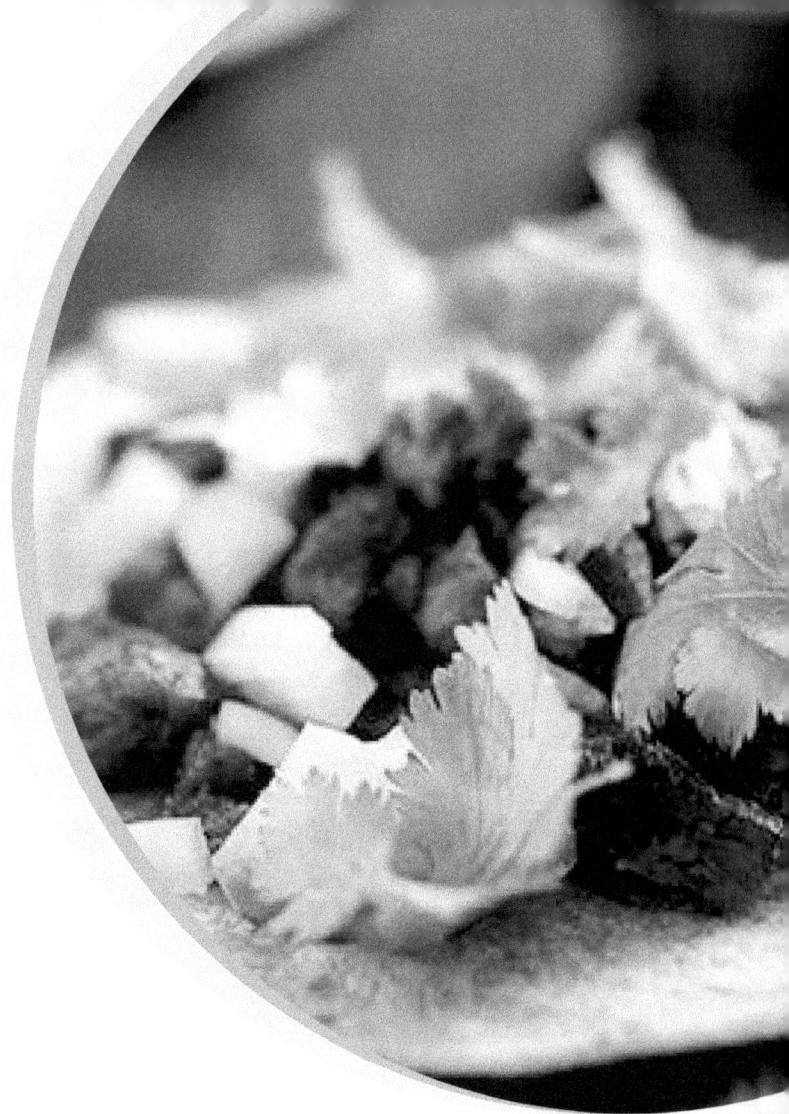

Calories: 230

Carbohydrate: 19.5 g

Protein: 15 g

Fat: 11 g

Sodium: 486.75 g

Potassium: 240 mg

Phosphorus: 268 mg

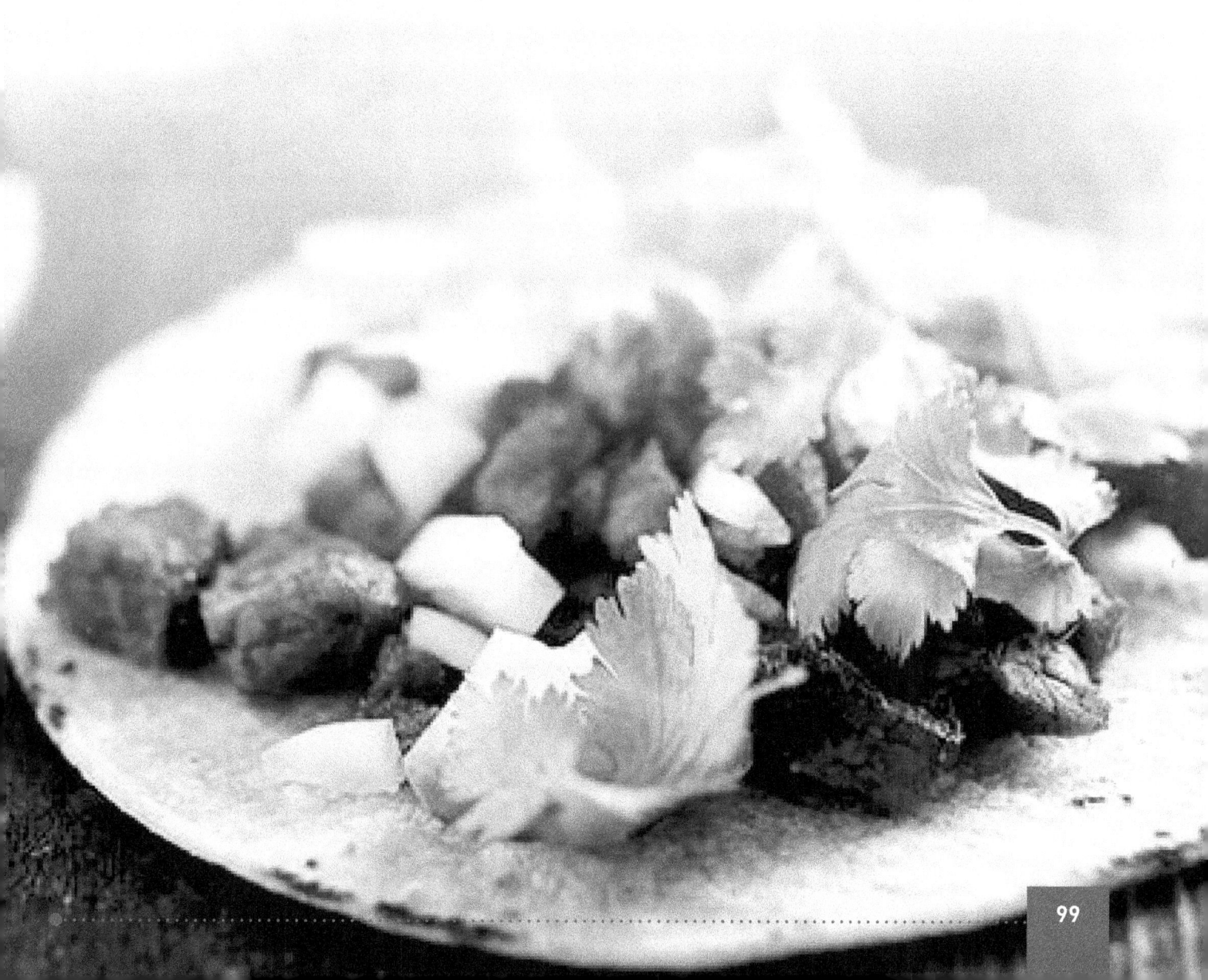

38 | BEER PORK RIBS

Preparation Time: 10 minutes

Cooking Time: 8 hours

Servings: 1

INGREDIENTS:

- 2 pounds of pork ribs, cut into two units/racks
- 18 oz. of root beer
- 2 cloves of garlic, minced
- 2 tbsp of onion powder
- 2 tbsp of vegetable oil (optional)

DIRECTIONS:

1. Wrap the pork ribs with vegetable oil and place one unit on the bottom of your slow cooker with half of the minced garlic and the onion powder.
2. Place the other rack on top with the rest of the garlic and onion powder.
3. Pour over the root beer and cover the lid.
4. Let simmer for 8 hours on low heat.
5. Take off and finish optionally in a grilling pan for a nice sear.

NUTRITION:

Calories: 301
Carbohydrate: 36 g
Protein: 21 g
Fat: 18 g
Sodium: 729 mg
Potassium: 200 mg
Phosphorus: 209 mg

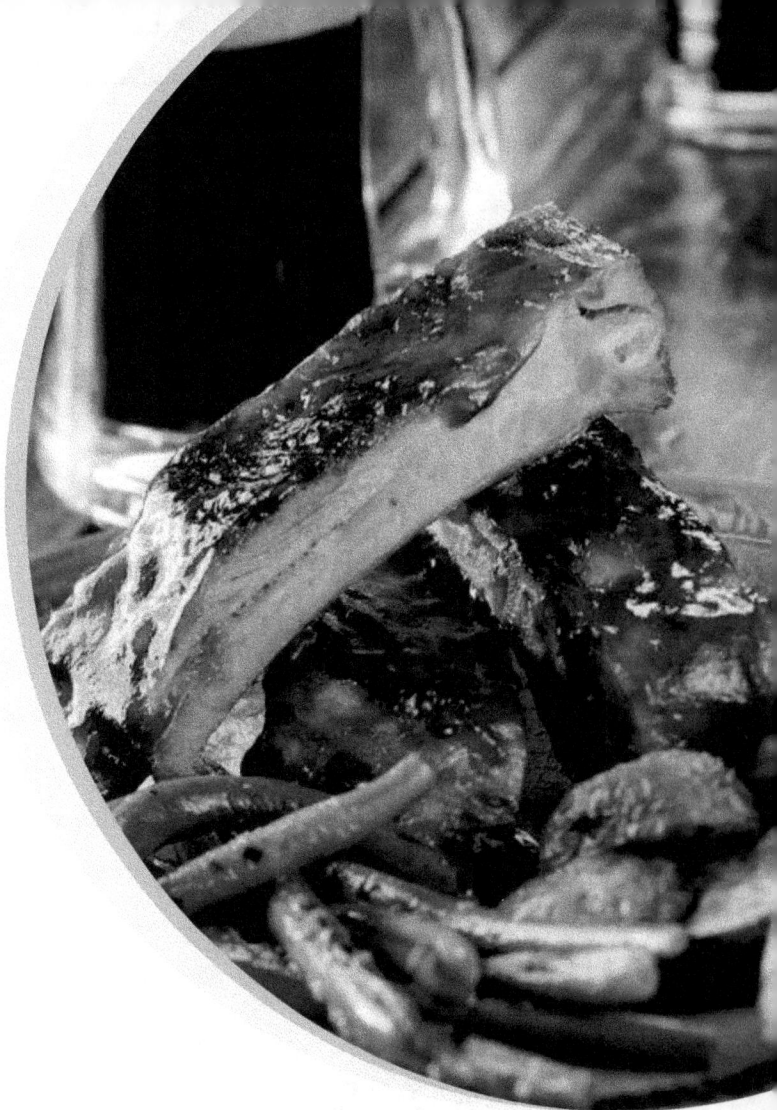

39 MEXICAN CHORIZO SAUSAGE

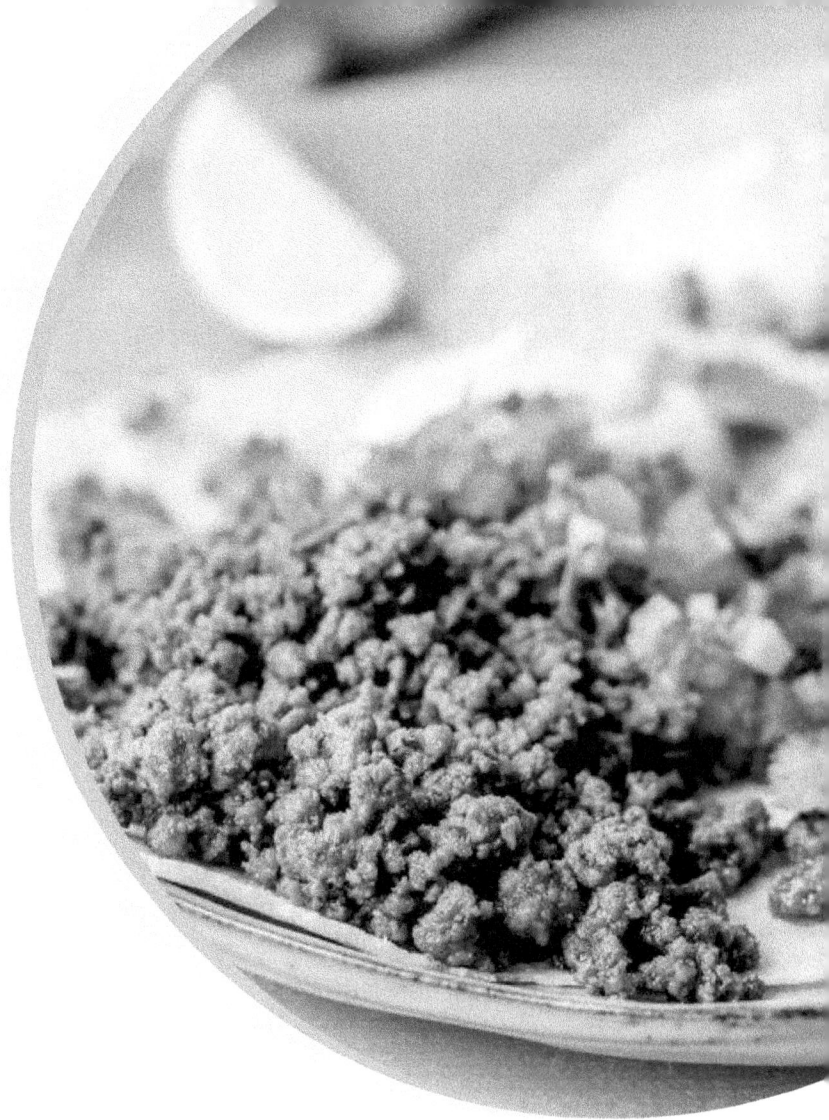

Preparation Time: 10 minutes

Cooking Time: 15 minutes

Servings: 1

INGREDIENTS:

- 2 pounds of boneless pork but coarsely ground
- 3 tbsp of red wine vinegar
- 2 tbsp of smoked paprika
- ½ tsp of cinnamon
- ½ tsp of ground cloves
- ¼ tsp of coriander seeds
- ¼ tsp ground ginger
- 1 tsp of ground cumin
- 3 tbsp of brandy

DIRECTIONS:

1. In a large mixing bowl, combine the ground pork with the seasonings, brandy, and vinegar and mix with your hands well.
2. Place the mixture into a large Ziploc bag and leave in the fridge overnight.
3. Form into 15-16 patties of equal size.
4. Heat the oil in a large pan and fry the patties for 5-7 minutes on each side, or until the meat inside is no longer pink and there is a light brown crust on top.
5. Serve hot.

NUTRITION:

Calories: 134
Carbohydrate: 0 g
Protein: 10 g
Fat: 7 g

Sodium: 40 mg
Potassium: 138 mg
Phosphorus: 128 mg

40 EGGPLANT CASSEROLE

Preparation Time: 10 minutes

Cooking Time: 25 – 30 minutes

Servings: 4

INGREDIENTS:

- 3 cups of eggplant, peeled and cut into large chunks
- 2 egg whites
- 1 large egg, whole
- ½ cup of unsweetened vegetable
- ¼ tsp of sage
- ½ cup of breadcrumbs
- 1 tbsp of margarine, melted
- 1/4 tsp garlic salt

DIRECTIONS:

1. Preheat the oven at 350F/180C.
2. Place the eggplants chunks in a medium pan, cover with a bit of water and cook with the lid covered until tender. Drain from the water and mash with a tool or fork.
3. Beat the eggs with the non-dairy vegetable cream, sage, salt, and pepper. Whisk in the eggplant mush.
4. Combine the melted margarine with the breadcrumbs.
5. Bake in the oven for 20-25 minutes or until the casserole has a golden-brown crust.

NUTRITION:

Calories: 186
Carbohydrate: 19 g
Protein: 7 g
Fat: 9 g

Sodium: 503 mg
Potassium: 230 mg
Phosphorus: 62 mg

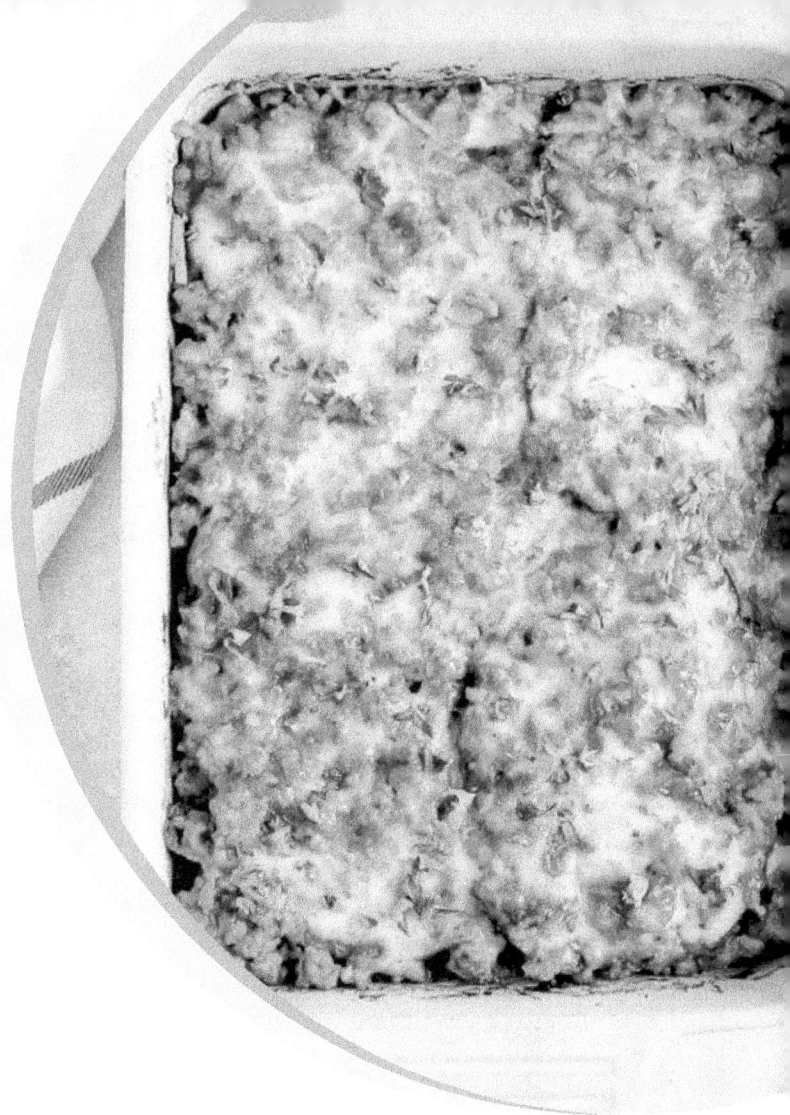

41 PIZZA WITH CHICKEN AND PESTO

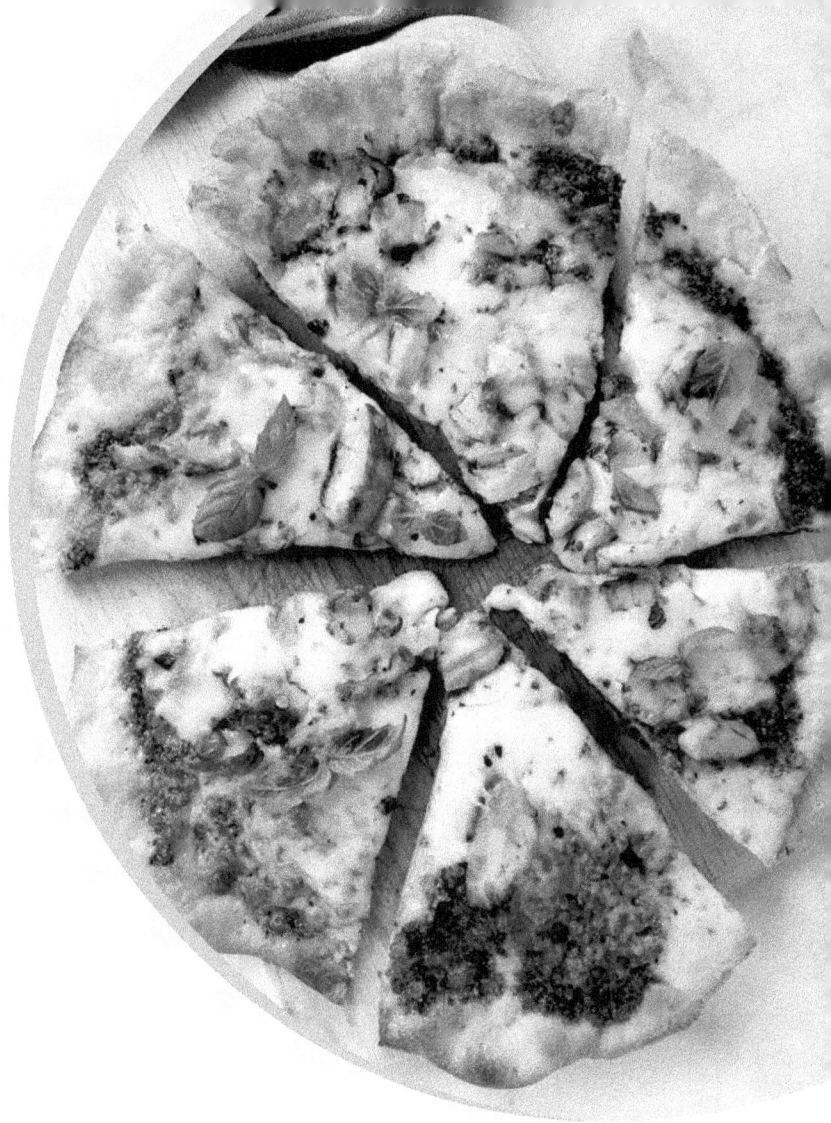

Preparation Time: 10 minutes

Cooking Time: 25 minutes

Servings: 4

INGREDIENTS:

- 1 ready-made frozen pizza dough
- 2/3 cup cooked chicken, chopped
- 1/2 cup of orange bell pepper, diced
-
  1/2 cup of green bell pepper, diced
- 1/4 cup of purple onion, chopped
- 2 tbsp of green basil pesto
- 1 tbsp of chives, chopped
- 1/3 cup of parmesan or Romano cheese, grated
- 1/4 cup of mozzarella cheese
- 1 tbsp of olive oil

DIRECTIONS:

1. Thaw the pizza dough according to instructions on the package.
2. Heat the olive oil in a pan and sauté the peppers and onions for a couple of minutes. Set aside
3. Once the pizza dough has thawed, spread the Bali pesto over its surface.
4. Top with half of the cheese, the peppers, the onions, and the chicken. Finish with the rest of the cheese.

5. Bake at 350F/180C for approx. 20 minutes (or until crust and cheese are baked).
6. Slice in triangles with a pizza cutter or sharp knife and serve.

NUTRITION:

Calories: 225
Carbohydrate: 13.9 g
Protein: 11.1 g
Fat: 12 g
Sodium: 321 mg
Potassium: 174 mg
Phosphorus: 172 mg

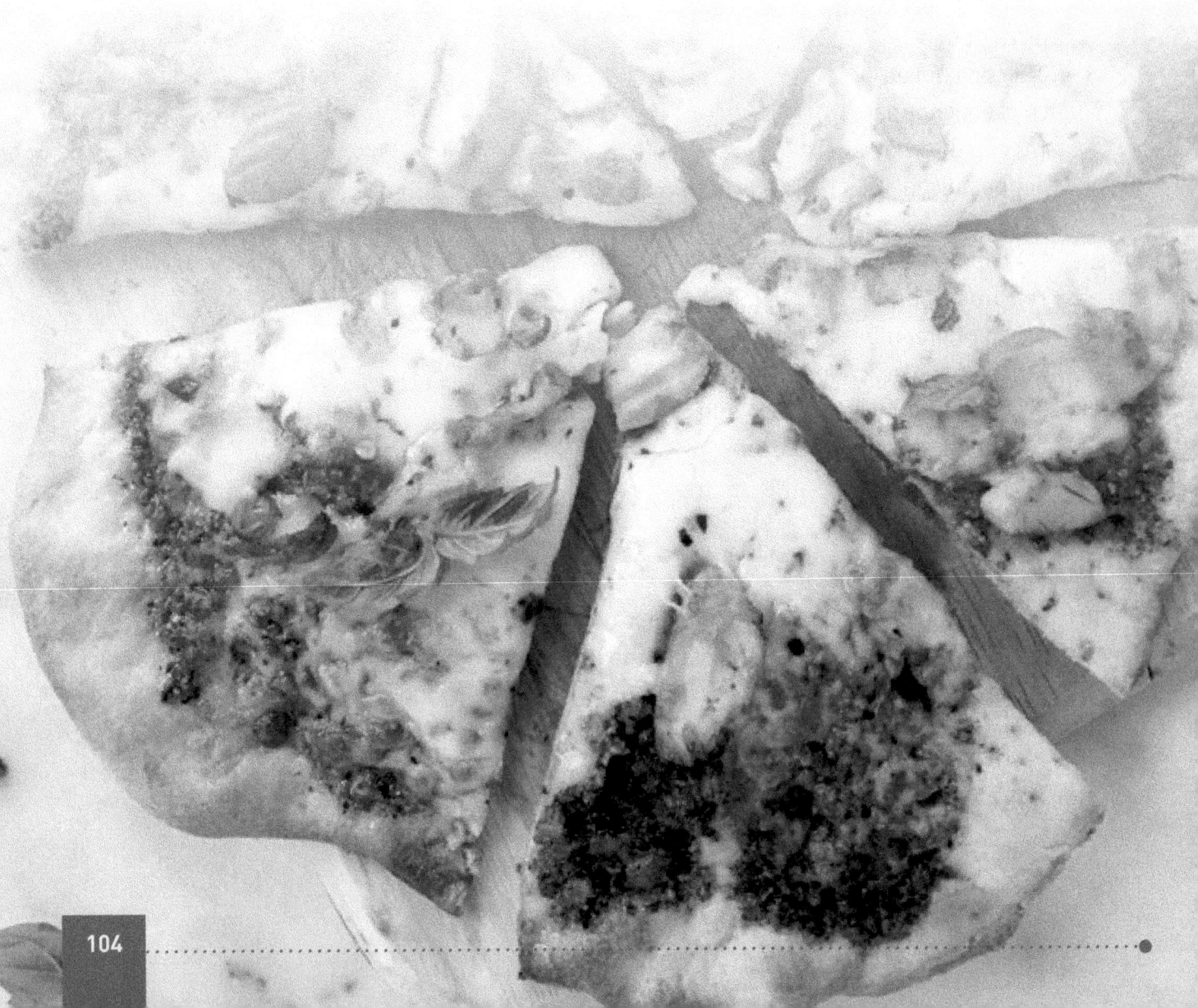

42 SHRIMP QUESADILLA

Preparation Time: 10 minutes

Cooking Time: 10 minutes

Servings: 2

INGREDIENTS:

- 5 oz of shrimp, shelled and deveined
- 4 tbsp of Mexican salsa
- 2 tbsp of fresh cilantro, chopped
- 1 tbsp of lemon juice
- 1 tsp of ground cumin
- 1 tsp of cayenne pepper
- 2 tbsp of unsweetened soy yogurt or creamy tofu
- 2 medium corn flour tortillas
- 2 tbsp of low-fat cheddar cheese

DIRECTIONS:

1. Mix the cilantro, cumin, lemon juice, and cayenne in a Ziploc bag to make your marinade.
2. Put the shrimps and marinate for 10 minutes.
3. Heat a pan over medium heat with some olive oil and toss in the shrimp with the marinade. Let cook for a couple of minutes or as soon as shrimps have turned pink and opaque.
4. Add the soy cream or soft tofu to the pan and mix well. Remove from the heat and keep the marinade aside.
5. Heat tortillas in the grill or microwave for a few seconds.
6. Place 2 tbsp of salsa on each tortilla. Top one tortilla with the shrimp mixture and add the cheese on top.
7. Stack one tortilla against each other (with the spread salsa layer facing the shrimp mixture).

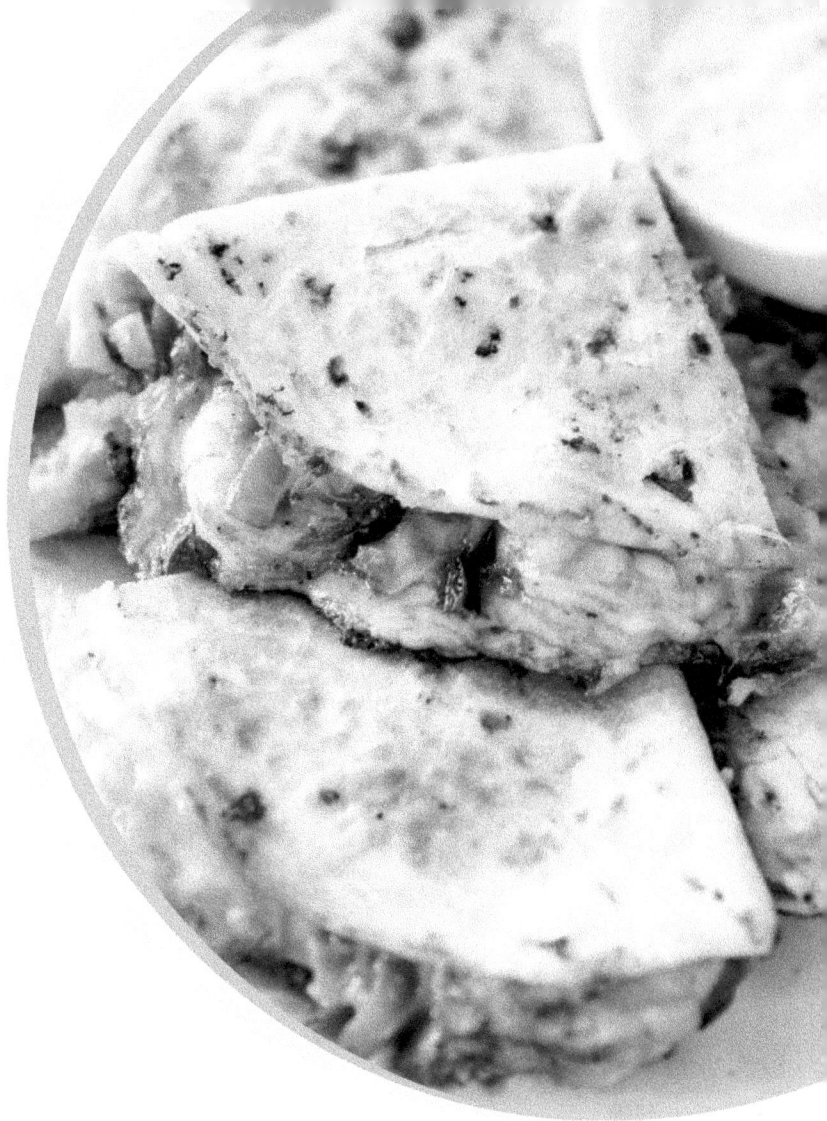

8. Transfer this on a baking tray and cook for 7-8 minutes at 350F/180C to melt the cheese and crisp up the tortillas.
9. Serve warm.

NUTRITION:

Calories: 255
Carbohydrate: 21 g
Fat: 9 g
Protein: 24 g
Sodium: 562 g
Potassium: 235 mg
Phosphorus: 189 mg

43 GRILLED CORN ON THE COB

Preparation Time: 5 minutes

Cooking Time: 20 minutes

Servings: 4

INGREDIENTS:

- 4 frozen corn on the cob, cut in half
- ½ tsp of thyme
- 1 tbsp of grated parmesan cheese
- ¼ tsp of black pepper

DIRECTIONS:

1. Combine the oil, cheese, thyme, and black pepper in a bowl.
2. Place the corn in the cheese/oil mix and roll to coat evenly.
3. Fold all 4 pieces in aluminum foil, leaving a small open surface on top.
4. Place the wrapped corns over the grill and let cook for 20 minutes.
5. Serve hot.

NUTRITION:

Calories: 125
Carbohydrate: 29.5 g
Protein: 2 g
Fat: 1.3 g
Sodium: 26 g
Potassium: 145 mg
Phosphorus: 91.5 mg

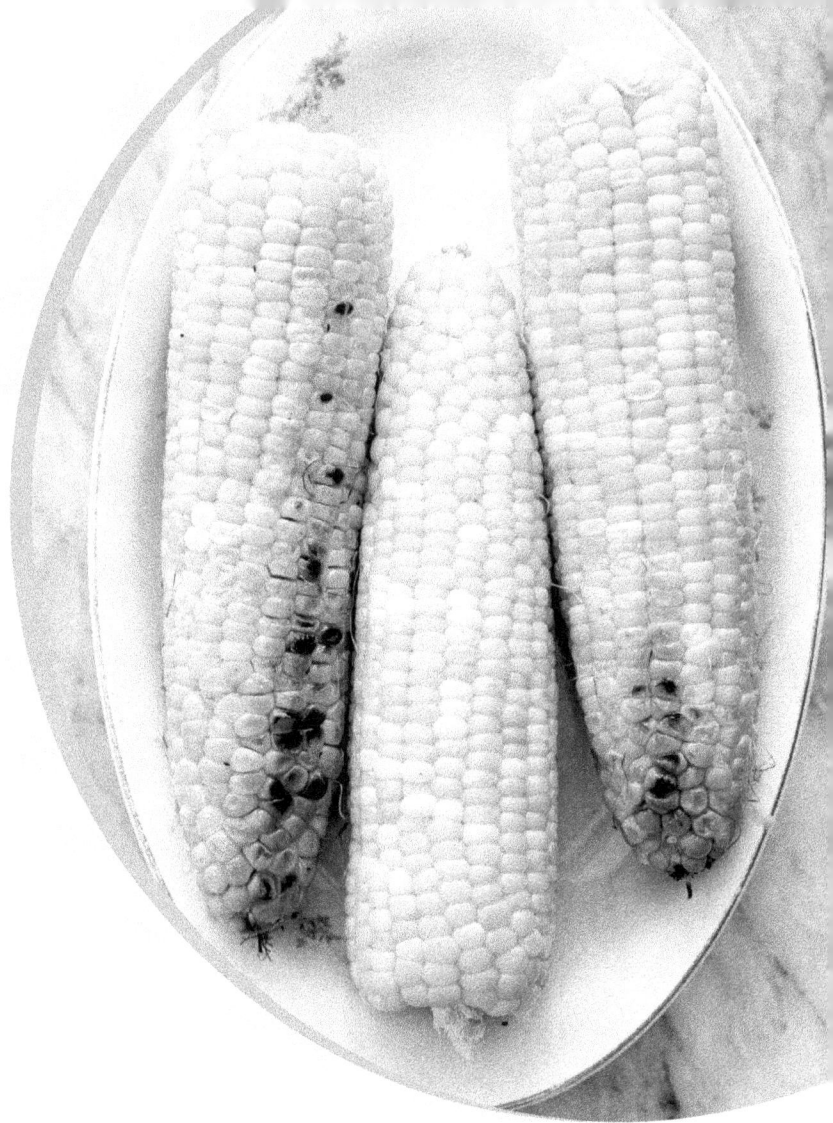

44 COUSCOUS WITH VEGGIES

Preparation Time: 10 minutes

Cooking Time: 10 minutes

Servings: 5

INGREDIENTS:

- ½ cup of uncooked couscous
- ¼ cup of white mushrooms, sliced
- ½ cup of red onion, chopped
- 1 garlic clove, minced
- ½ cup of frozen peas
- 2 tbsp of dry white wine
- ½ tsp of basil
- 2 tbsp of fresh parsley, chopped
- 1 cup water or vegetable stock
- 1 tbsp of margarine or vegetable oil

DIRECTIONS:

1. Thaw the peas by setting them aside at room temperature for 15-20 minutes.
2. In a medium pan, heat the margarine or vegetable oil.
3. Add the onions, peas, mushroom, and garlic and sauté for around 5 minutes. Add the wine and let it evaporate.
4. Add all the herbs and spices and toss well. Take off the heat and keep aside.
5. In a small pot, cook the couscous with 1 cup of hot water or vegetable stock. Bring to a boil, take off the heat, and sit for a few minutes with a lid covered.
6. Add the sauté veggies to the couscous and toss well.
7. Serve in a serving bowl warm or cold.

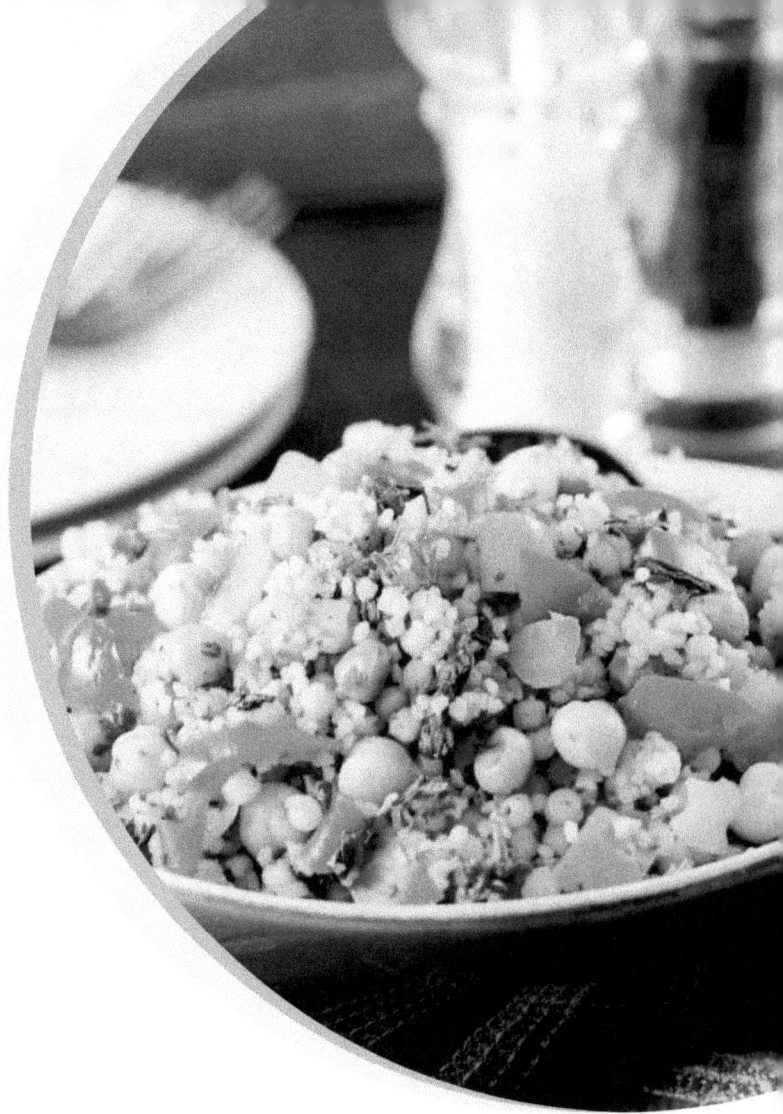

Calories: 110.4

Carbohydrate: 18 g

Protein: 3 g

Fat: 2 g

Sodium: 112.2 mg

Potassium: 69.6 mg

Phosphorus: 46.8 mg

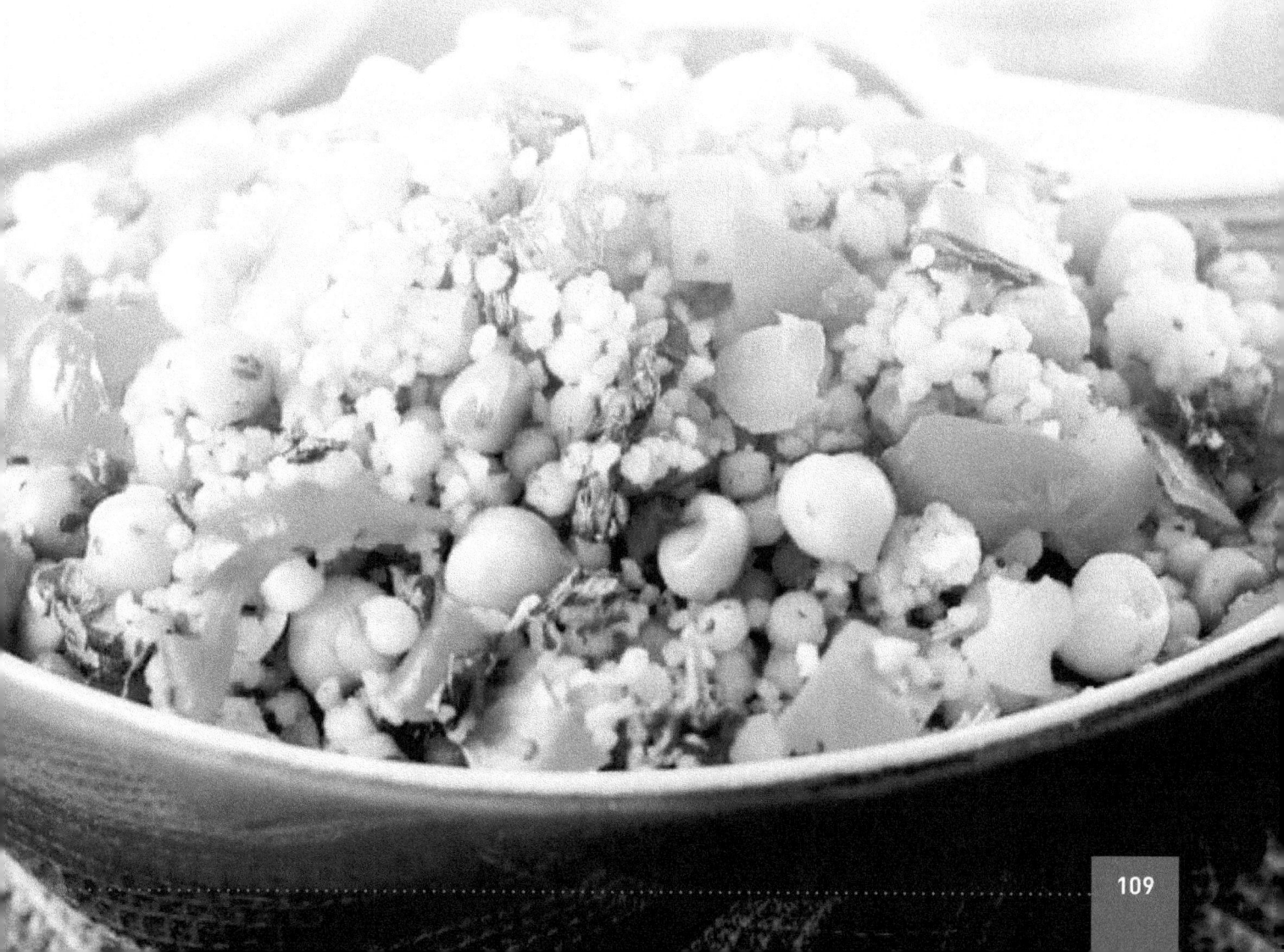

45 EASY EGG SALAD

Preparation Time: 5 minutes

Cooking Time: 8 minutes

Servings: 4

INGREDIENTS:

- 4 large eggs
- ½ cup of sweet onion, chopped
- ¼ cup of celery, chopped
- 2 tbsp of pickle relish
- 1 tbsp of yellow mustard
- 1 tsp of smoked paprika
- 3 tbsp of mayo

DIRECTIONS:

1. Hard boil the eggs in a small pot filled with water for approx. 7-8 minutes. Leave the eggs in the water for an extra couple of minutes before peeling.
2. Peel the eggs and chop finely with a knife or tool.
3. Combine all the chopped veggies with the mayo and mustard. Add in the eggs and mix well.
4. Sprinkle with some smoked paprika on top.
5. Serve cold with pitta, white bread slices, or lettuce wraps.

NUTRITION:

Calories: 127
Carbohydrate: 6 g
Protein: 7 g
Fat: 13 g
Sodium: 170.7 mg
Potassium: 87.5 mg
Phosphorus: 101 mg

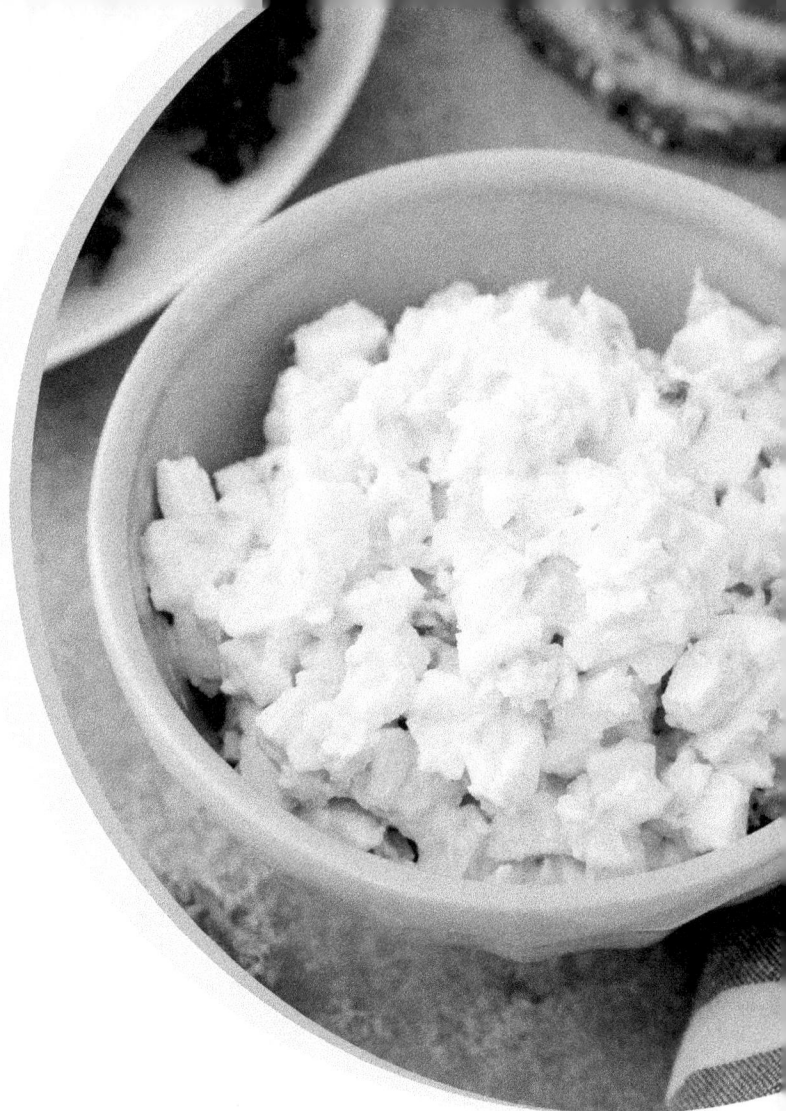

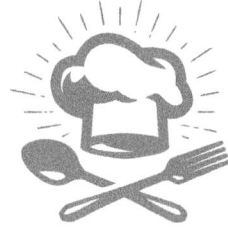

CHAPTER 14

DINNER RECIPES

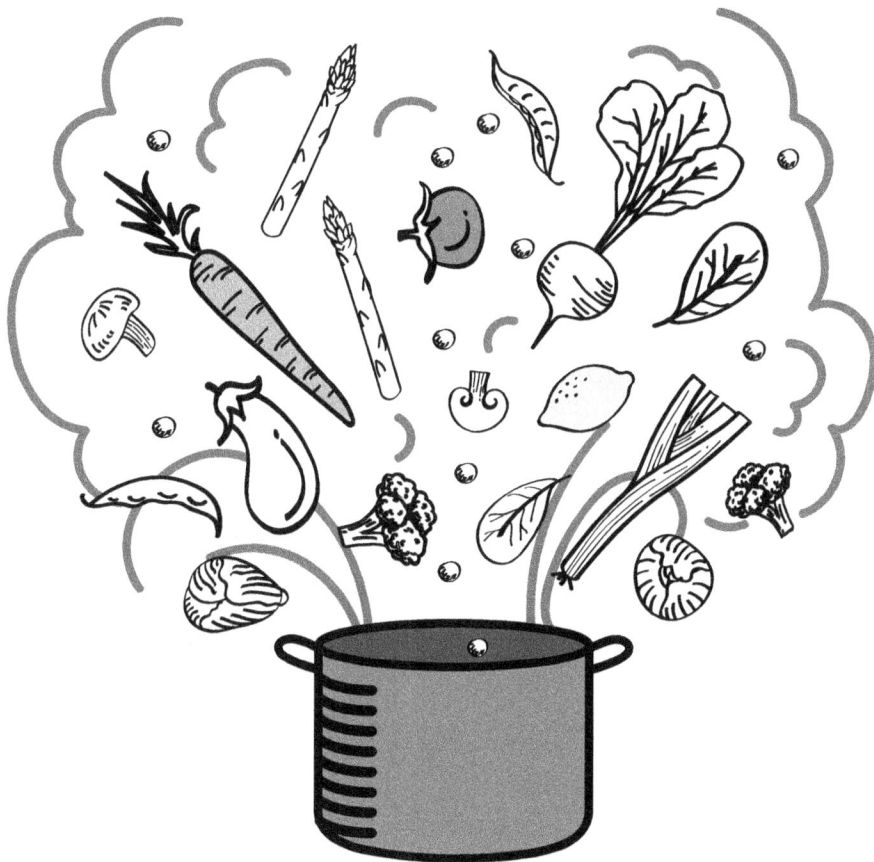

46 GREEN TUNA SALAD

Preparation Time: 10 minutes

Cooking Time: 15 -20 minutes

Servings: 2

INGREDIENTS:

- 5 ounces of tuna (in freshwater only)
- 2-3 cups of lettuce
- 1/2 cup of Italian tomatoes
- 1 cup of baby marrows
- 1/2 cup of red bell pepper
- 1/4 cup of red onion
- 1/4 cup of fresh thyme
- 2 tbsp olive oil
- 1/8 tsp of black pepper
- 2 tbsp of red wine vinegar

DIRECTIONS:

1. Chop the bell pepper, onion, baby marrow, and thyme into small pieces.
2. Add a 3/4 cup of water to a saucepan and add the bell pepper, onion, baby marrow, and thyme to the pan. Let it boil, steam the vegetables by adding a lid on top of the saucepan—steam for 10 minutes.
3. Remove the vegetables and drain them.
4. Combine the vegetables (once cooled down) with the chopped tomatoes and tuna.
5. Mix olive oil, red wine vinegar, and black pepper to create a salad dressing.
6. Add the mixture on a bed of lettuce and drizzle the dressing on top.

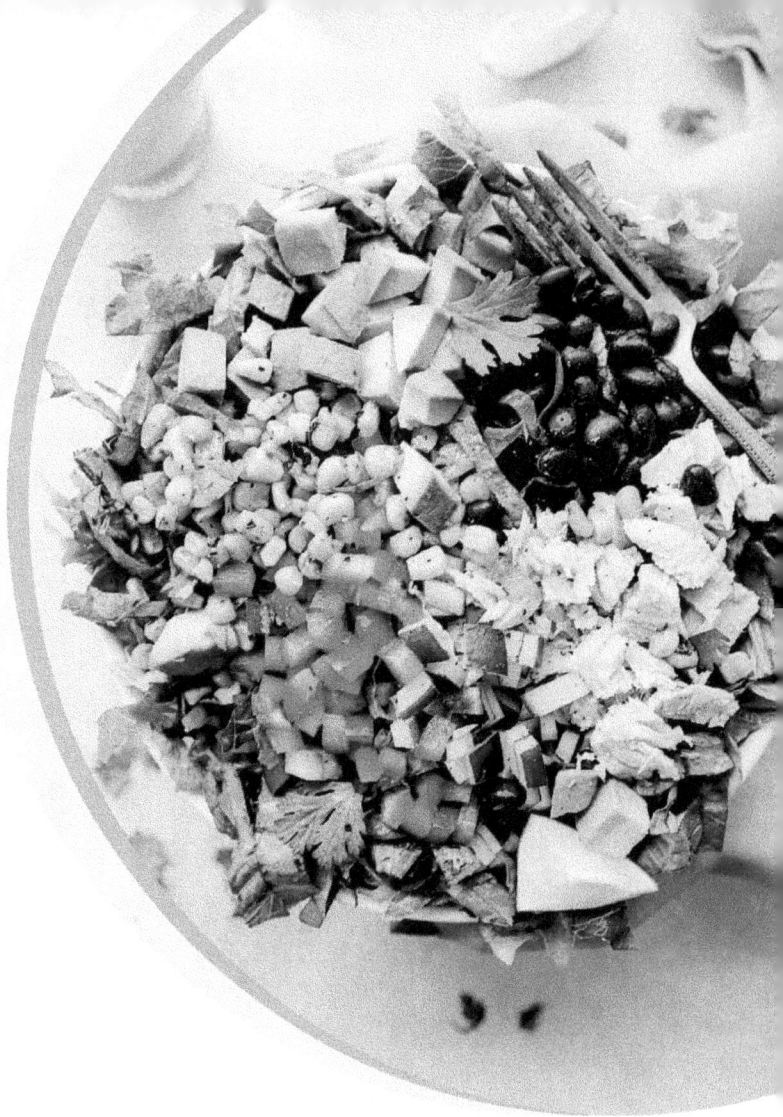

Calories: 210
Fat: 1.5g
Carbs: 4g
Protein: 43.3g
Sodium: 726mg
Potassium: 582mg
Phosphorus: 296mg

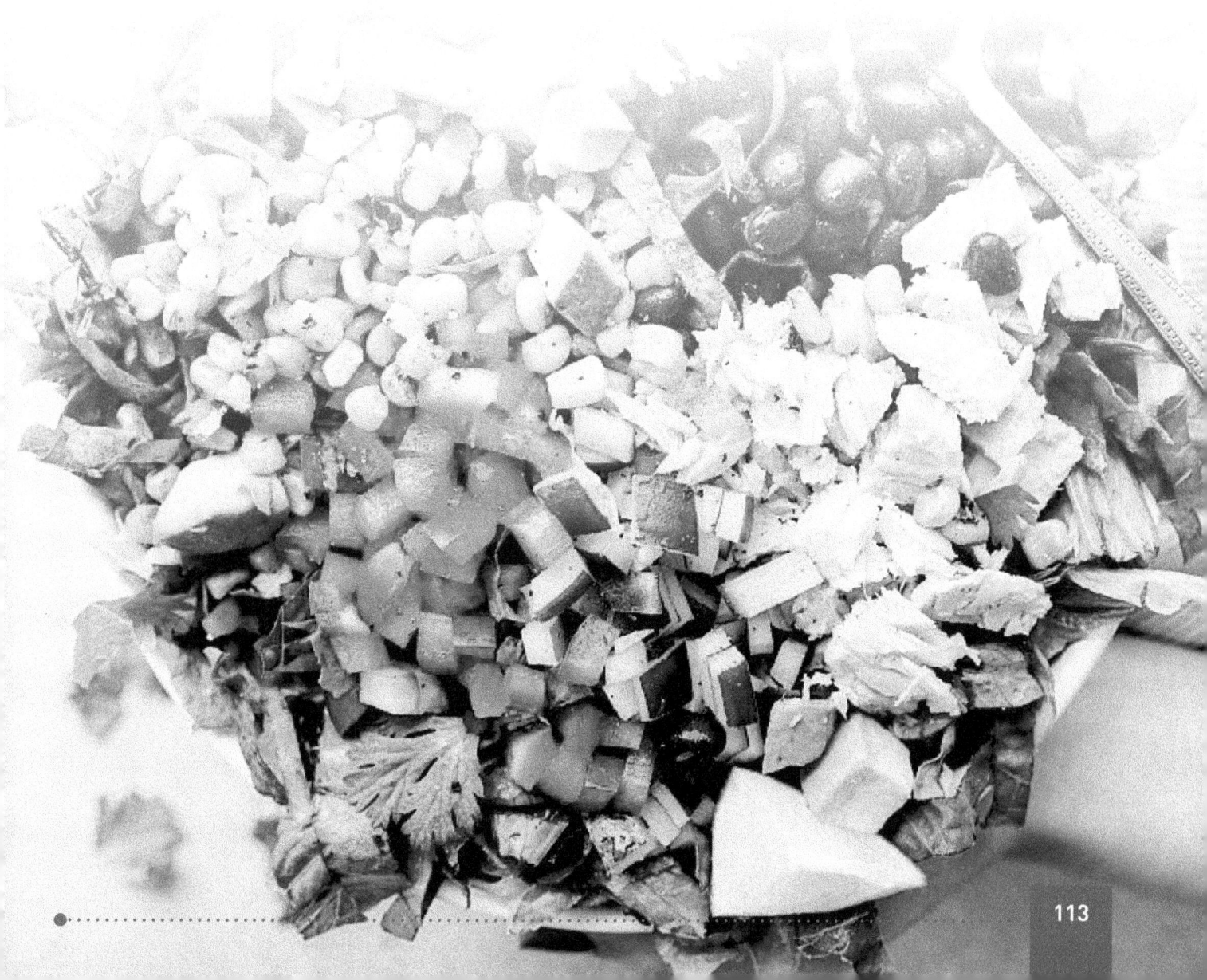

47 ROASTED CHICKEN AND VEGETABLES

Preparation Time: 10 minutes

Cooking Time: 45 minutes

Servings: 2

INGREDIENTS:

- 8 oz chicken strips
- 1 ½ cups baby potatoes
- 5 oz green beans
- 2 tbsp sesame seed oil
- 1 tsp of Cajun chicken spice
- ½ tbsp Italian herb dressing

DIRECTIONS:

1. Heat the oven to 400 degrees-Fahrenheit
2. Fill up a large pot with water until it is ¾ full. Add the baby potatoes to the pot and cook for 10 minutes.
3. Drain the baby potatoes.
4. Chop off the tips of the green beans.
5. Line a 9 x 13-inch oven tray with parchment paper or spray the oven tray with cooking spray.
6. Place the chicken strips on the tray side, with the green beans and baby potatoes.
7. Add Cajun chicken spice to the chicken breasts and drizzle sesame seed oil over the chicken and vegetables.
8. Roast for 20 minutes.
9. Drizzle Italian herb dressing on top of the chicken and vegetables and roast for another 5-10 minutes.

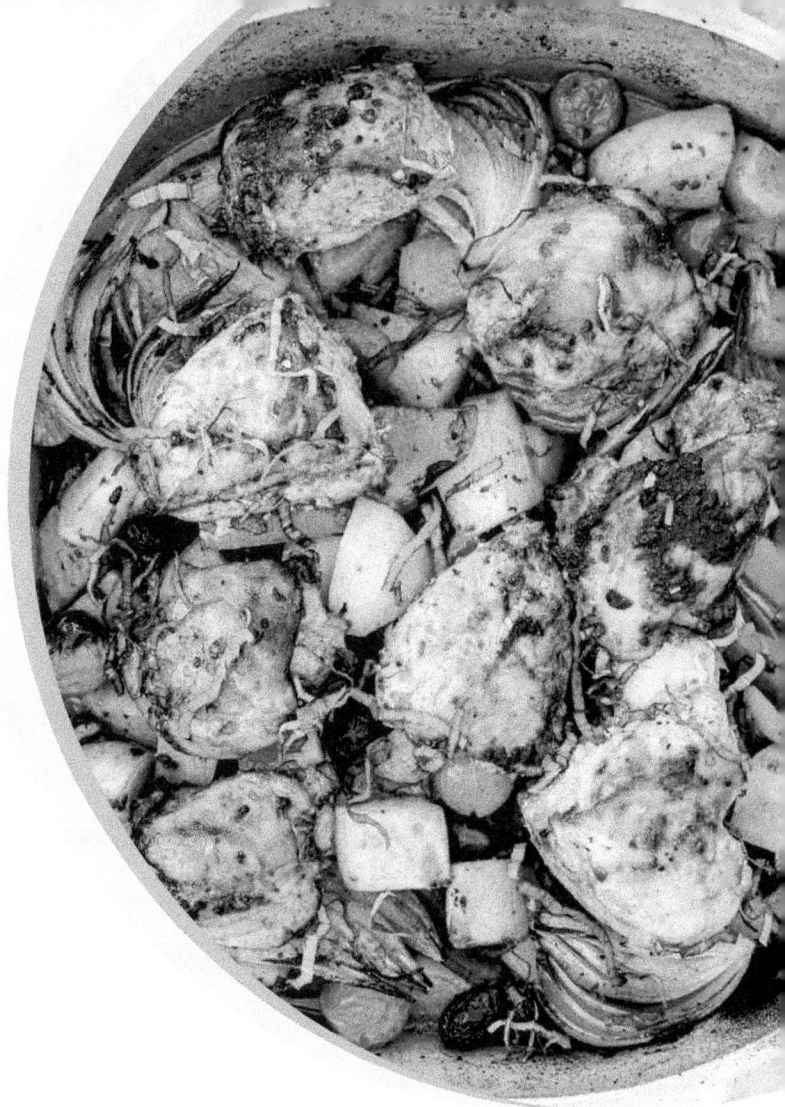

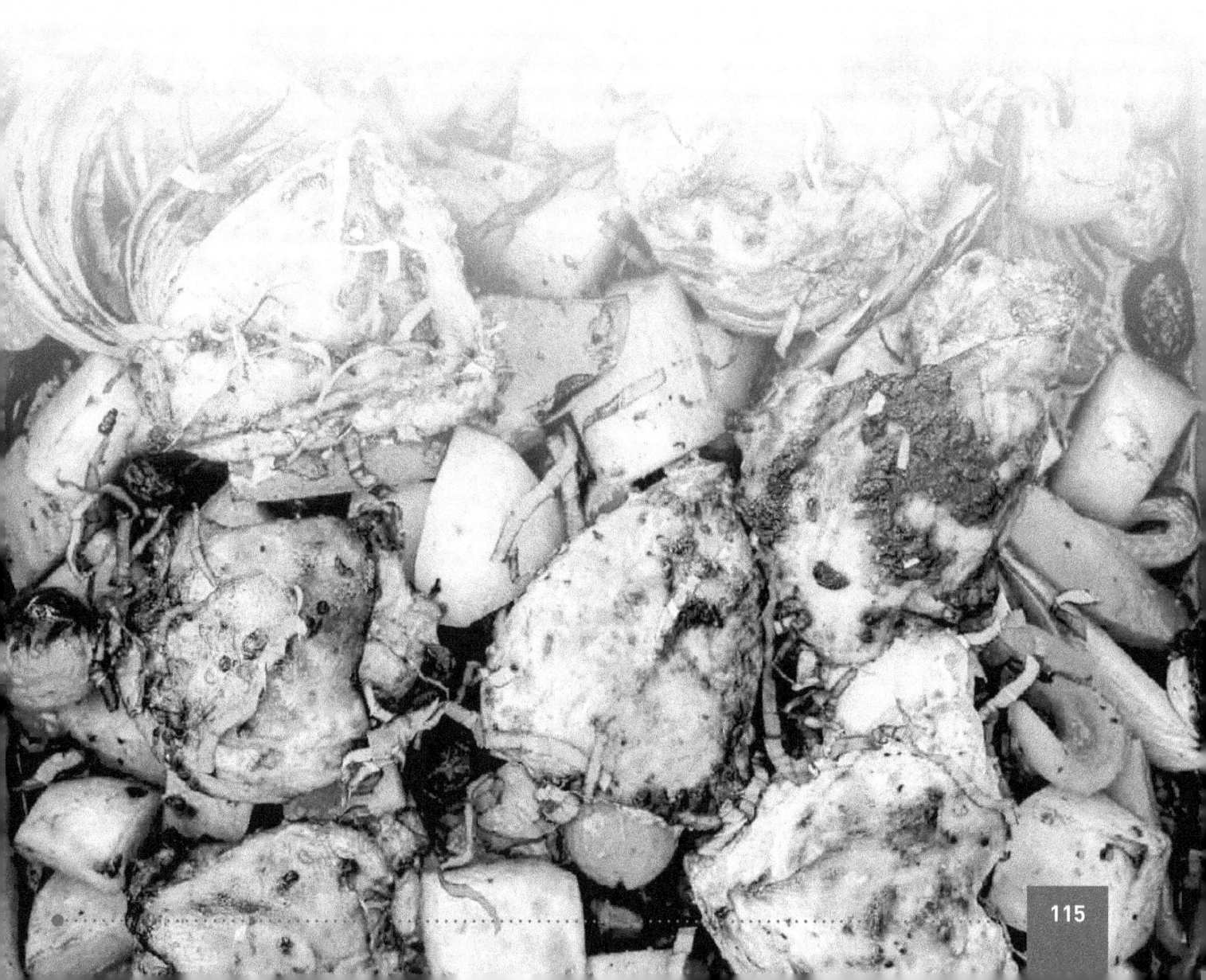

Calories: 263
Fat: 6g
Sodium: 366mg
Potassium: 879mg
Phosphorus: 275mg
Carbs: 28.6g
Protein: 23g

48 SIRLOIN MEDALLIONS, GREEN SQUASH, AND PINEAPPLE

Preparation Time: 10 minutes

Cooking Time: 40 minutes

Servings: 4

INGREDIENTS:

- 1 lb. of sirloin medallions
- 1 medium baby marrows
- 1 yellow squash
- ½ onion
- 8 oz of thinly sliced pineapple
- 3 tbsp of olive oil
- 2 tsp of ginger
- ½ tsp of salt
- 1 garlic clove

DIRECTIONS:

1. Retrieve thinly sliced pineapple rings from a can and drain. Set the juice aside.
2. Slice garlic and ginger into fine pieces.
3. Mix the pineapple juice, ginger, garlic, salt, and olive oil together in a bowl to create a dressing for the sirloin medallions.
4. Add the sirloin medallions to the marinade and let it sit for 10-15 minutes.
5. Heat the oven to 450 degrees-Fahrenheit and line 2 oven trays with parchment paper.
6. Chop the squash into little ½-inch circles and place it on the parchment paper—drizzle 1tbsp of olive oil on top of it.
7. Cut the onion into small wedges, add to the tray and drizzle with olive oil.
8. Add pineapple rings next to the squash on the first tray and roast for 6 minutes.

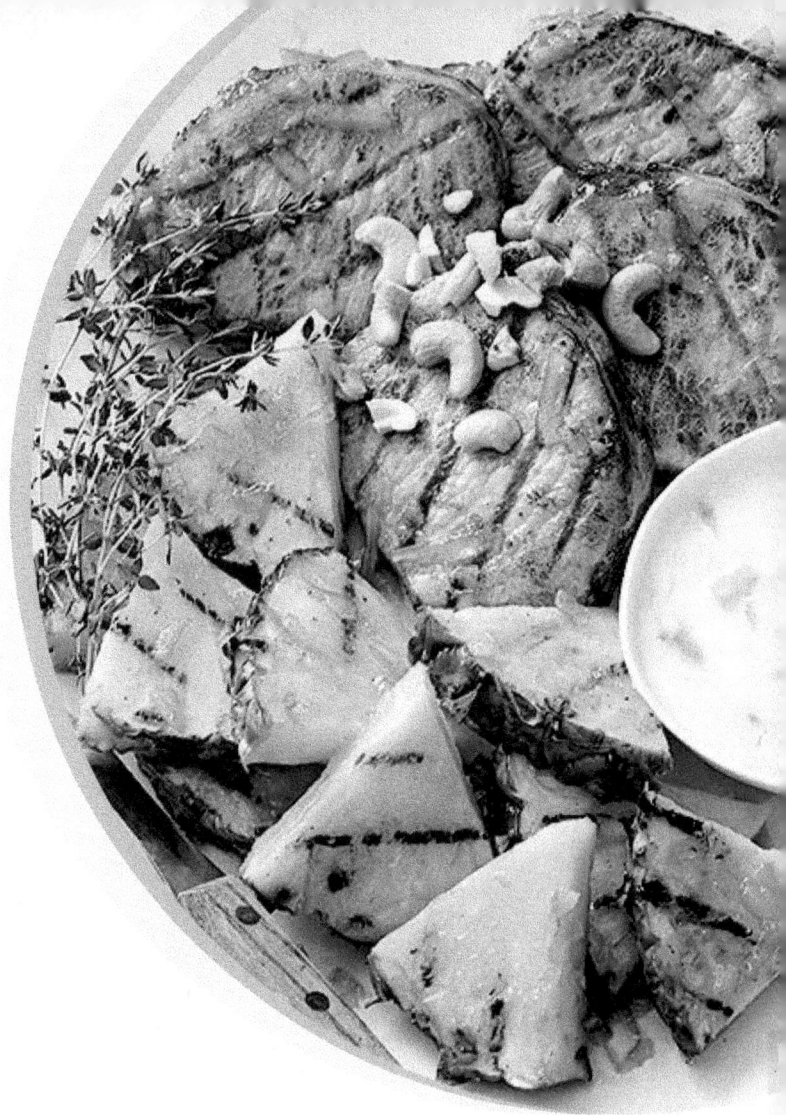

9. Remove the pan and turn the squash and pineapple over. Add the onion onto the tray and roast it for another 5 minutes. Close the fruit and vegetables with foil to lock in the heat and set aside.
10. Remove sirloin medallions from the marinade. Line another oven tray pan with parchment paper and place the sirloin medallions on top.
11. Cook for 5 minutes and flip the sirloin to cook for another 5 minutes on the other side.
12. Serve the sirloin medallions with the vegetables and pineapple on a platter.

NUTRITION:

Calories: 264
Fat: 12g
Carbs: 14g
Protein: 25g
Sodium: 150mg
Potassium: 685mg
Phosphorus: 257mg

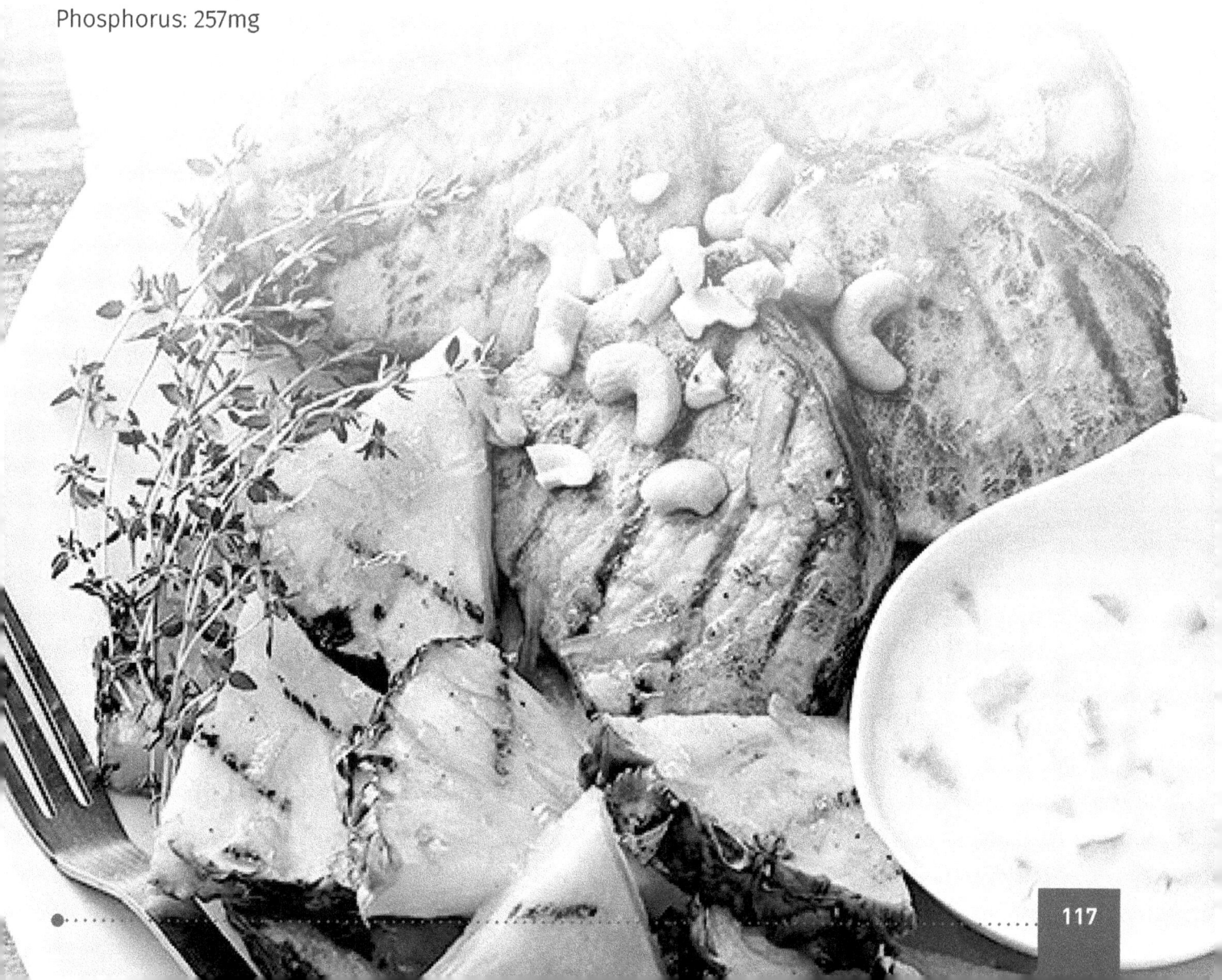

49 CHICKEN AND SAVORY RICE

Preparation Time: 15 minutes

Cooking Time: 45 minutes

Servings: 4

INGREDIENTS:

- 4 medium chicken breasts
- 1 baby marrow (chopped)
- 1 red bell pepper (chopped)
- 3 tbsp olive oil
- 1 onion
- 1 garlic clove (minced)
- ½ tsp of black pepper
- 1 tbsp of cumin
- ¼ tsp cayenne pepper
- 2 cups of brown rice

DIRECTIONS:

1. Add 2 tbsp of olive oil to medium heat and place the chicken breasts into the pan. Cook for 15 minutes and remove from the pan.
2. Add another tbsp of olive oil to the pan, and add the baby marrow, onion, red pepper, and corn.
3. Sauté the vegetables on medium heat for 10 minutes or until golden brown.
4. Add minced garlic, black pepper, cumin, and cayenne pepper to the vegetables. Stir the vegetables and spices together well.
5. Cut the chicken into cube and add it back to the pan. Mix it with the vegetables for 5 minutes.
6. In a medium pot, fill it up with water until it is 2/3 full. Add the rice to the pot and cook it for 35-40 minutes.
7. Serve the chicken and vegetable mixture on a bed of rice with extra black pepper.

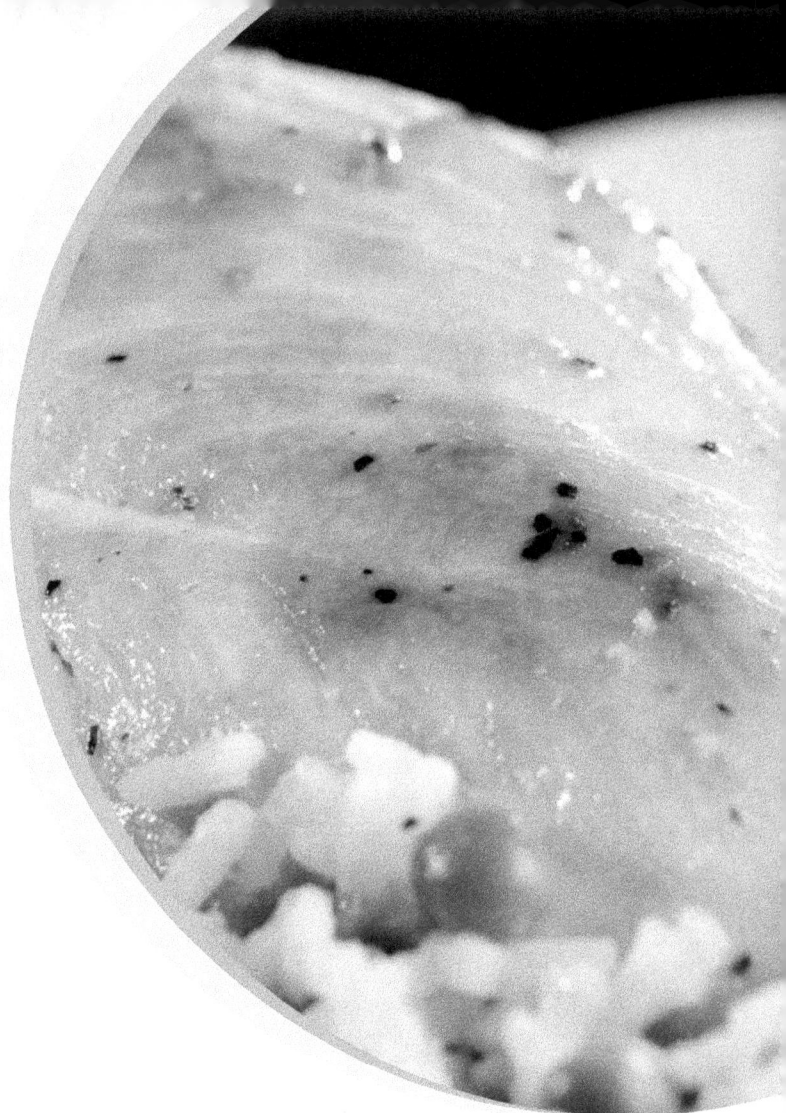

NUTRITION:

Calories: 374
Fat: 6.2g
Carbs: 65g
Protein: 15g
Sodium: 520mg
Potassium: 645mg
Phosphorus: 268mg

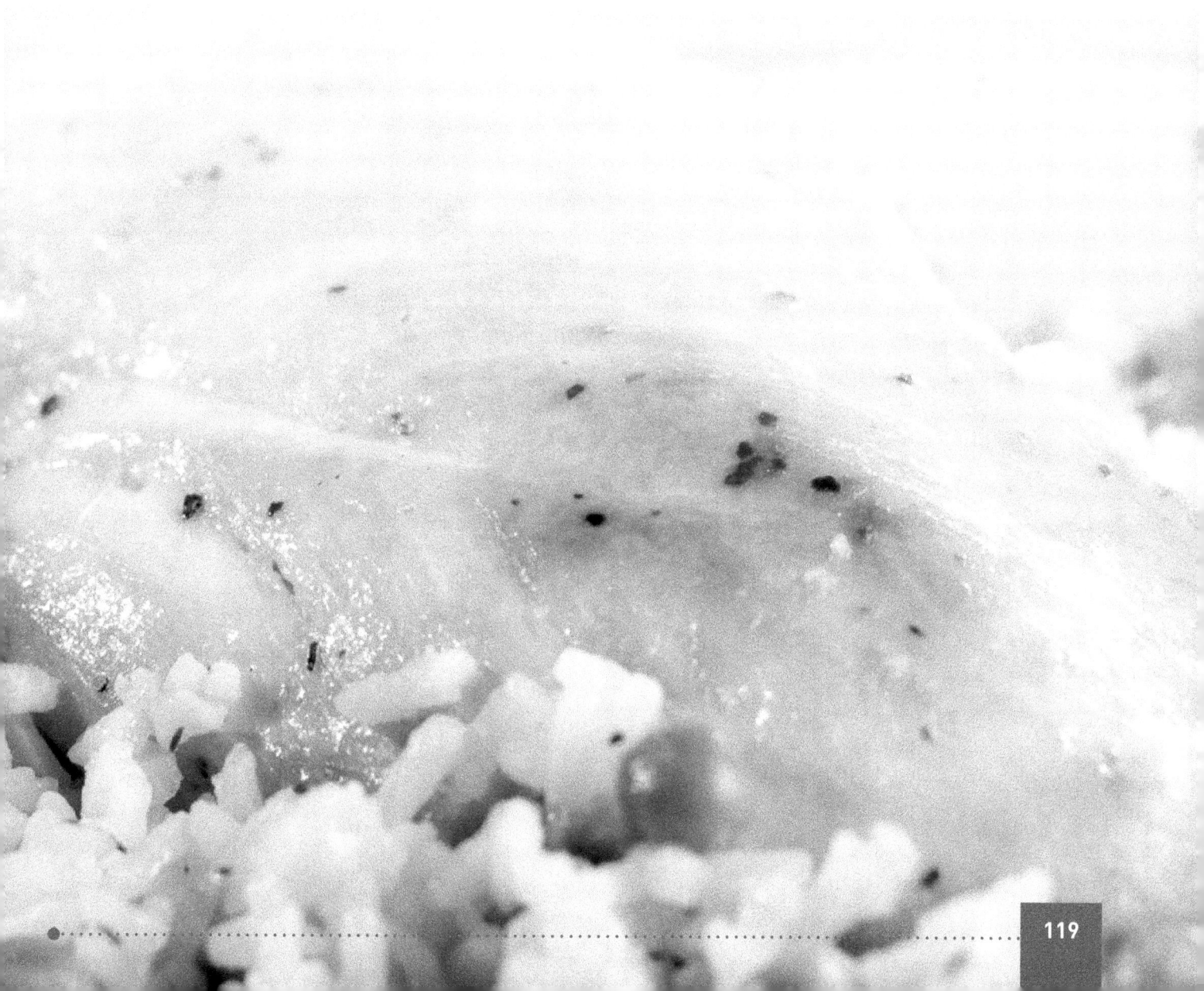

50 | SALMON AND GREEN BEANS

Preparation Time: 10 minutes

Cooking Time: 20 minutes

Servings: 4

INGREDIENTS:

- 3 oz x 4 salmon fillets
- ½ lb. of green beans
- 2 tbsp of dill
- 2 tbsp of coriander
- 2 lemons
- 2 tbsp olive oil
- 4 tbsp of mayonnaise

DIRECTIONS:

1. Rinse and salmon fillets and wait for it to dry. Don't remove the skin.
2. Wash green beans and chop the tips of the green beans.
3. Heat the oven up to 425 degrees-Fahrenheit.
4. Spray an oven sheet pan with cooking spray and place the salmon fillets on the sheet pan.
5. Chop up the dill and combine it with the mayonnaise.
6. Put mayo mixture on top of the salmon fillets.
7. Place the green beans next to the salmon fillets and drizzle olive oil on top of everything.
8. Place the oven baking sheet in the middle of the oven and cook for 15 minutes.
9. Slice the lemons into wedges and serve with the salmon fillets and green beans.

NUTRITION:

Calories: 399
Fat: 21g
Carbs: 8g
Protein: 38g

Sodium: 229mg
Potassium: 1000mg
Phosphorus: 723mg

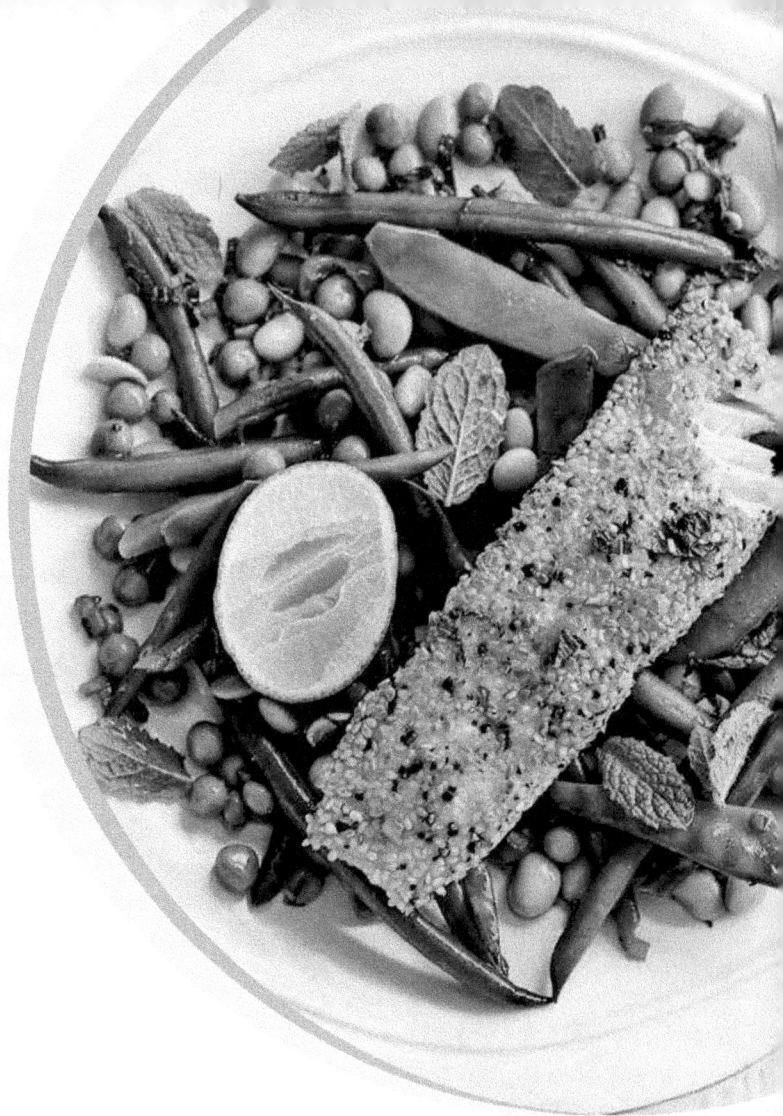

51 BAKED MACARONI & CHEESE

Preparation Time: 10 minutes

Cooking Time: 40 – 45 minutes

Servings: 1

INGREDIENTS:

- 3 cups of macaroni
- 2 cups of milk
- 2 tbsp of butter (unsalted)
- 2 tbsp of flour (all-purpose)
- 2 ½ cups of cheddar
- 2 tbsp of blanched almonds
- 1 tbsp of thyme
- 1 tbsp of olive oil
-

1 cheese sauce (quick make packets)

DIRECTIONS:

1. Preheat the oven to 350 degrees-Fahrenheit.
2. Prepare a medium-sized pot on the stove and fill it up with water.
3. Add the macaroni to the pot with a tbsp of olive oil for 8-10 minutes. Stir until cooked.
4. In a measuring cup, measure your butter and flour and mix it. Place it in the microwave for 1 minute. Then stir in the milk, spices, and herbs—microwave for 2-3 minutes, or until the mixture is thick.
5. Drain the noodles and add to a casserole dish that has been sprayed with cooking spray, the sauce, and cheese. Mix it well, followed with more cheese on top.
6. Put and bake casserole dish into the oven for 15-20 minutes.
7. Serve with blanched almonds on top.

NUTRITION:

Calories: 314
Fat: 14g
Carbs: 34g
Protein: 19g
Sodium: 373mg
Potassium: 120mg
Phosphorus: 222mg

52 | KOREAN PEAR SALAD

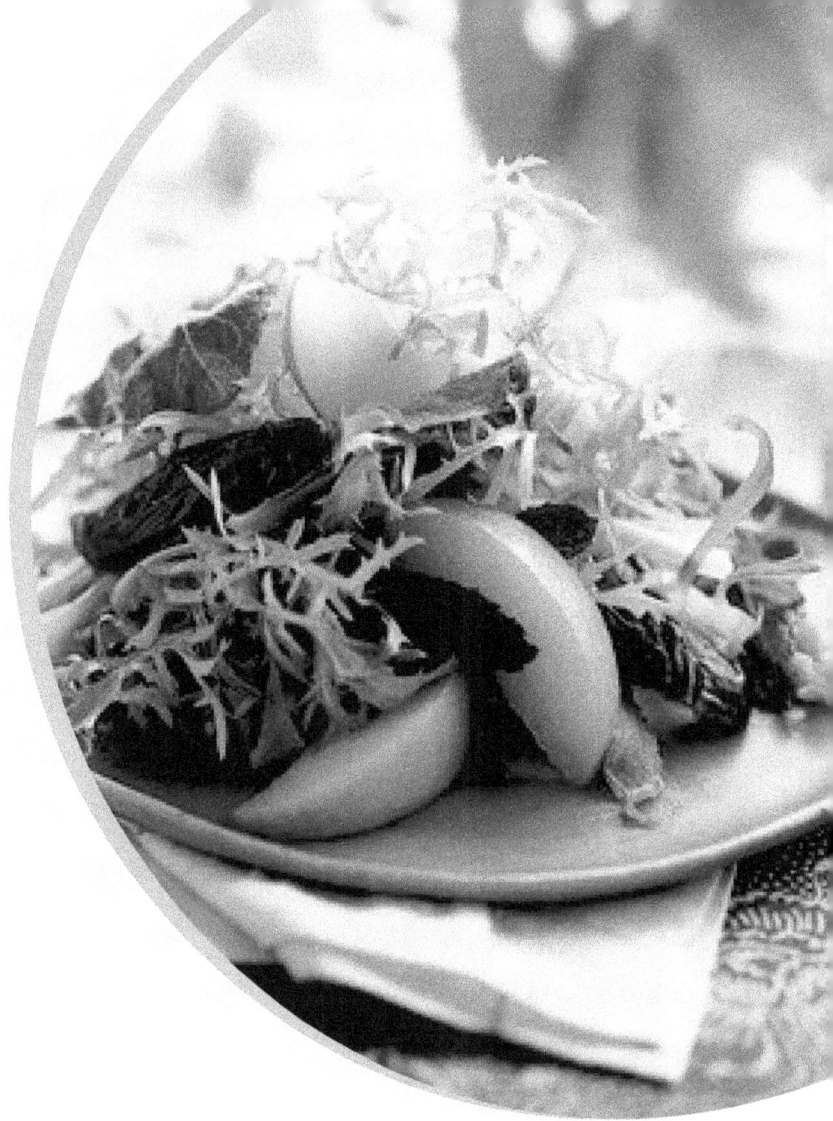

Preparation Time: 5 minutes

Cooking Time: 15 minutes

Servings: 2

INGREDIENTS:

- 6 cups green lettuce
- 4 medium-sized pears (peeled, cored, and diced)
- ½ cup of sugar
- ½ cup of pecan nuts
- ½ cup of water
- 2 oz of blue cheese
- ½ cup of cranberries
- ½ cup of dressing

DIRECTIONS:

1. Dissolve the water and sugar in a frying pan (non-stick).
2. Heat the mixture until it turns into a syrup, and then add the nuts immediately.
3. Place the syrup with the nuts on a piece of parchment paper and separate the nuts while the mixture is hot. Let it cool down.
4. Prepare lettuce in a salad bowl and add the pears, blue cheese, and cranberries to the salad.
5. Add the caramelized nuts to the salad and serve it with a dressing of choice on the side.

NUTRITION:

Calories: 112
Fat: 9g
Carbs: 5.5g
Protein: 2g

Sodium: 130mg
Potassium: 160mg
Phosphorus: 71.7mg

53 BEEF ENCHILADAS

Preparation Time: 10 minutes

Cooking Time: 30 minutes

Servings: 1

INGREDIENTS:

- 1 pound of lean beef
- 12 whole-wheat tortillas
- 1 can of low-sodium enchilada sauce
- ½ cup of onion (diced)
- ½ tsp of black pepper
- 1 garlic clove
- 1 tbsp of olive oil
- 1 tsp of cumin

DIRECTIONS:

1. Heat the oven to 375 degrees-Fahrenheit
2. In a medium-sized frying pan, cook the beef in olive oil until completely cooked.
3. Add the minced garlic, diced onion, cumin, and black pepper to the pan and mix everything in with the beef.
4. In a separate pan, cook the tortillas in olive oil and dip each cooked tortilla in the enchilada sauce.
5. Fill the tortilla with the meat mixture and roll it up.
6. Put the finished product in a slightly heated pan with cheese on top.
7. Bake the tortillas in the pan until crispy, golden brown, and the cheese is melted.

NUTRITION:

Calories: 177
Fat: 6g
Carbs: 15g

Protein: 15g
Sodium: 501mg

Potassium: 231mg
Phosphorus: 98mg

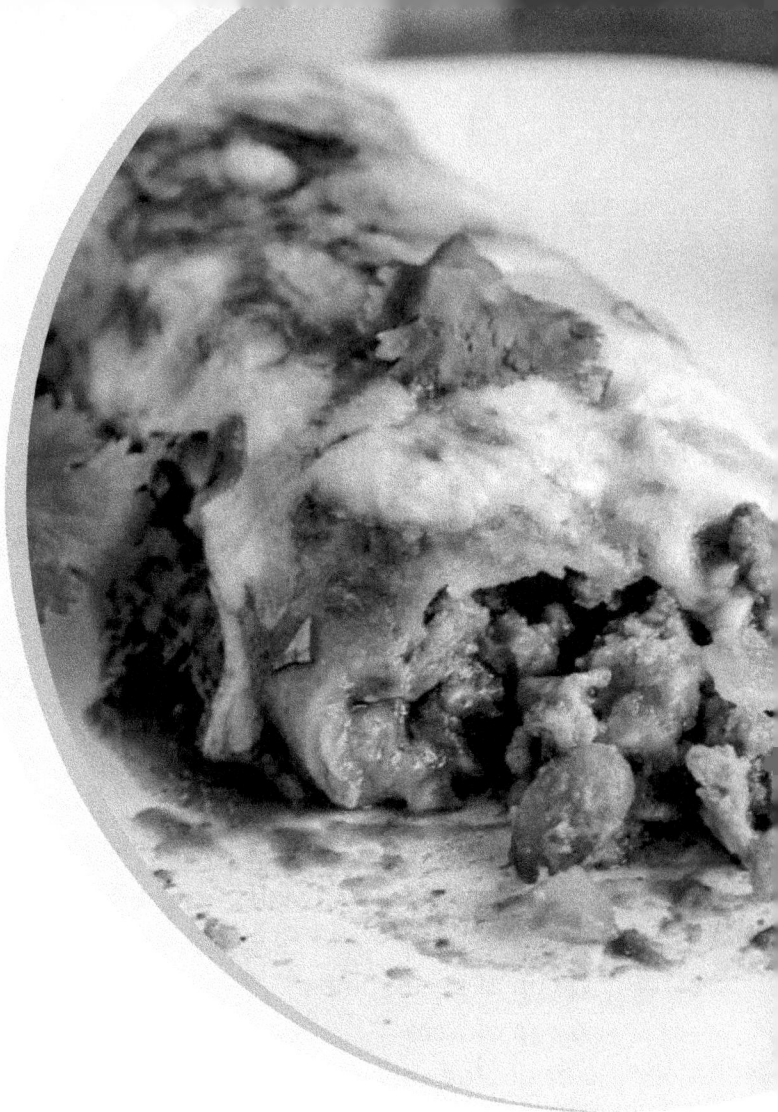

54 CHICKEN AND BROCCOLI CASSEROLE

Preparation Time: 15 minutes

Cooking Time: 45 minutes – 1 hour

Servings: 1

INGREDIENTS:

- 2 cups of rice (cooked)
- 3 chicken breasts
- 2 cups of broccoli
- 1 onion (diced)
- 2 eggs
- 2 cups of cheddar cheese
- 2 tbsp of butter
- 1-2 tbsp of parmesan cheese

DIRECTIONS:

1. Heat the oven to 350 degrees-Fahrenheit
2. Add the broccoli to a bowl and cover it with plastic wrap. Microwave the broccoli for 2-3 minutes.
3. Dice the onion and add it with the chicken and the butter in the pa.
4. Cook the chicken for 15 minutes.
5. Once the chicken is cooked, mix it, broccoli, and rice together, and add to a greased casserole dish.
6. Add the grated cheese into the casserole dish and stir well.
7. Add the parmesan cheese on top.
8. Place the casserole dish in the oven for 30-45 minutes.

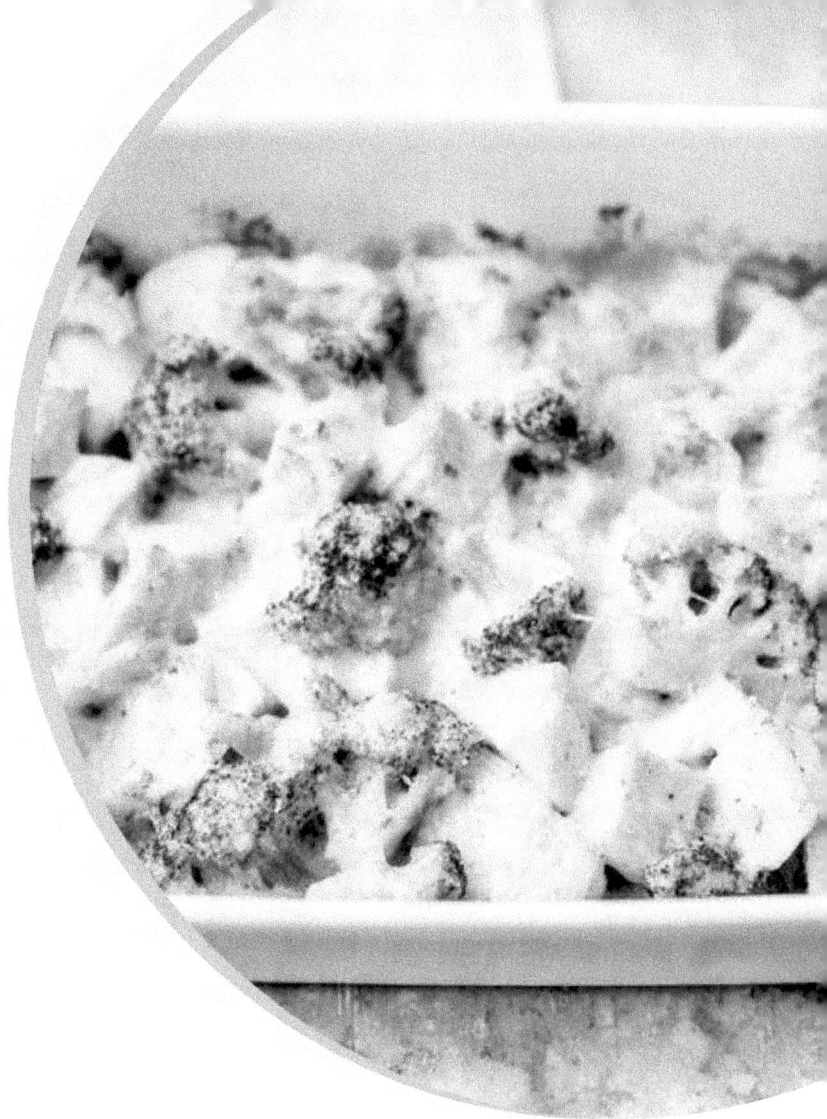

Calories: 349
Fat: 12g
Carbs: 14g
Protein: 44g
Sodium: 980mg
Potassium: 713mg
Phosphorus: 451mg

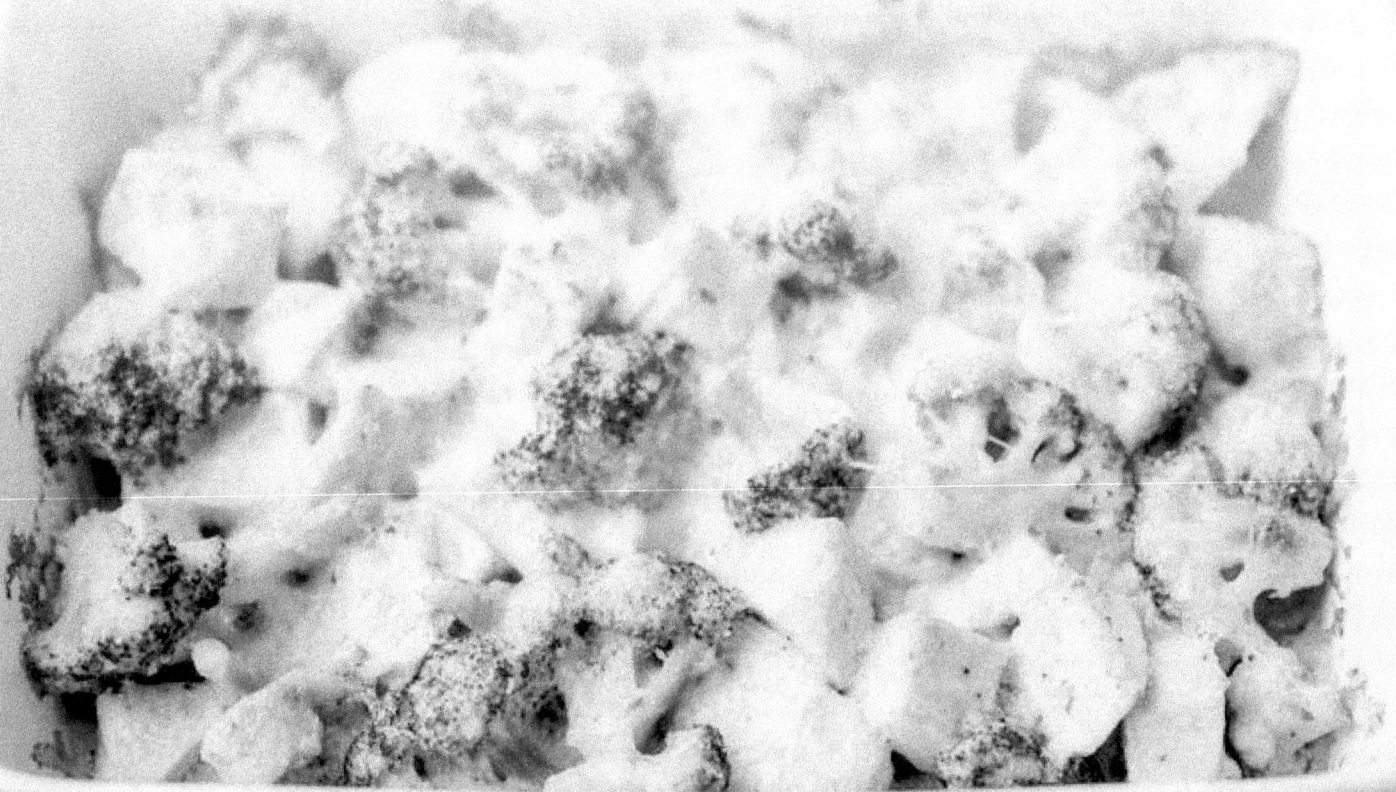

55 FETA BEAN SALAD

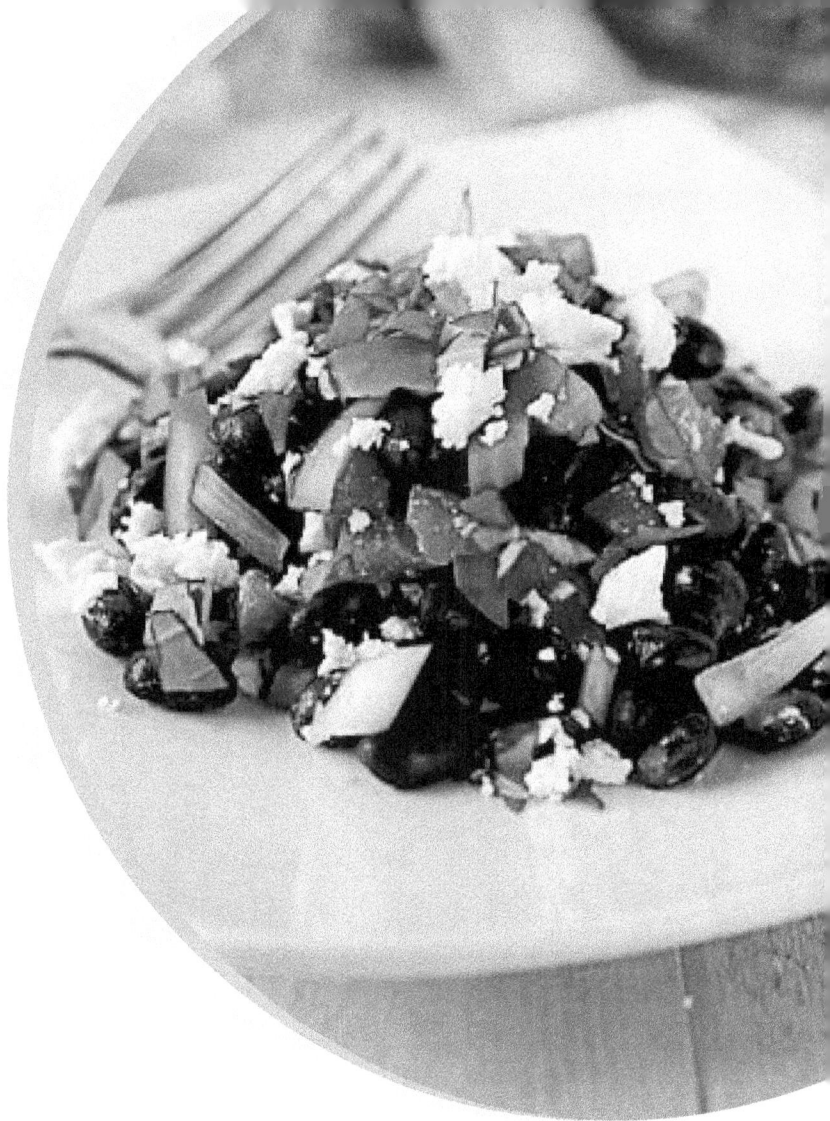

Preparation Time: 5 minutes

Cooking Time: 20 minutes

Servings: 2

INGREDIENTS:

- 1 tbsp of olive oil
- 2 egg whites (boiled)
- 1 cup of green beans (8 oz)
- 1 tbsp of onion
- 1/2 red chili
- 1/8 cup of cilantro
- 1 1/2 tbsp lime juice
- 1/4 tbsp of black pepper

DIRECTIONS:

1. Remove the ends off the green beans and cut them into small pieces.
2. Chop the onion, cilantro, and chili and mix it.
3. Use a steamer to cook green beans for 5- 10 minutes and rinse with cold water once done.
4. Place all the mixed dry ingredients together in two serving bowls.
5. Chop the egg whites up and place them on top of the salad with crumbled feta.
6. Drizzle a pinch of olive oil with black pepper on top.

NUTRITION:

Calories: 255

Fat: 24g

Carbs: 8g

Protein: 5g

Sodium: 215.6mg

Potassium: 211mg

Phosphorus: 125mg

56 SEAFOOD CASSEROLE

Preparation Time: 20 minutes

Cooking Time: 45 minutes

Servings: 1

INGREDIENTS:

- 2 cups, peeled and diced into 1-inch pieces Eggplant
- Butter, for greasing the baking dish
- 1 tbsp. Olive oil
- ½, chopped Sweet onion
- 1 tsp. Minced garlic
- 1 chopped Celery stalk
- ½ boiled and chopped Red bell pepper
- 3 tbsps. Freshly squeezed lemon juice
- 1 tsp. Hot sauce
- ¼ tsp. Creole seasoning mix
- ½ cup, uncooked White rice
- 1 large Egg
- 4 ounces Cooked shrimp
- 6 ounces Queen crab meat

DIRECTIONS:

1. Preheat the oven to 350f.
2. Boil the eggplant in a saucepan for 5 minutes. Drain and set aside.
3. Grease a 9-by-13-inch baking dish with butter and set aside.
4. Heat the olive oil in a large skillet over medium heat.
5. Sauté the garlic, onion, celery, and bell pepper for 4 minutes or until tender.
6. Add the sautéed vegetables to the eggplant, along with the lemon juice, hot sauce, seasoning, rice, and egg.

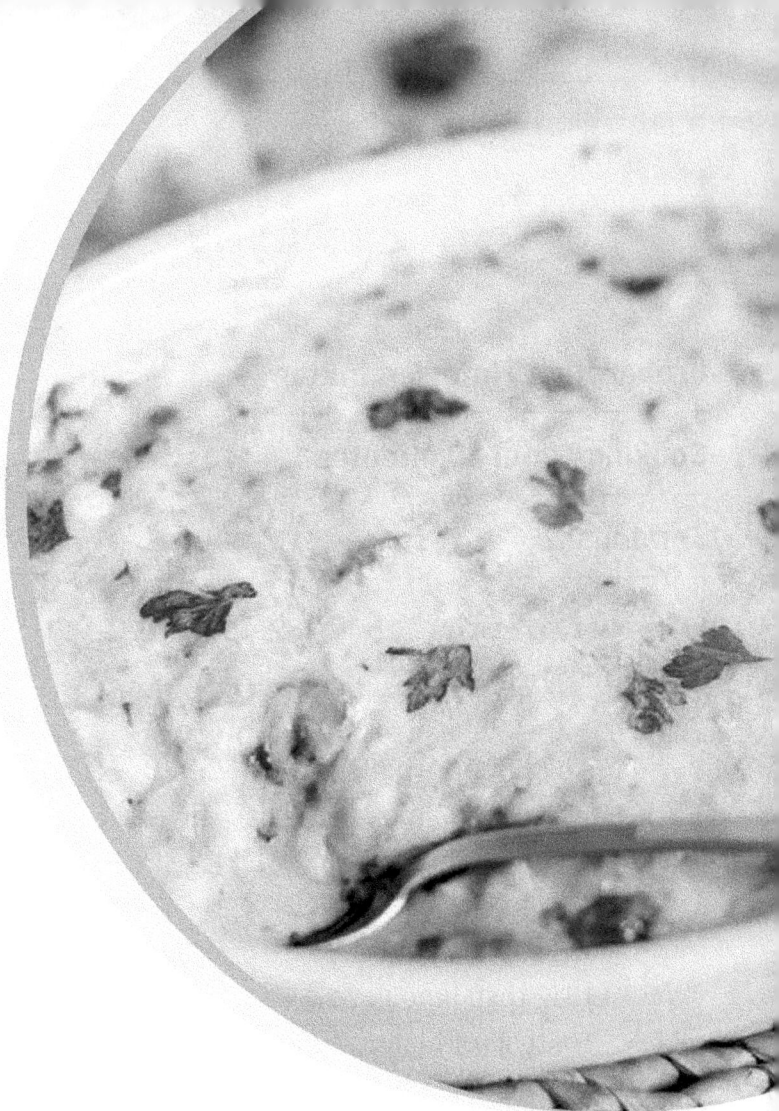

7. Stir to combine.
8. Fold in the shrimp and crab meat.
9. Spoon the casserole mixture into the casserole dish, patting down the top.
10. Bake for 25 to 30 minutes or until casserole is heated through and rice is tender. Serve warm.

NUTRITION:

Calories: 118
Fat: 4g
Carb: 9g
Protein: 12g
Sodium: 235mg
Potassium: 199mg
Phosphorus: 102mg

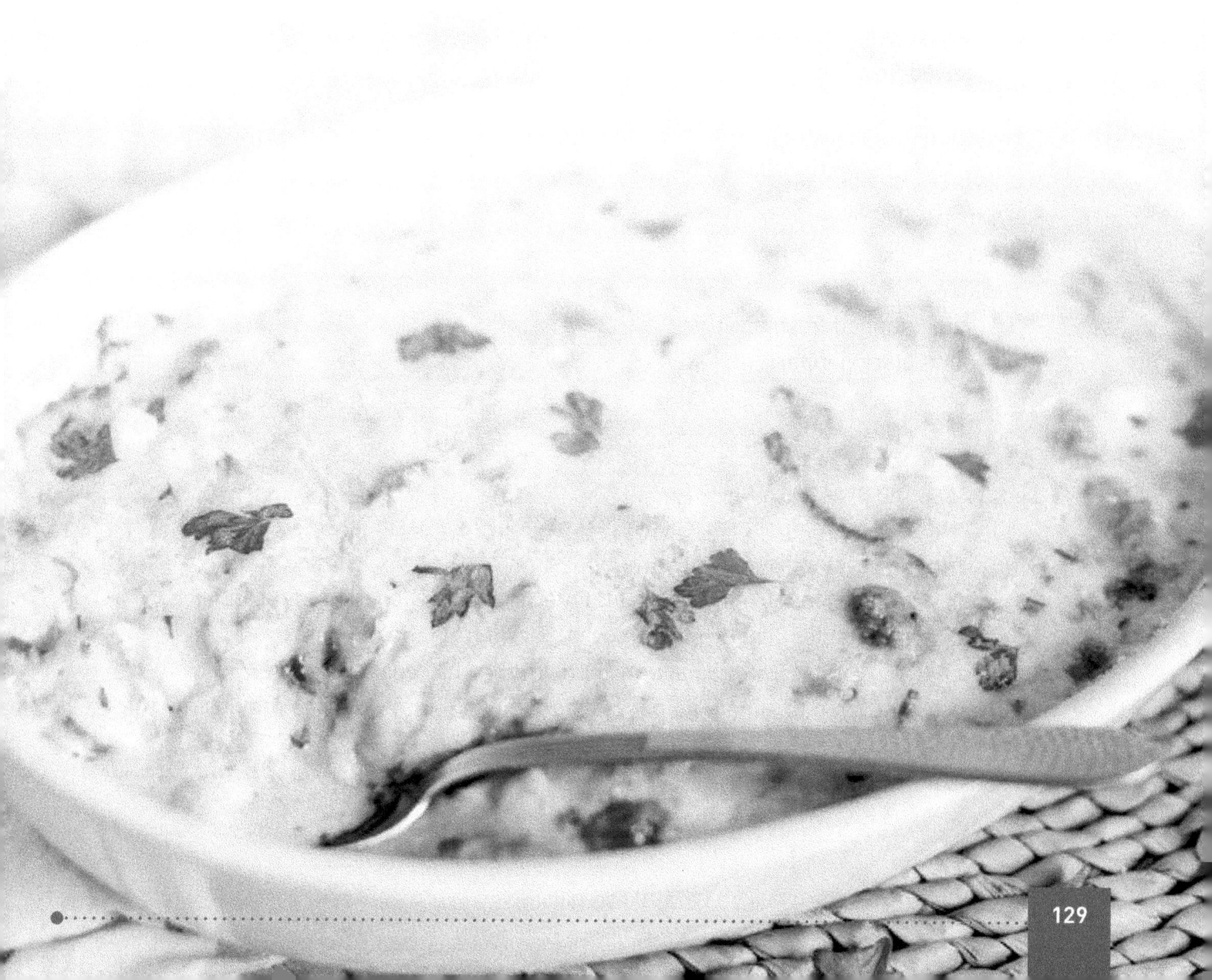

57 EGGPLANT AND RED PEPPER SOUP

Preparation Time: 20 minutes

Cooking Time: 40 minutes

Servings: 1

INGREDIENTS:

- 1 small, cut into quarters Sweet onion
- 2, halved Small red bell peppers
- 2 cups Cubed eggplant
- 2 cloves, crushed Garlic
- 1 tbsp. Olive oil
- 1 cup Chicken stock
- Water
- ¼ cup Chopped fresh basil
- Ground black pepper

DIRECTIONS:

1. Preheat the oven to 350f.
2. Put the onions, red peppers, eggplant, and garlic in a baking dish.
3. Drizzle the vegetables with the olive oil.
4. Cook vegetables for 30 minutes or until they are slightly charred and soft.
5. Cool the vegetables slightly and remove the skin from the peppers.
6. Puree the vegetables with a hand mixer (with the chicken stock).
7. Transfer the soup to a medium pot and add enough water to reach the desired thickness.
8. Heat the soup to a simmer and add the basil.
9. Season with pepper and serve.

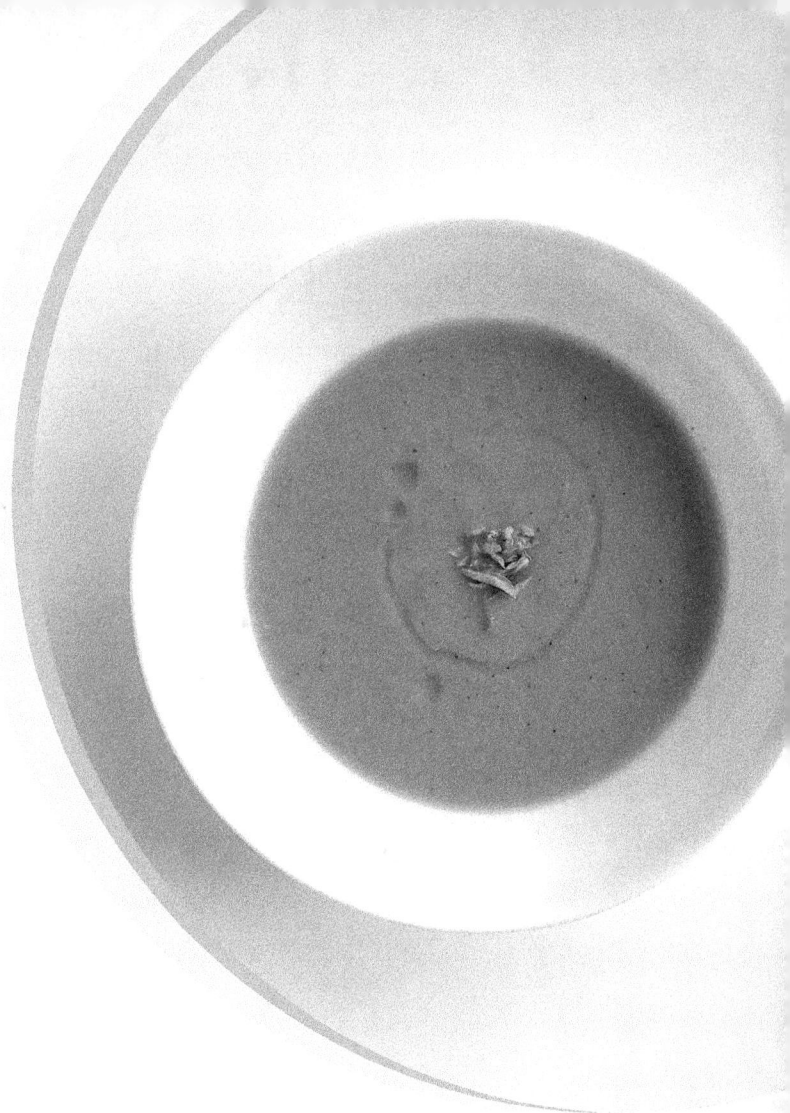

Calories: 61
Fat: 2g
Carb: 9g
Protein: 2g
Sodium: 98mg
Potassium: 198mg
Phosphorus: 33mg

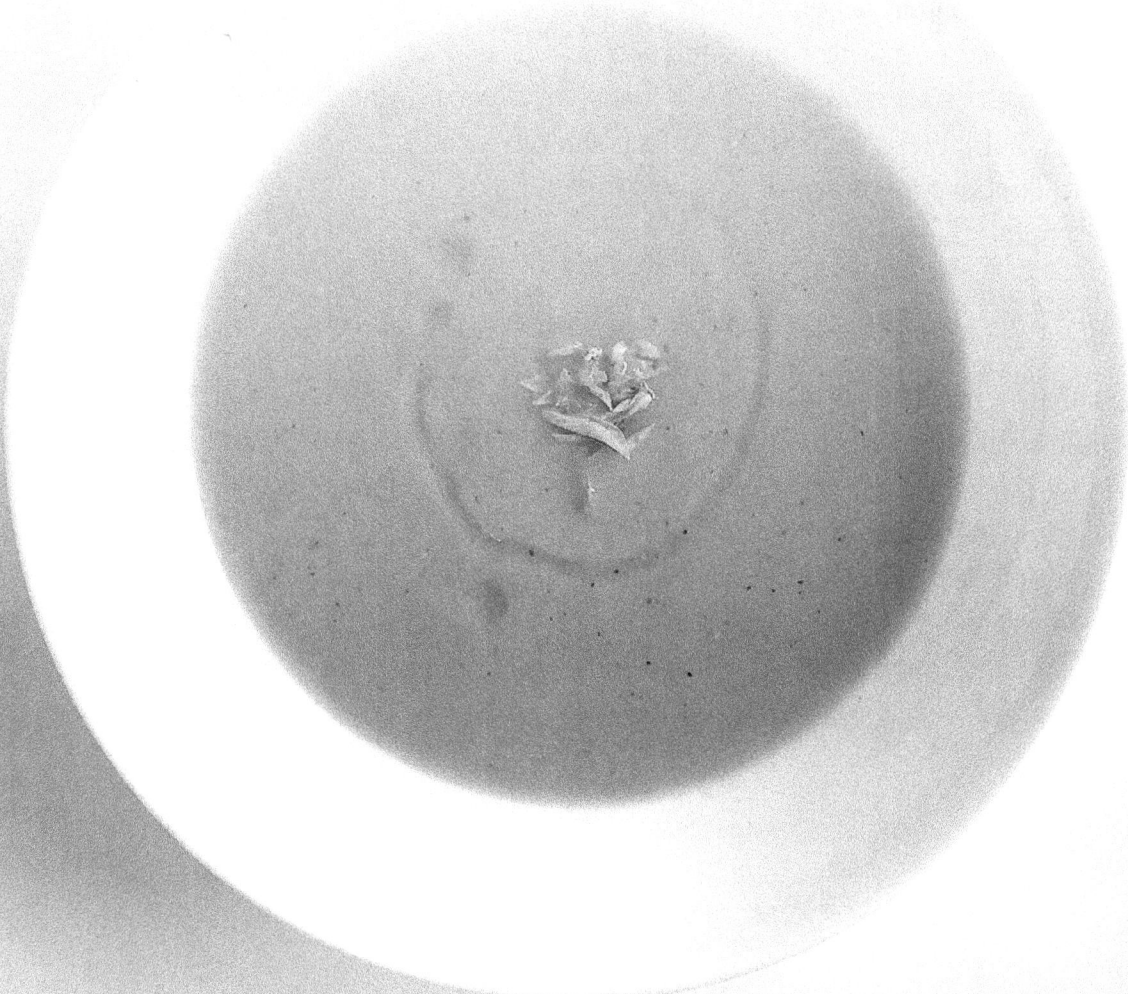

58 GROUND BEEF AND RICE SOUP

Preparation time: 15 minutes

cooking time: 40 minutes

Servings: 1

INGREDIENTS:

- ½ pound Extra-lean ground beef
- ½, chopped Small sweet onion
- 1 tsp. Minced garlic
- 2 cups Water
- 1 cup Low-sodium beef broth
- ½ cup, uncooked Long-grain white rice
- 1, chopped Celery stalk
- ½ cup, cut into – 1-inch pieces Fresh green beans
- 1 tsp. Chopped fresh thyme
- Ground black pepper

DIRECTIONS:

1. Sauté the ground beef in a saucepan for 6 minutes or until the beef is completely browned.
2. Drain off the excess fat and add the onion and garlic to the saucepan.
3. Sauté the vegetables for about 3 minutes, or until they are softened.
4. Add the celery, rice, beef broth, and water.
5. Let it boil, reduce the heat to low, and simmer for 30 minutes or until the rice is tender.
6. Add the green beans and thyme and simmer for 3 minutes.
7. Remove the soup from the heat and season with pepper.

NUTRITION:

Calories: 154

Fat: 7g

Carb: 14g

Protein: 9g

Sodium: 133mg

Potassium: 179mg

Phosphorus: 76mg

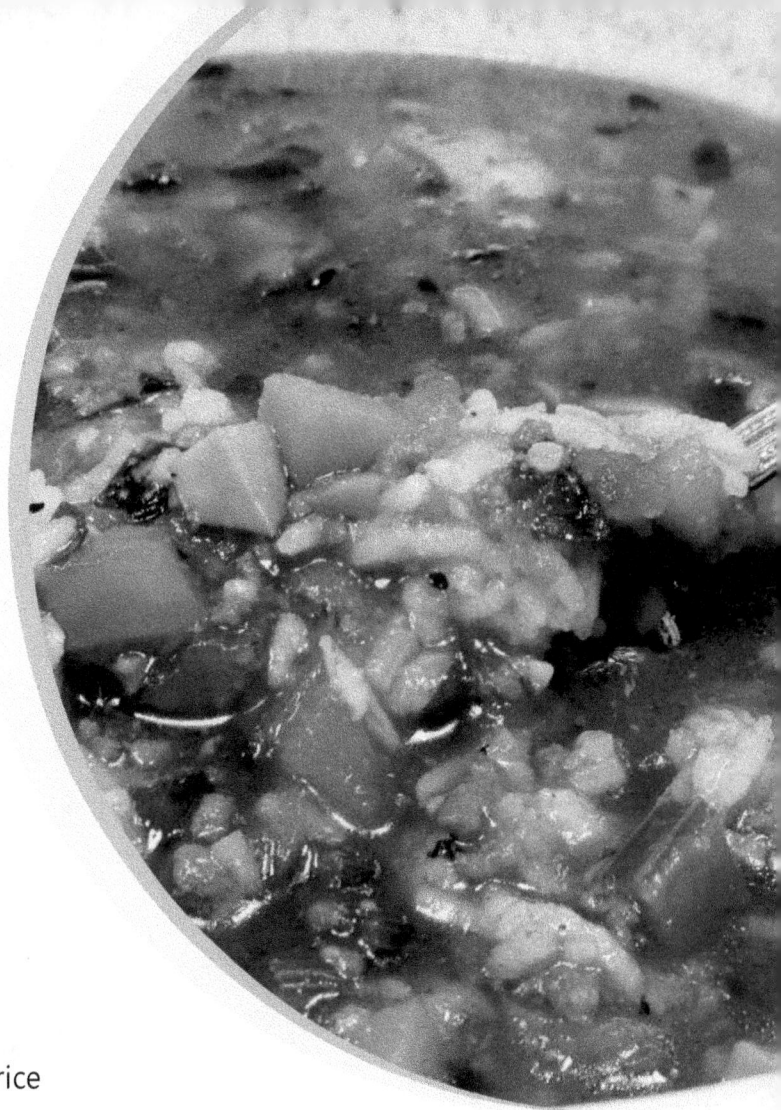

59 COUSCOUS BURGERS

Preparation Time: 20 minutes

Cooking Time: 10 minutes

Servings: 4

INGREDIENTS:

- ½ cup, rinsed and drained Canned chickpeas
- 2 tbsps. Chopped fresh cilantro
- Chopped fresh parsley
- 1 tbsp. Lemon juice
- 2 tsp. Lemon zest
- 1 tsp. Minced garlic
- 2 ½ cups Cooked couscous
- 2 lightly beaten Eggs
- 2 tbsps. Olive oil

DIRECTIONS:

1. Put the cilantro, chickpeas, parsley, lemon juice, lemon zest, and garlic in a food processor and pulse until a paste form.
2. Put chickpea mixture to a bowl. Add the eggs and couscous. Mix well.
3. Refrigerate the mixture for 1 hour.
4. Form the couscous mixture into 4 patties.
5. Heat olive oil in a skillet.
6. Place and cook two patties in the skillet, gently pressing them down with a spatula for 5 minutes or until golden and flip the patties over.
7. Repeat with the remaining burgers.

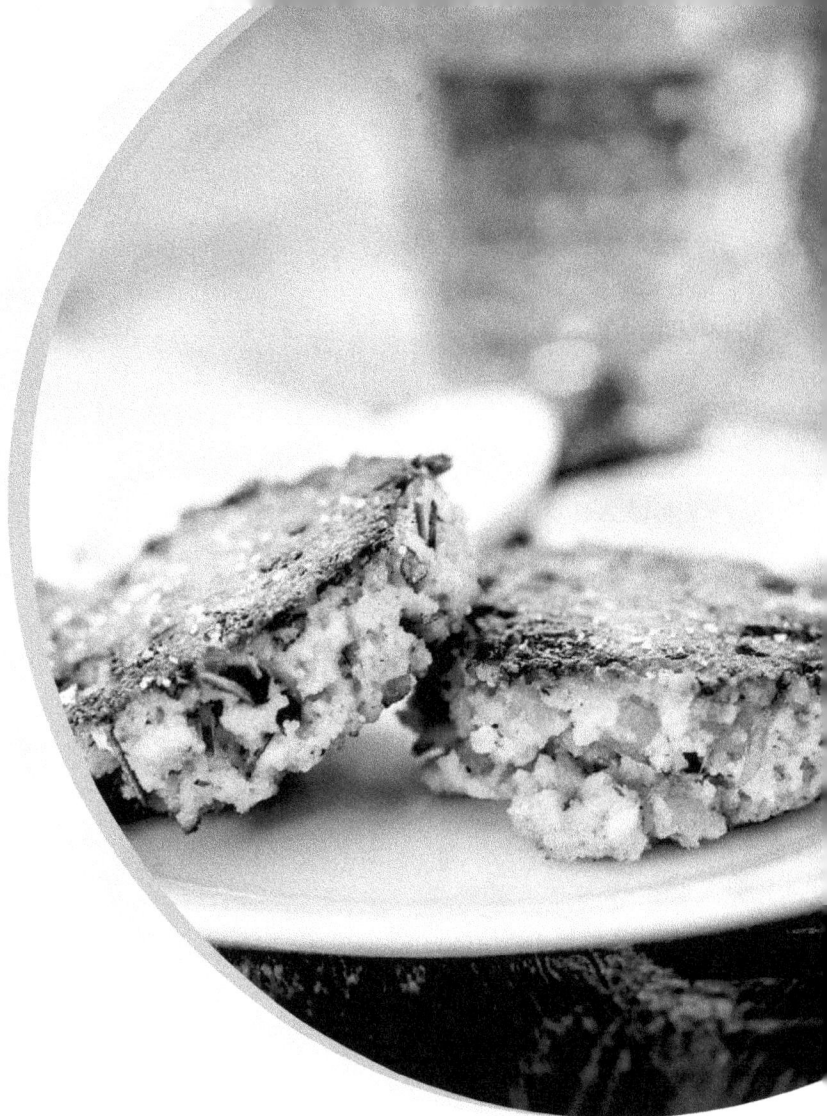

Calories: 242
Fat: 10g
Carb: 29g
Protein: 9g
Sodium: 43mg
Potassium: 168mg
Phosphorus: 108mg

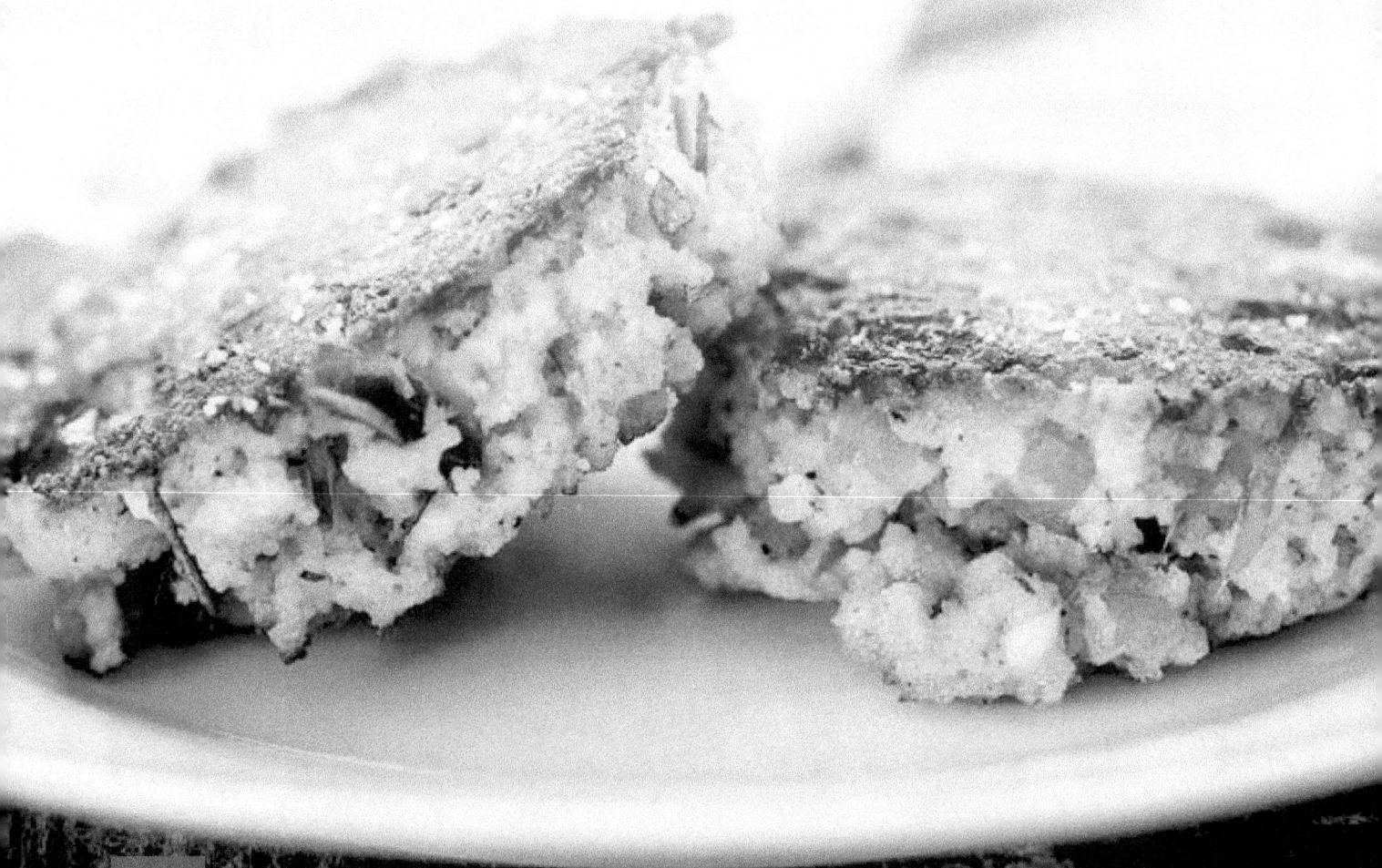

60 | PORK SOUVLAKI

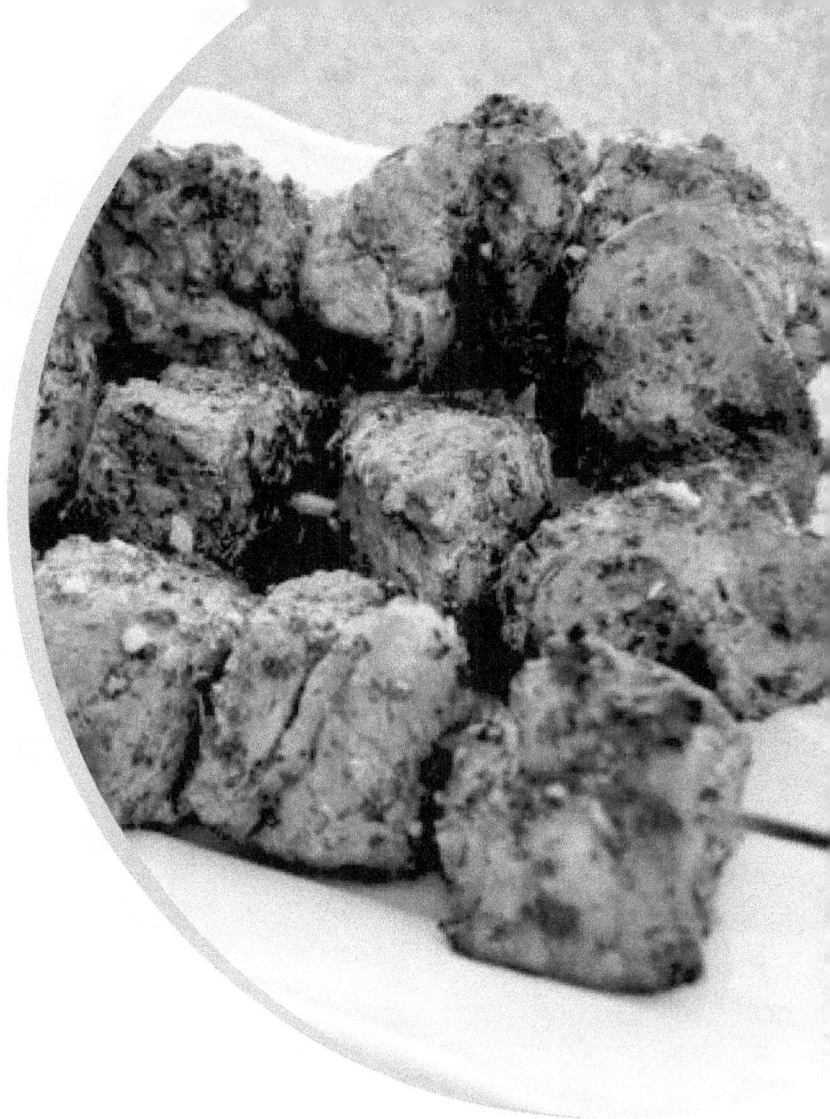

Preparation Time: 20 minutes

Cooking Time: 12 minutes

Servings: 8

INGREDIENTS:

- 3 tbsps. Olive oil
- 2 tbsps. Lemon juice
- 1 tsp. Minced garlic
- 1 tbsp. Chopped fresh oregano
- ¼ tsp. Ground black pepper
- 1 pound, cut into 2-inch cubes Pork leg

DIRECTIONS:

1. In a bowl, stir together the lemon juice, olive oil, garlic, oregano, and pepper.
2. Add the pork cubes and toss to coat.
3. Place the bowl in the refrigerator, covered, for 2 hours to marinate.
4. Thread the pork chunks onto 8 wooden skewers that have been soaked in water.
5. Preheat the barbecue to medium-high heat.
6. Grill the pork skewers for about 12 minutes, turning once, until just cooked through but still juicy.

NUTRITION:

Calories: 95
Fat: 4g
Carb: 0g
Protein: 13g
Sodium: 29mg
Potassium: 230mg
Phosphorus: 125mg

BAKED FLOUNDER

Preparation Time: 20 minutes

Cooking Time: 5 minutes

Servings: 4

INGREDIENTS:

- ¼ cup Homemade mayonnaise
- Juice of 1 lime
- Zest of 1 lime
- ½ cup Chopped fresh cilantro
- 4 (3-ounce) Flounder fillets
- Ground black pepper

DIRECTIONS:

1. Preheat the oven to 400f.
2. In a bowl, stir together the cilantro, lime juice, lime zest, and mayonnaise.
3. Prepare foil on a clean work surface.
4. Place a flounder fillet in the center of each square.
5. Top the fillets evenly with the mayonnaise mixture.
6. Season the flounder with pepper.
7. Fold the foil's sides over the fish, and place on baking sheet.
8. Bake for 4 - 5 minutes.
9. Unfold the packets and serve.

NUTRITION:

Calories: 92
Fat: 4g
Carb: 2g
Protein: 12g

Sodium: 267mg
Potassium: 137mg
Phosphorus: 208mg

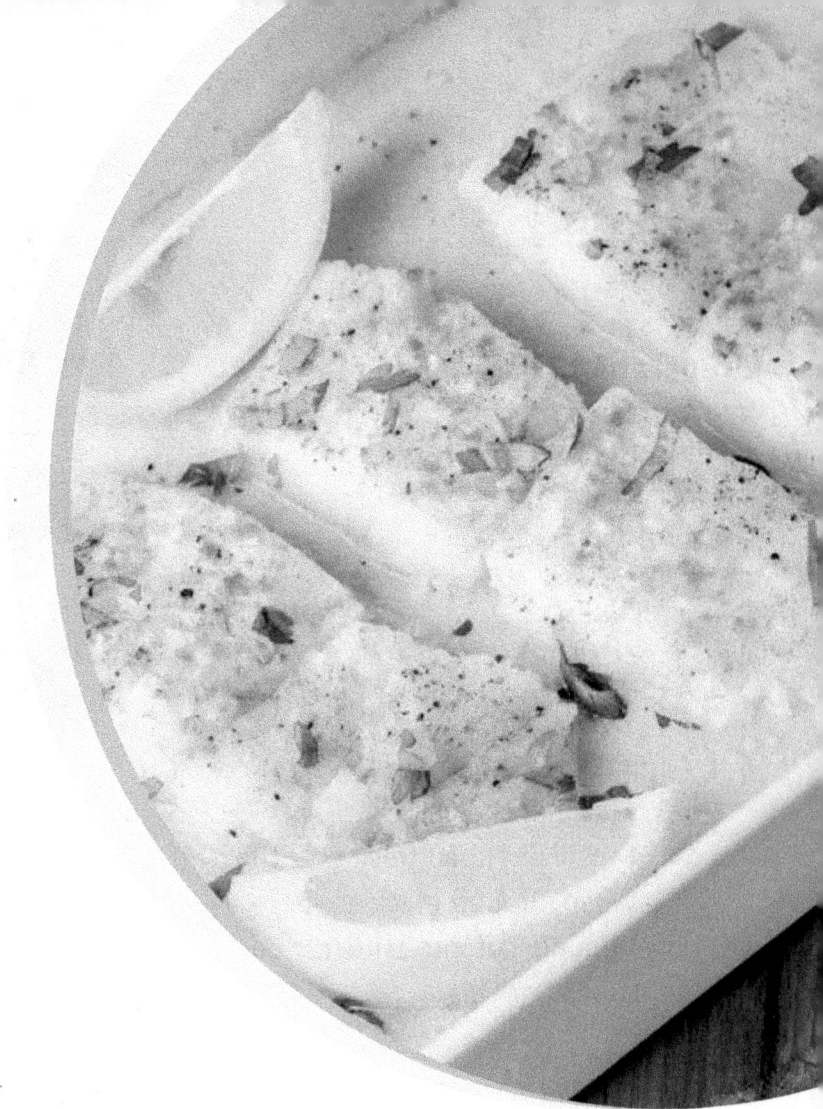

62 PERSIAN CHICKEN

Preparation Time: 10 minutes

Cooking Time: 20 minutes

Servings: 5

INGREDIENTS:

- ½, chopped Sweet onion
- ¼ cup Lemon juice
- 1 tbsp. Dried oregano
- 1 tsp. Minced garlic
- 1 tsp. Sweet paprika
- ½ tsp. Ground cumin
- ½ cup Olive oil
- 5 Boneless, skinless chicken thighs

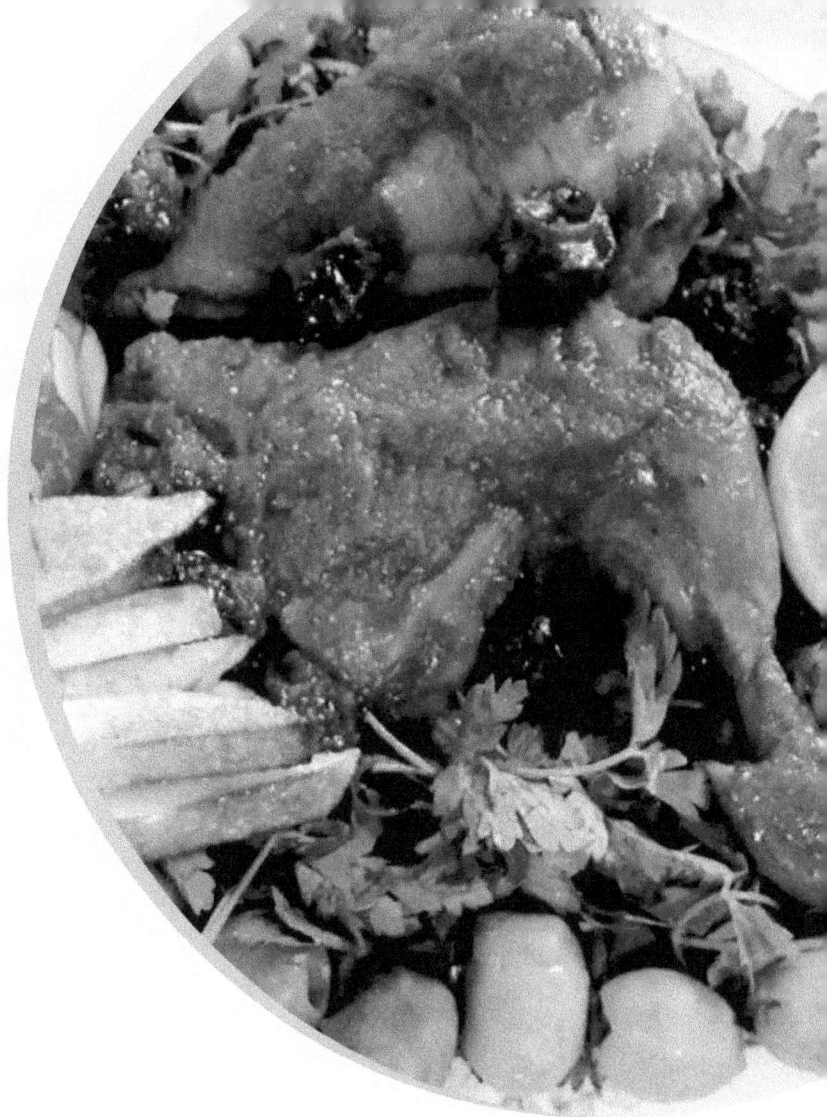

DIRECTIONS:

1. Put the cumin, paprika, garlic, oregano, lemon juice, and onion in a food processor and pulse to mix the ingredients.
2. Put olive oil until the mixture is smooth.
3. Put chicken thighs in a large Ziploc and add the marinade for 2 hours.
4. Remove the thighs from the marinade.
5. Preheat the barbecue to medium.
6. Grill the chicken for about 20 minutes, turning once, until it reaches 165F.

NUTRITION:

Calories: 321
Fat: 21g
Carb: 3g
Protein: 22g

Sodium: 86mg
Potassium: 220mg
Phosphorus: 131mg

63 BEEF CHILI

Preparation Time: 10 minutes

Cooking Time: 30 minutes

Servings: 2

INGREDIENTS:

- 1 diced Onion
- 1 diced Red bell pepper
- 2 cloves, minced Garlic
- 6 oz. Lean ground beef
- 1 tsp. Chili powder
- 1 tsp. Oregano
- 2 tbsps. Extra virgin olive oil
- 1 cup Water
- 1 cup Brown rice
- 1 tbsp. Fresh cilantro to serve

DIRECTIONS:

1. Soak vegetables in warm water.
2. Boil pan of water and add rice for 20 minutes.
3. Meanwhile, add the oil to a pan and heat on medium-high heat.
4. Add the pepper, onions, and garlic and sauté for 5 minutes until soft.
5. Remove and set aside.
6. Add the beef to the pan and stir until browned.
7. Put and stir vegetables back into the pan.
8. Now add the chili powder and herbs and the water, cover, and turn the heat down a little to simmer for 15 minutes.
9. Meanwhile, drain the water from the rice and the lid and steam while the chili is cooking.
10. Serve hot with the fresh cilantro sprinkled over the top.

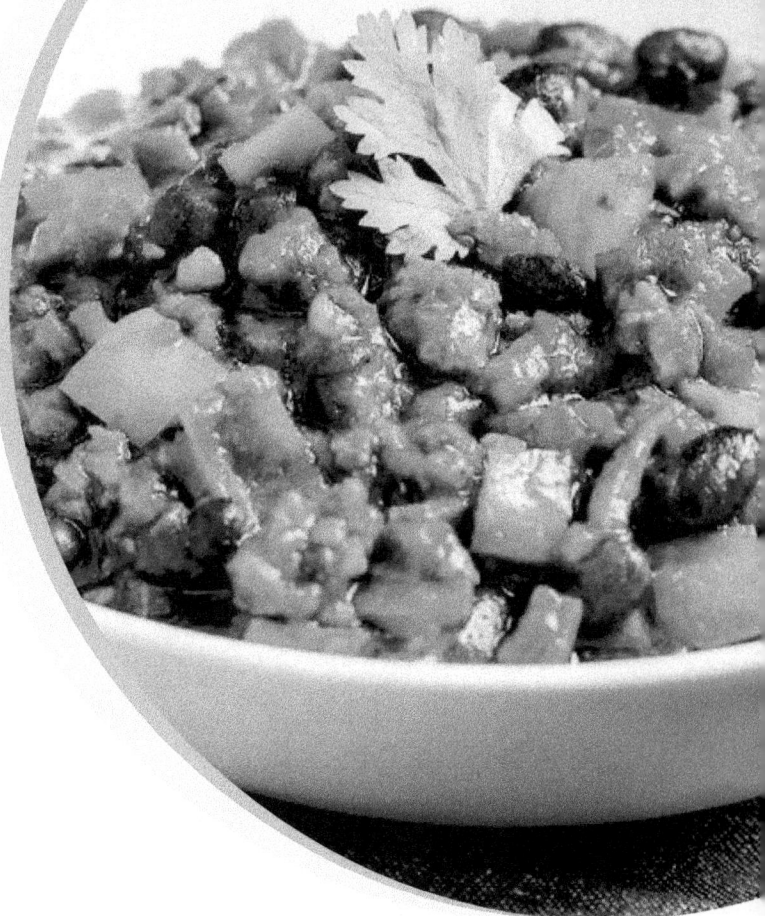

Calories: 459
Fat: 22g
Carb: 36g
Protein: 22g
Sodium: 33mg
Potassium: 360mg
Phosphorus: 332mg

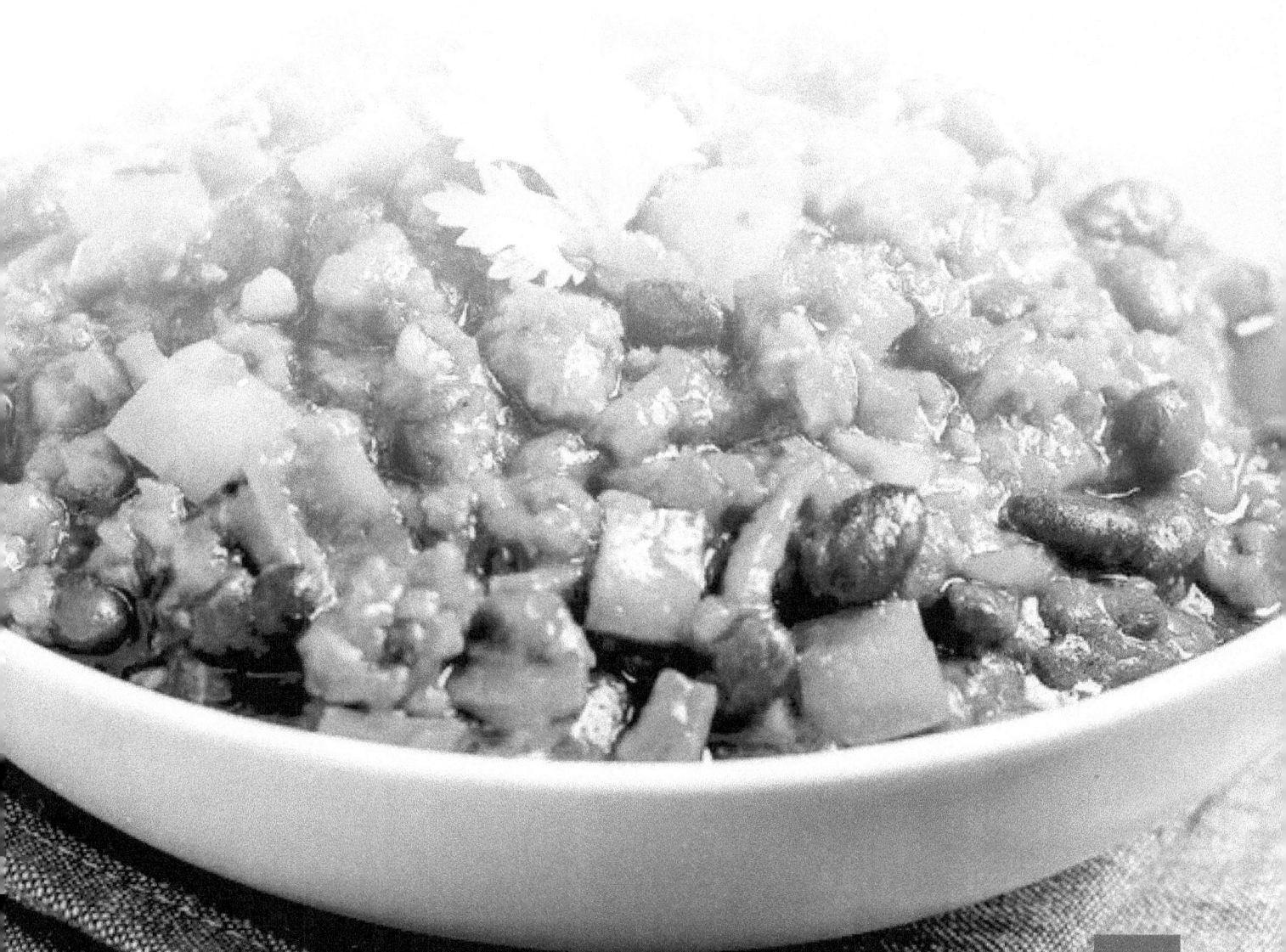

PORK MEATLOAF

Preparation Time: 10 minutes

Cooking Time: 50 minutes

Servings: 1

INGREDIENTS:

- 1-pound lean ground beef
- ½ cup Breadcrumbs
- ½ cup Chopped sweet onion
- 1 Egg
- 2 tbsps. Chopped fresh basil
- 1 tsp. Chopped fresh thyme
- 1 tsp. Chopped fresh parsley
- ¼ tsp. Ground black pepper
- 1 tbsp. Brown sugar
- 1 tsp. White vinegar
- ¼ tsp. Garlic powder

DIRECTIONS:

1. Preheat the oven to 350f.
2. Mix well the breadcrumbs, beef, onion, basil, egg, thyme, parsley, and pepper.
3. Stir the brown sugar, vinegar, and garlic powder in a small bowl.
4. Put the brown sugar mixture evenly over the meat.
5. Bake the meatloaf for about 50 minutes or until it is cooked through.
6. Let the meatloaf stand for 10 minutes and then pour out any accumulated grease.

NUTRITION:

Calories: 103

Fat: 3g

Carb: 7g

Protein: 11g

Sodium: 87mg

Potassium: 190mg

Phosphorus: 112mg

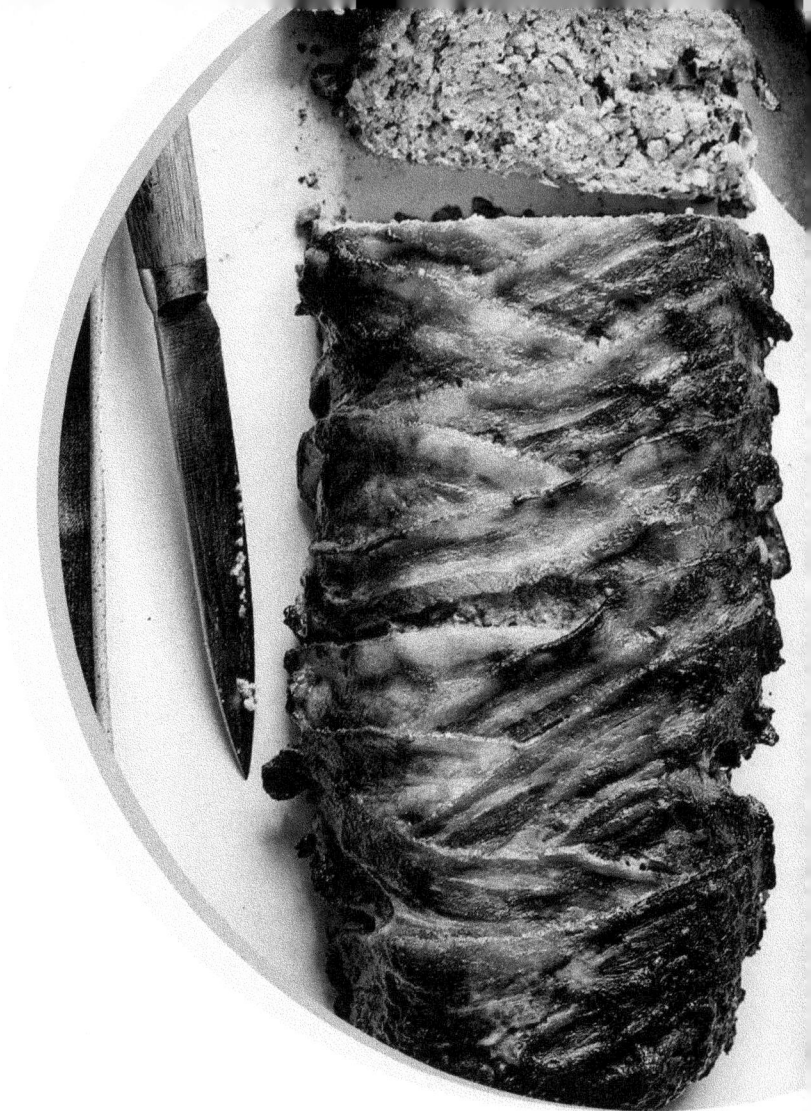

65 CHICKEN STEW

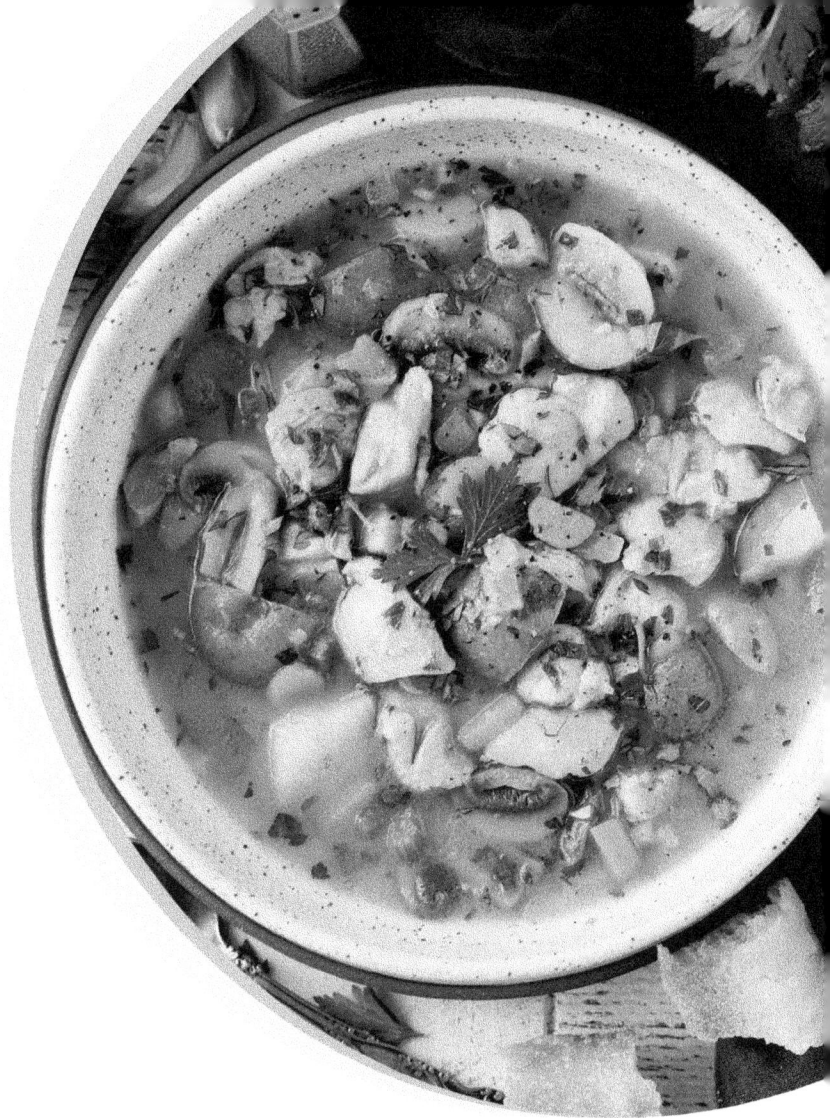

Preparation Time: 20 minutes

Cooking Time: 50 minutes

Servings: 1

INGREDIENTS:

- 1 tbsp. Olive oil
- 1 pound, cut into 1-inch cubes Boneless, skinless chicken thighs
- ½, chopped Sweet onion
- 1 tbsp. Minced garlic
- 2 cups Chicken stock
- 1 cup, plus 2 tbsps. Water
- 1 sliced Carrot
- 2 stalks, sliced Celery
- 1, sliced thin Turnip
- 1 tbsp. Chopped fresh thyme
- 1 tsp. Chopped fresh rosemary
- 2 tsp. Cornstarch
- Ground black pepper to taste

DIRECTIONS:

1. Prepare a large saucepan on medium heat and add the olive oil.
2. Sauté the chicken for 6 minutes or until it is lightly browned, stirring often.
3. Add the onion and garlic, and sauté for 3 minutes.
4. Add 1-cup water, chicken stock, carrot, celery, and turnip and bring the stew to a boil.
5. Simmer for 30 minutes or until cooked and tender.
6. Add the thyme and rosemary and simmer for 3 minutes more.
7. In a small bowl, stir together the 2 tbsps. Of water and the cornstarch

8.   add the mixture to the stew.

9.   Stir to incorporate the cornstarch mixture and cook for 3 to 4 minutes or until the stew thickens.

10. Remove from the heat once done and season with pepper.

NUTRITION:

Calories: 141
Fat: 8g
Carb: 5g
Protein: 9g
Sodium: 214mg
Potassium: 192mg
Phosphorus: 53mg

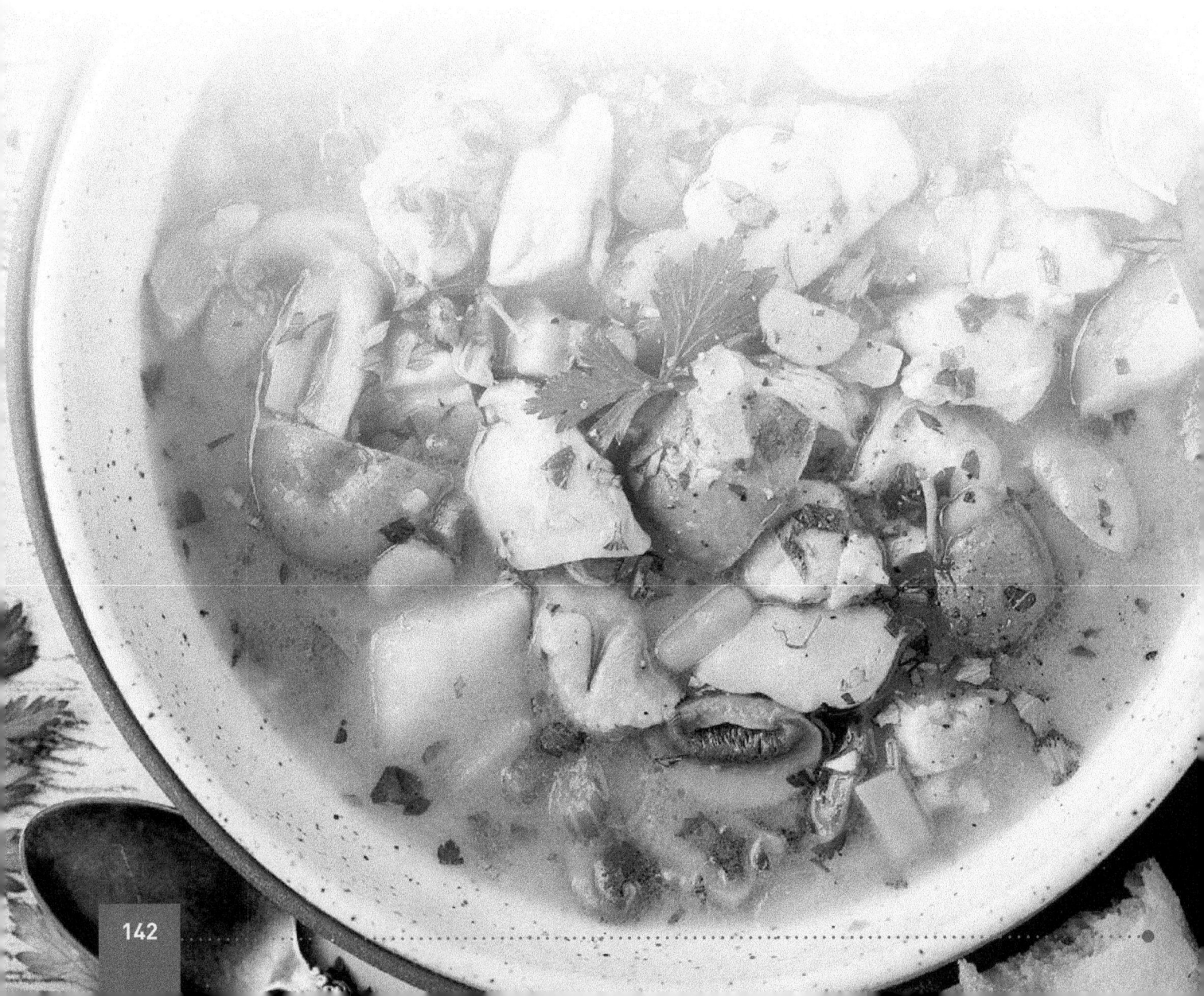

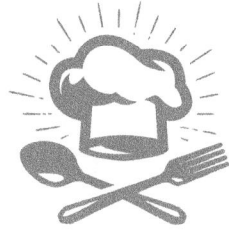

CHAPTER 15

SOUP RECIPES

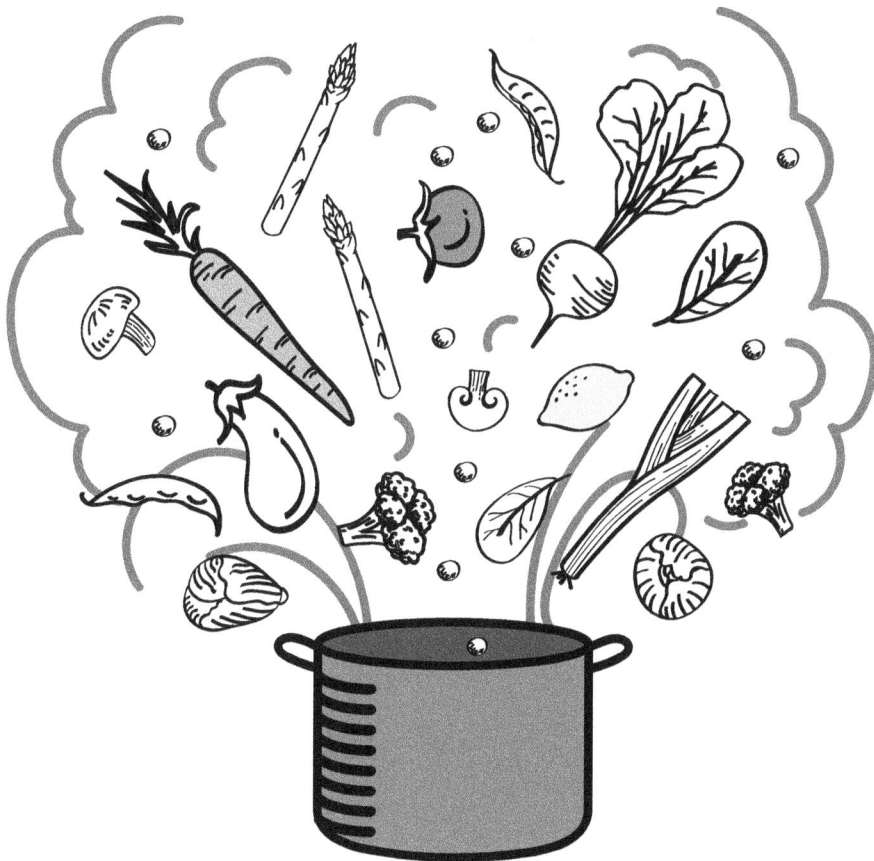

PESTO GREEN
VEGETABLE SOUP

Preparation Time: 10 minutes

Cooking Time: 15 minutes

Servings: 1

INGREDIENTS:

- 2 teaspoons olive oil
- 1 sliced leek, white and light green
- 2 celery stalks, diced
- 1 teaspoon minced garlic
- 2 cups sodium-free chicken stock
- 1 cup chopped snow peas
- 1 cup shredded spinach
- 1 tablespoon chopped fresh thyme
- Juice and zest of ½ lemon
- ¼ teaspoon freshly ground black pepper
- 1 tablespoon Basil Pesto

DIRECTIONS:

1. Add olive oil in a large saucepan.
2. Add the leek, celery, and garlic, and sauté until tender, about 3 minutes.
3. Stir in the stock and bring to a boil.
4. Stir in the snow peas, spinach, and thyme, and simmer for about 5 minutes.
5. Remove the pan from the heat, and stir in the lemon juice, lemon zest, pepper, and pesto.
6. Serve immediately.

NUTRITION:

Calories: 170

Fat: 13g

Carbohydrates: 8g

Protein: 3g

Sodium: 333mg

Phosphorus: 42mg

Potassium: 200mg

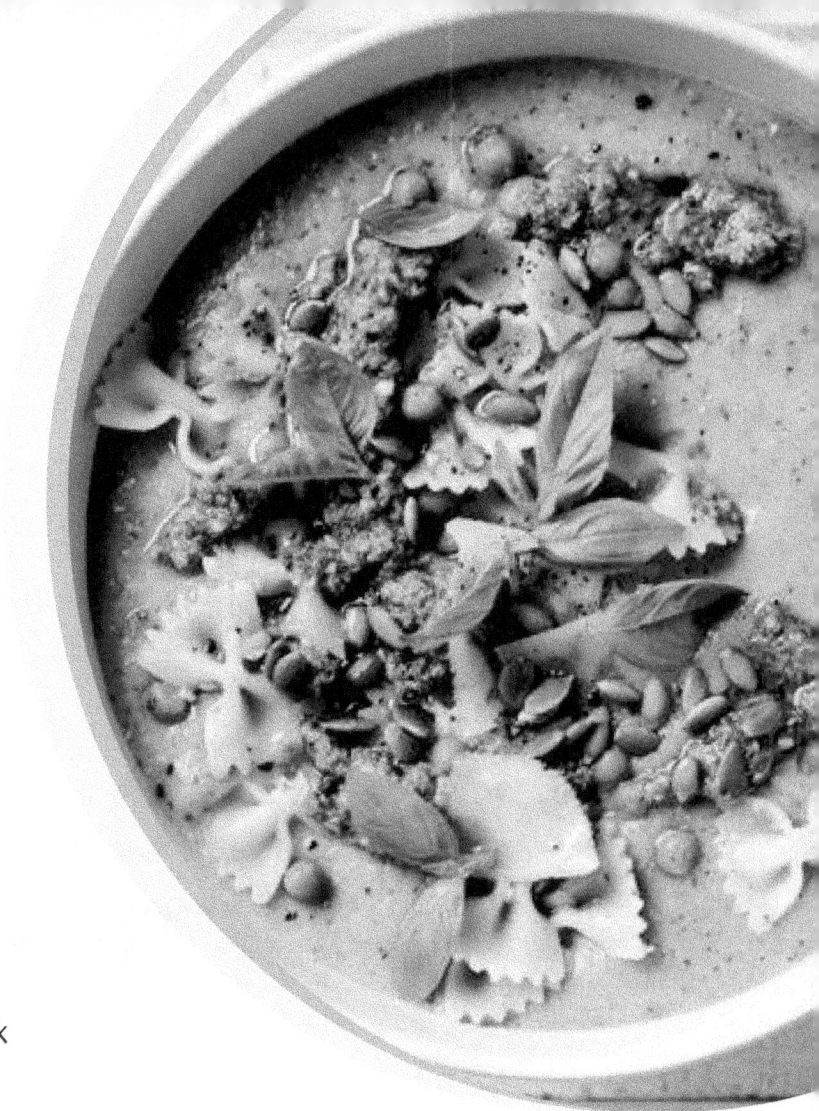

67 EASY LOW-SODIUM CHICKEN BROTH

Preparation Time: 10 minutes

Cooking Time: 4 hours

Servings: 1

INGREDIENTS:

- 2 pounds skinless whole chicken, cut into pieces
- 4 garlic cloves, lightly crushed
- 2 celery stalks, with greens, roughly chopped
- 2 carrots, roughly chopped
- 1 sweet onion, cut into quarters
- 10 peppercorns
- 4 fresh thyme sprigs
- 2 bay leaves
- Water

DIRECTIONS:

1. In a large stockpot, place the chicken, garlic, celery, carrots, onion, peppercorns, thyme, and bay leaves, and cover with water by about 3 inches.
2. Let the water boil over high heat. Simmer for about 4 hours in low heat.
3. Skim off any foam on top of the stock and pour the stock through a fine-mesh sieve.
4. Pick off all the usable chicken meat for another recipe, discard the bones and other solids, and allow the stock to cool for about 30 minutes before transferring it to sealable containers.
5. You can put the stock in the refrigerator for 1 week or up to 2 months in the freezer.

NUTRITION:

Calories: 32
Carbohydrates: 8g

Protein: 1g
Sodium: 57mg

Potassium: 187mg
Phosphorus: 50mg

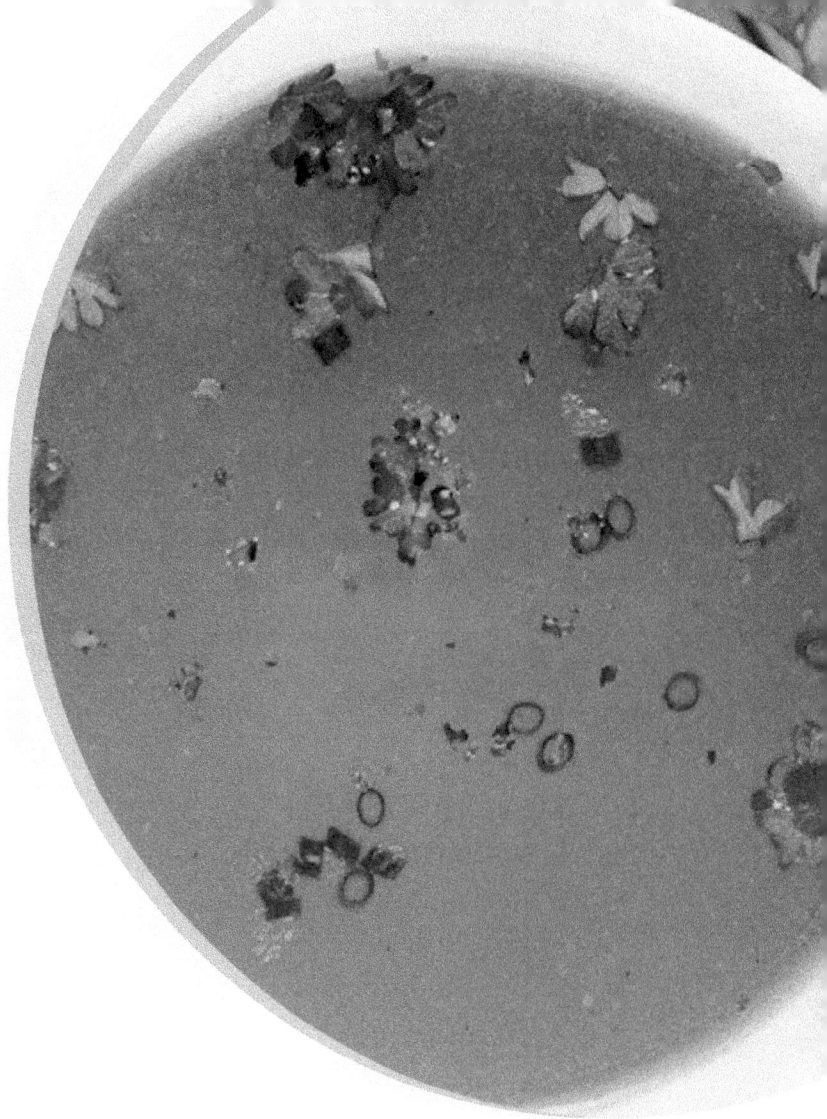

CREAM OF SPINACH SOUP

Preparation Time: 15 minutes

Cooking Time: 30 minutes

Servings: 4

INGREDIENTS:

- 1 tablespoon olive oil
- ½ sweet onion, chopped
- 2 teaspoons minced garlic
- 4 cups fresh spinach
- ¼ cup chopped fresh parsley
- 3 cups of water
- ¼ cup heavy (whipping) cream
- 1 tablespoon freshly squeezed lemon juice
- Freshly ground black pepper

DIRECTIONS:

1. On a heated olive oil, sauté the onion and garlic in a large saucepan for 3 minutes.
2. Add the spinach and parsley, and sauté for 5 minutes.
3. Stir in the water, bring to a boil, then reduce the heat to low. Simmer the soup until the vegetables are tender, about 20 minutes.
4. Let it cool for 5 minutes, then, along with the heavy cream, purée the soup in batches in a food processor (or a blender or a handheld immersion blender).
5. Return the soup to the pot and cook through on low heat.
6. Add the lemon juice, season with pepper, and stir to combine. Serve hot.

NUTRITION:

Calories: 141

Fat: 14g

Carbohydrates: 3g

Protein: 2g

Sodium: 36mg

Phosphorus: 38mg

Potassium: 200mg

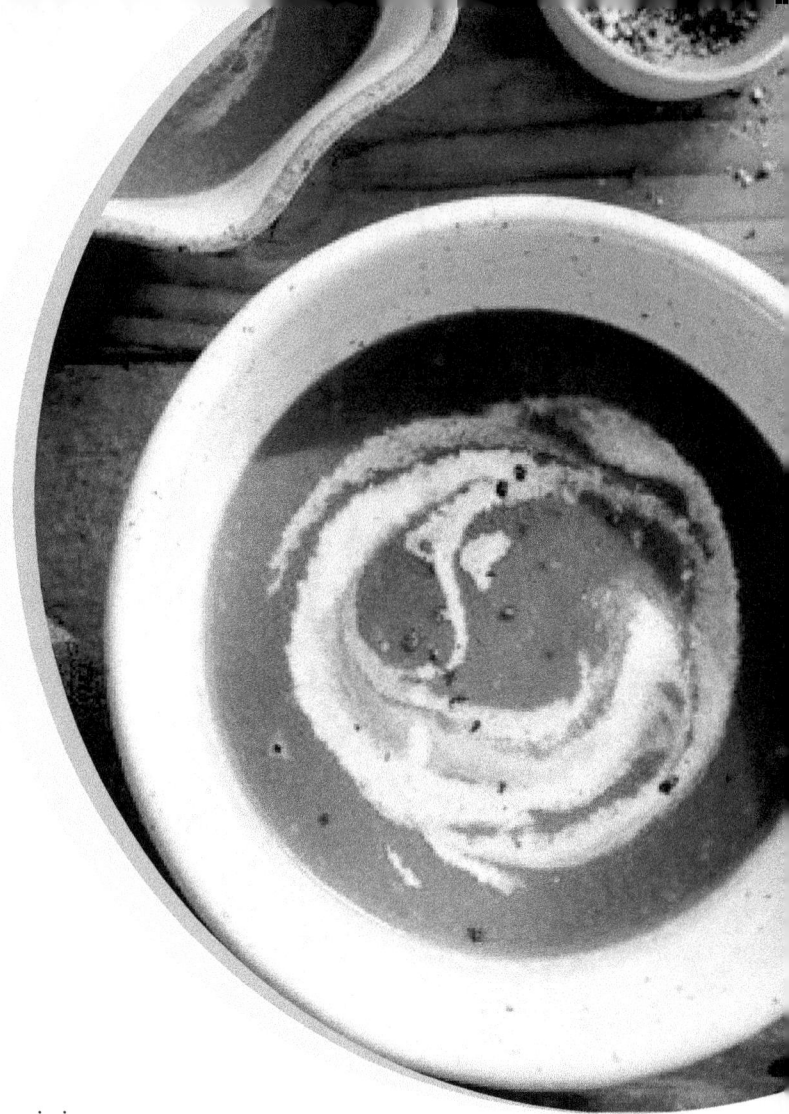

69 VEGETABLE MINESTRONE

Preparation Time: 20 minutes

Cooking Time: 20 minutes

Servings: 6

INGREDIENTS:

- 1 teaspoon olive oil
- ½ sweet onion, chopped
- 1 celery stalk, diced
- 1 teaspoon minced garlic
- 2 cups sodium-free chicken stock
- 2 medium tomatoes, chopped
- 1 zucchini, diced
- ½ cup shredded stemmed kale
- Freshly ground black pepper
- 1-ounce grated Parmesan cheese

DIRECTIONS:

1. Prepare a large saucepan over medium-high heat.
2. Add the onion, celery, and garlic. Sauté until softened, about 5 minutes.
3. Stir in the stock, tomatoes, and zucchini, and bring to a boil. Let it simmer for 15 minutes.
4. Stir in the kale and season with pepper.
5. Garnish with the parmesan cheese and serve.

NUTRITION:

Calories: 100
Fat: 3g
Carbohydrates: 6g
Protein: 4g

Sodium: 195mg
Phosphorus: 70mg
Potassium: 200mg

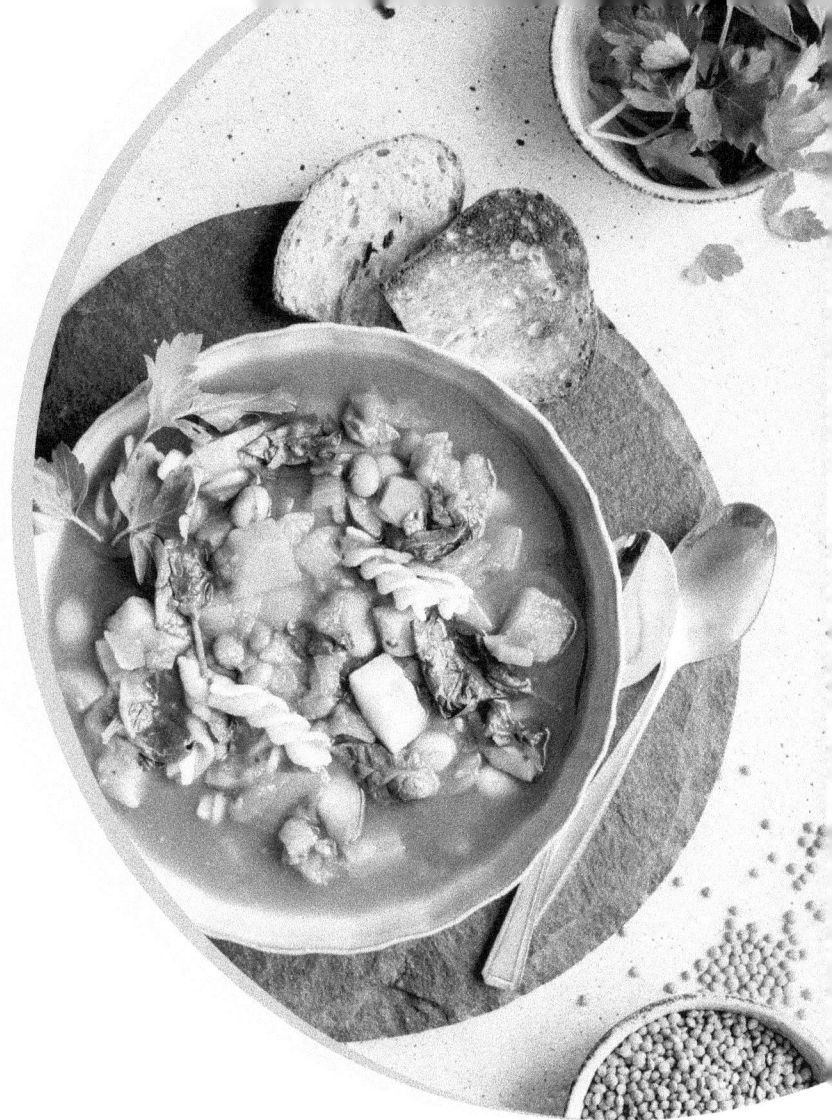

70 | VIBRANT CARROT SOUP

Preparation Time: 15 minutes

Cooking Time: 25 minutes

Servings: 4

INGREDIENTS:

- 1 tablespoon olive oil
- ½ sweet onion, chopped
- 2 teaspoons grated peeled fresh ginger
- 1 teaspoon minced fresh garlic
- 4 cups of water
- 3 carrots, chopped
- 1 teaspoon ground turmeric
- ½ cup of coconut milk
- 1 tablespoon chopped fresh cilantro

DIRECTIONS:

1. Heat the olive oil in a saucepan.
2. Sauté the onion, ginger, and garlic until softened.
3. Stir in the water, carrots, and turmeric. Bring the soup to a boil, reduce the heat to low, and simmer until the carrots are tender about 20 minutes.
4. Transfer the soup in batches to a food processor (or blender) and process with the coconut milk until the soup is smooth.
5. Reheat the soup in a pan.
6. Serve topped with the cilantro.

NUTRITION:

Calories: 113
Fat: 10g
Protein: 1g

Carbohydrates: 7g
Sodium: 30mg

Phosphorus: 50mg
Potassium: 200mg;

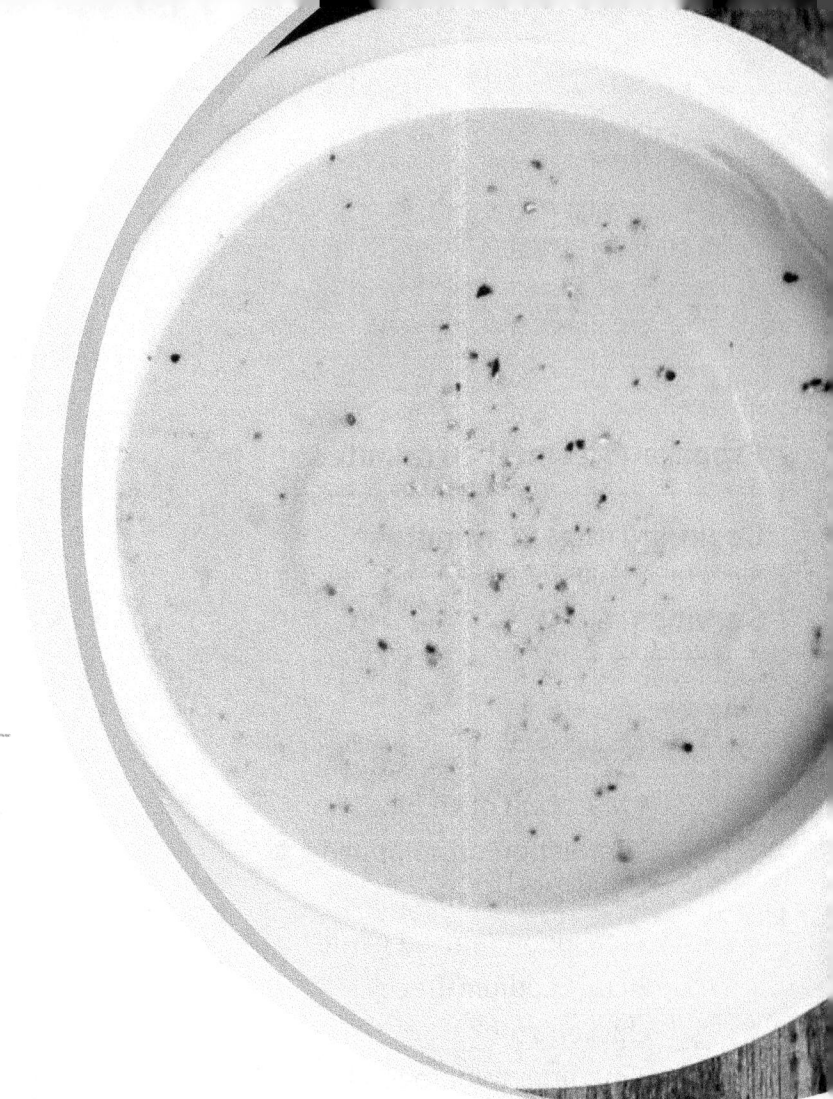

71 SIMPLE CABBAGE SOUP

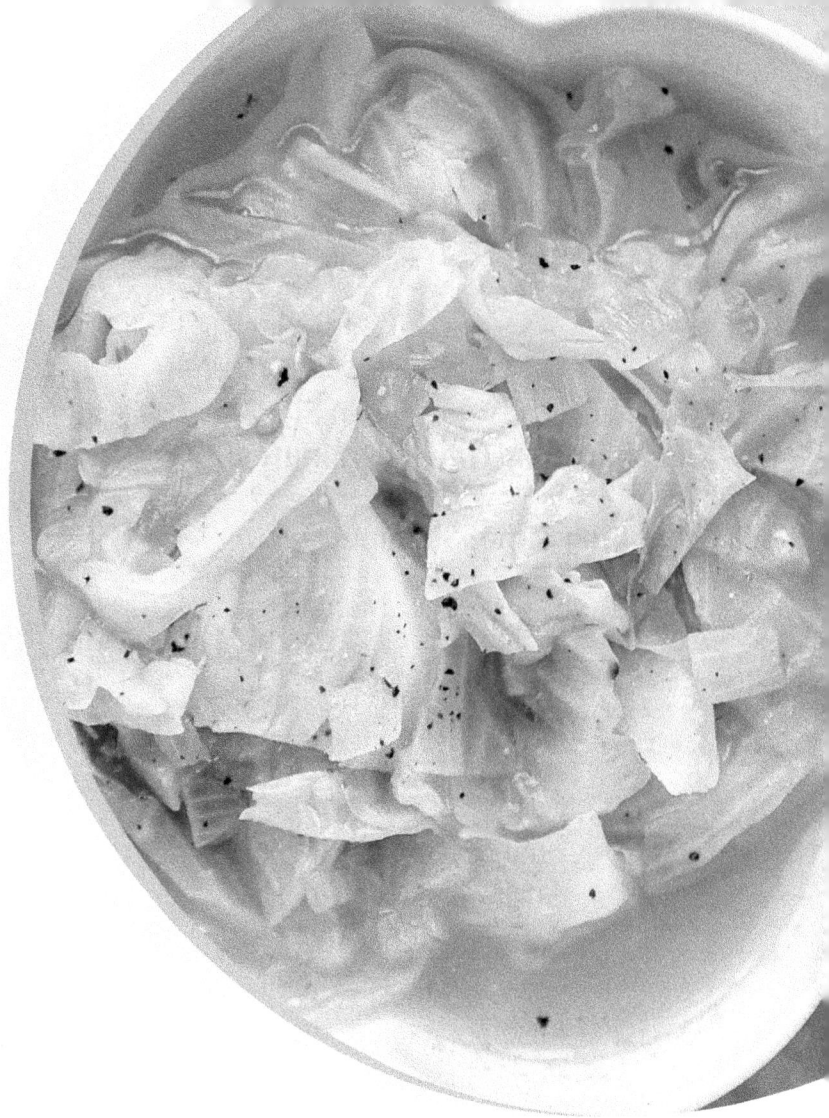

Preparation Time: 20 minutes

Cooking Time: 35 minutes

Servings: 8

INGREDIENTS:

- 1 tablespoon olive oil
- ½ sweet onion, chopped
- 2 teaspoons minced garlic
- 6 cups of water
- 1 cup sodium-free chicken stock
- ½ head green cabbage, shredded
- 2 carrots, diced
- 2 medium tomatoes, diced
- Freshly ground black pepper
- 2 tablespoons chopped fresh thyme

DIRECTIONS:

1. Prepare olive oil in a large saucepan over medium-high heat.
2. Sauté the onion and garlic until softened.
3. Add water, chicken stock, cabbage, carrots, and tomatoes. Let it bring it to a boil.
4. In medium-low heat, simmer the vegetables for 30 minutes or until tender.
5. Season the soup with black pepper. Serve hot, topped with the thyme.

NUTRITION:

Calories: 62
Fat: 2g
Carbohydrates: 6g
Protein: 2g

Sodium: 61mg
Phosphorus: 32mg
Potassium: 200mg

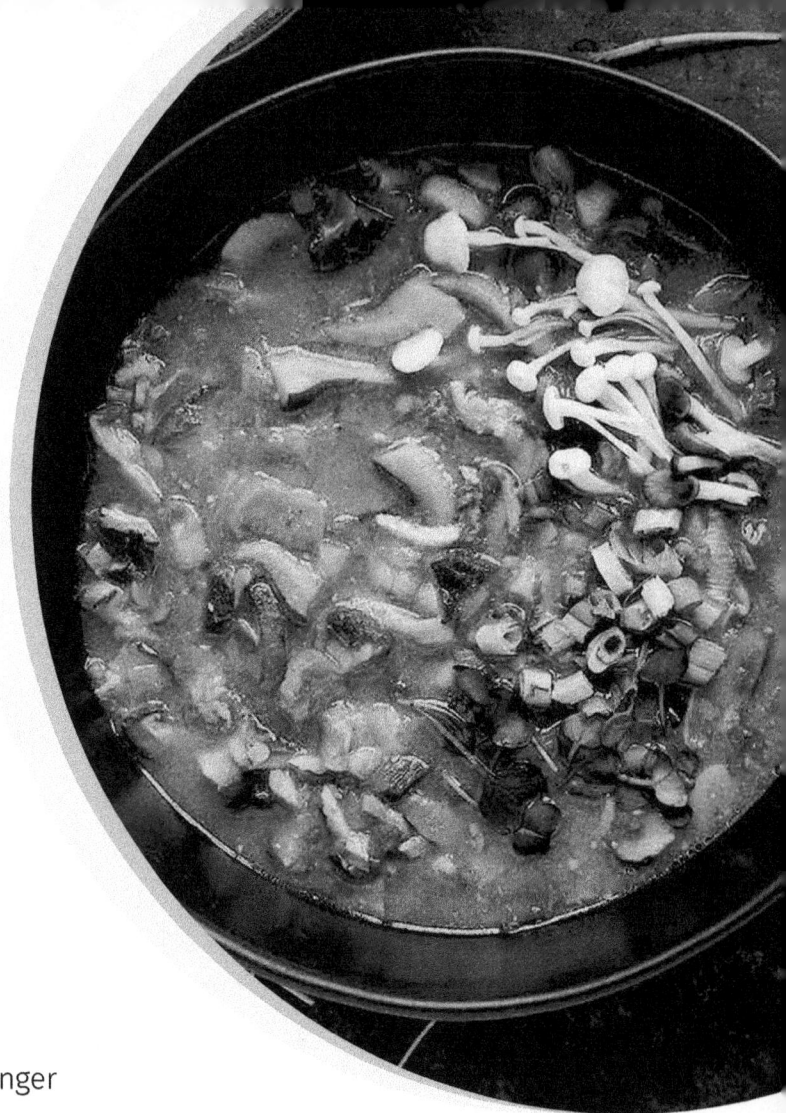

72 MUSHROOM MOCK MISO SOUP

Preparation Time: 10 minutes

Cooking Time: 35 minutes

Servings: 6

INGREDIENTS:

- 6 cups water, divided
- 2 ounces dried mixed mushrooms
- ¼ cup of seasoned rice vinegar
- 1 teaspoon low-sodium soy sauce
- 1 tablespoon grated peeled fresh ginger
- 1 cup julienned snow peas
- ½ cup grated carrot
- 2 scallions, green and white parts, chopped

DIRECTIONS:

1. Prepare 2 cups of water in a small saucepan over high heat and bring to a boil.
2. Place the dried mushrooms in a medium bowl and pour the boiling water over them. Let the mushrooms reconstitute for 30 minutes, then remove them from the water and slice them thinly.
3. Transfer the mushroom water, the remaining 4 cups of water, vinegar, soy sauce, ginger to a large saucepan, and place over medium-high heat.
4. Bring to a boil, then put mushrooms, snow peas, and carrot. Reduce the heat to low, and simmer for 5 minutes.
5. Serve hot, topped with the scallions.

Calories: 56
Fat: 0g
Carbohydrates: 9g
Protein: 2g
Sodium: 118mg
Phosphorus: 43mg
Potassium: 198mg

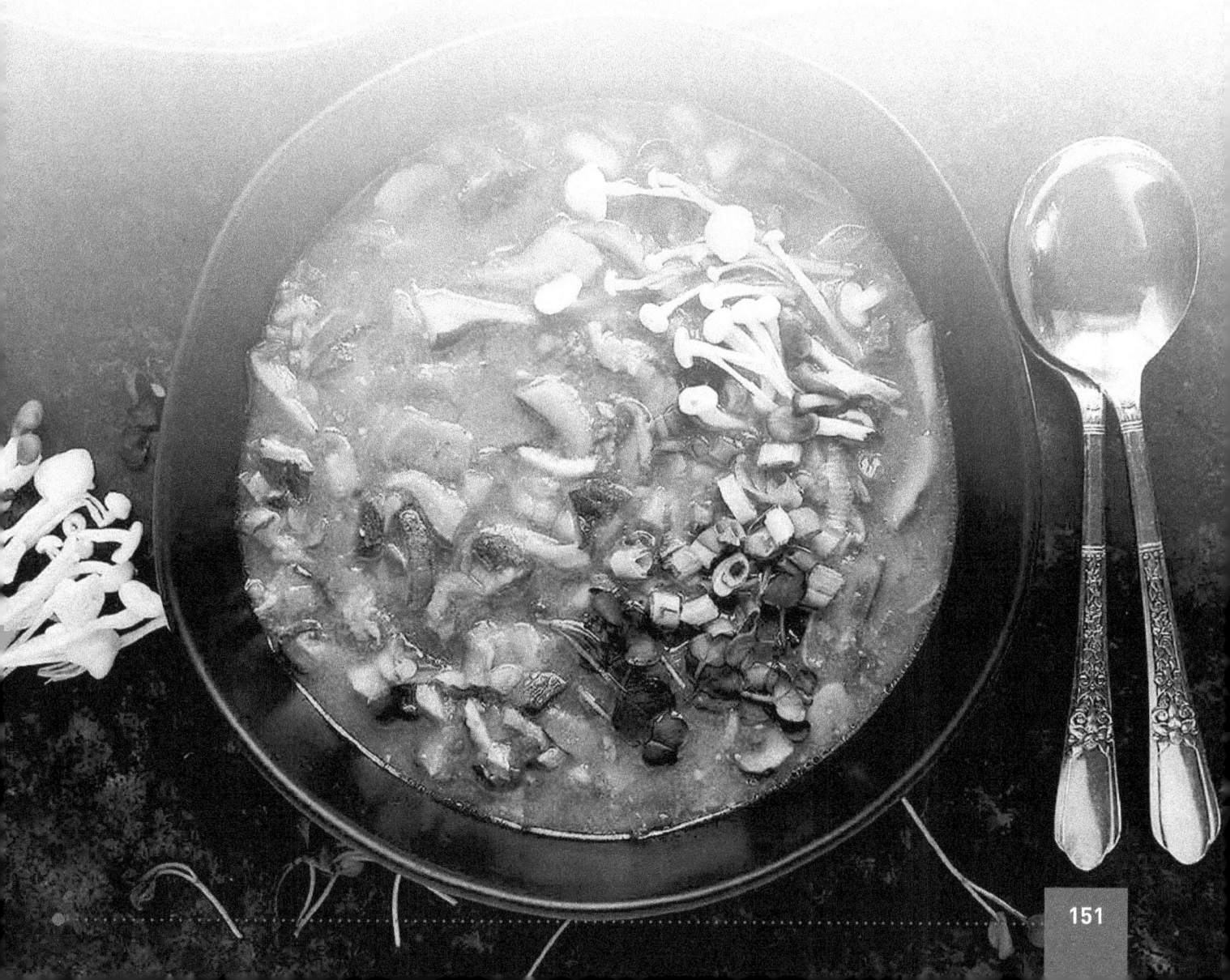

73 FENNEL CAULIFLOWER SOUP

Preparation Time: 20 minutes

Cooking Time: 30 minutes

Servings: 1

INGREDIENTS:

- 1 teaspoon olive oil
- 1 small sweet onion, chopped
- 2 teaspoons minced garlic
- ½ small head cauliflower, cut into small florets
- 2 cups chopped fresh fennel
- 4 cups of water
- 2 teaspoons chopped fresh thyme
- ¼ cup heavy (whipping) cream

DIRECTIONS:

1. Prepare a saucepan and heat the olive oil.
2. Put onion and garlic. Sauté until softened, about 3 minutes.
3. Add the cauliflower, fennel, and water. Let it boil, then reduce the heat to medium-low and simmer until the cauliflower is tender, about 20 minutes.
4. In batches, pour the soup into a food processor (or blender), and purée until smooth and creamy.
5. Return the soup to the pan. Stir in the thyme and cream—heat on medium-low until warmed through, about 5 minutes. Serve.

NUTRITION:

Calories: 105
Fat: 8g
Carbohydrates: 5g

Protein: 1g
Sodium: 30mg

Phosphorus: 41mg
Potassium: 200mg

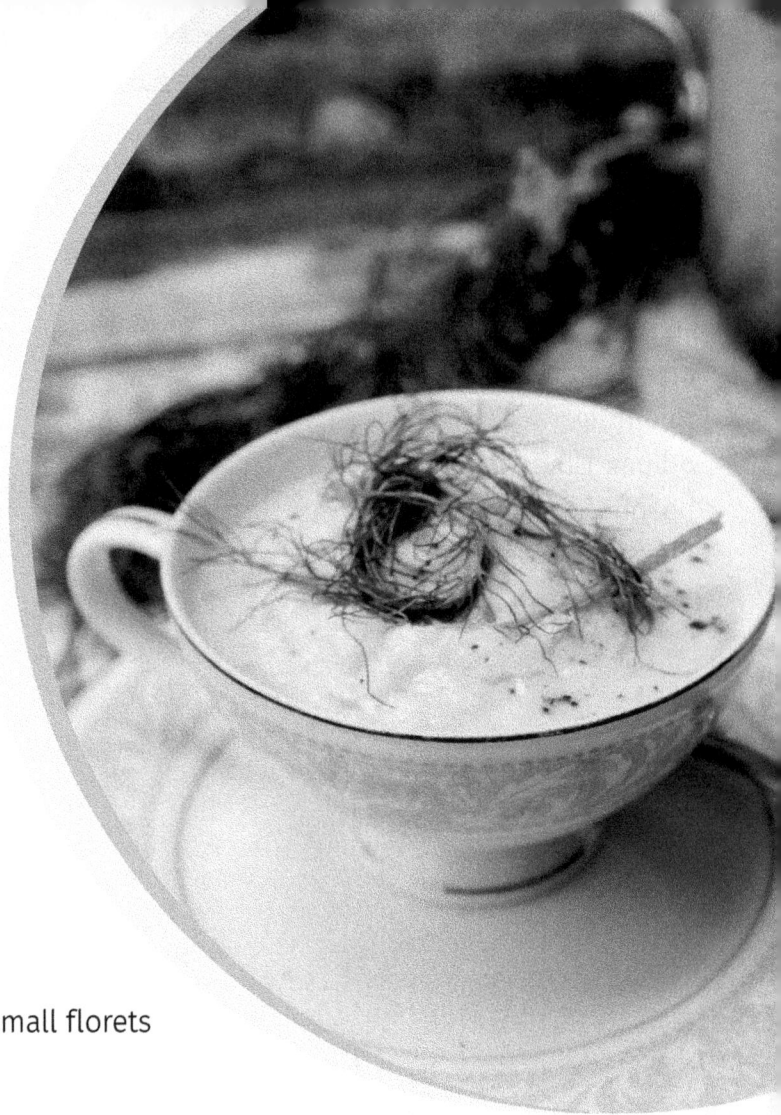

74 CHICKEN ALPHABET SOUP

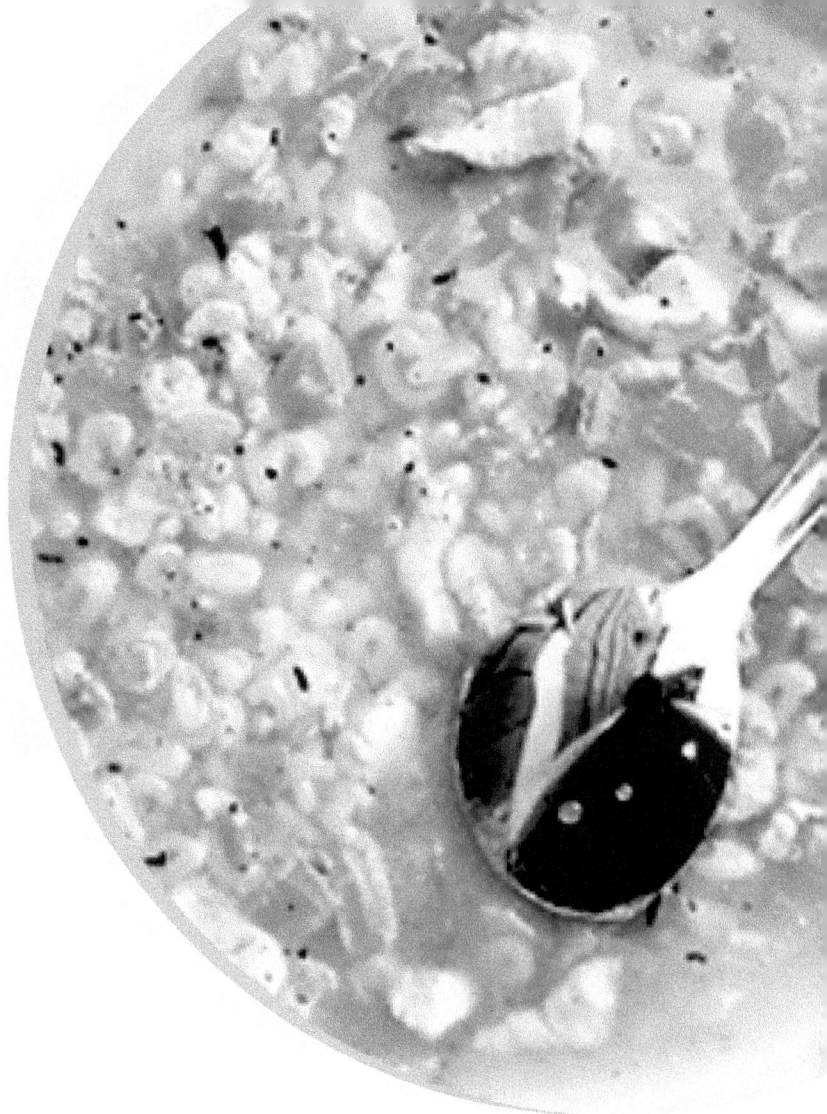

Preparation Time: 15 minutes

Cooking Time: 35 minutes

Servings: 6

INGREDIENTS:

- 1 tablespoon olive oil
- ½ sweet onion, diced
- 2 teaspoons minced garlic
- 4 cups of water
- 1½ cups chopped cooked chicken breast
- 1 cup sodium-free chicken stock
- 2 celery stalks, chopped
- 1 carrot, peeled and diced
- ½ cup dried alphabet noodles
- Freshly ground black pepper
- 2 tablespoons chopped fresh parsley

DIRECTIONS:

1. Put olive oil in a large saucepan with medium-high heat.
2. Add the onion and garlic. Cook until softened, about 3 minutes.
3. Add the water, chicken, chicken stock, celery, and carrot. Bring to a boil, then reduce the heat to medium-low and simmer until the vegetables are tender-crisp about 15 minutes.
4. Add the noodles, stir, and simmer the soup until the noodles are tender about 15 minutes.
5. Season with pepper. Serve hot with topped parsley.

NUTRITION:

Calories: 132

Fat: 3g

Carbohydrates: 10g

Protein: 13g

Sodium: 95mg

Phosphorus: 116mg

Potassium: 200mg

MEATBALL SOUP

Preparation Time: 20 minutes

Cooking Time: 40 minutes

Servings: 6

INGREDIENTS:

- ½ pound lean ground beef
- 2 tablespoons breadcrumbs
- 1 tablespoon chopped fresh parsley
- 1 teaspoon minced garlic
- 1 teaspoon olive oil
- ½ sweet onion, chopped
- 5 cups of water
- 2 tomatoes, chopped
- 2 celery stalks with the greens, chopped
- 1 carrot, diced
- Freshly ground black pepper

DIRECTIONS:

1. Mix the ground beef, breadcrumbs, parsley, and garlic in a large bowl. Roll the meat mixture into small (1-inch) meatballs.
2. Add the onion in a large saucepan, and sauté until softened, about 3 minutes.
3. Add the water, tomatoes, celery, and carrot, and bring to a boil. Add the meatballs, reduce the heat to medium-low, and simmer until the vegetables are tender and the meatballs are cooked through about 35 minutes.
4. Season the soup with pepper and serve hot.

NUTRITION:

Calories: 106   Protein: 9g   Phosphorus: 92mg

Total fat: 3g   Sodium: 53mg   Potassium: 200mg

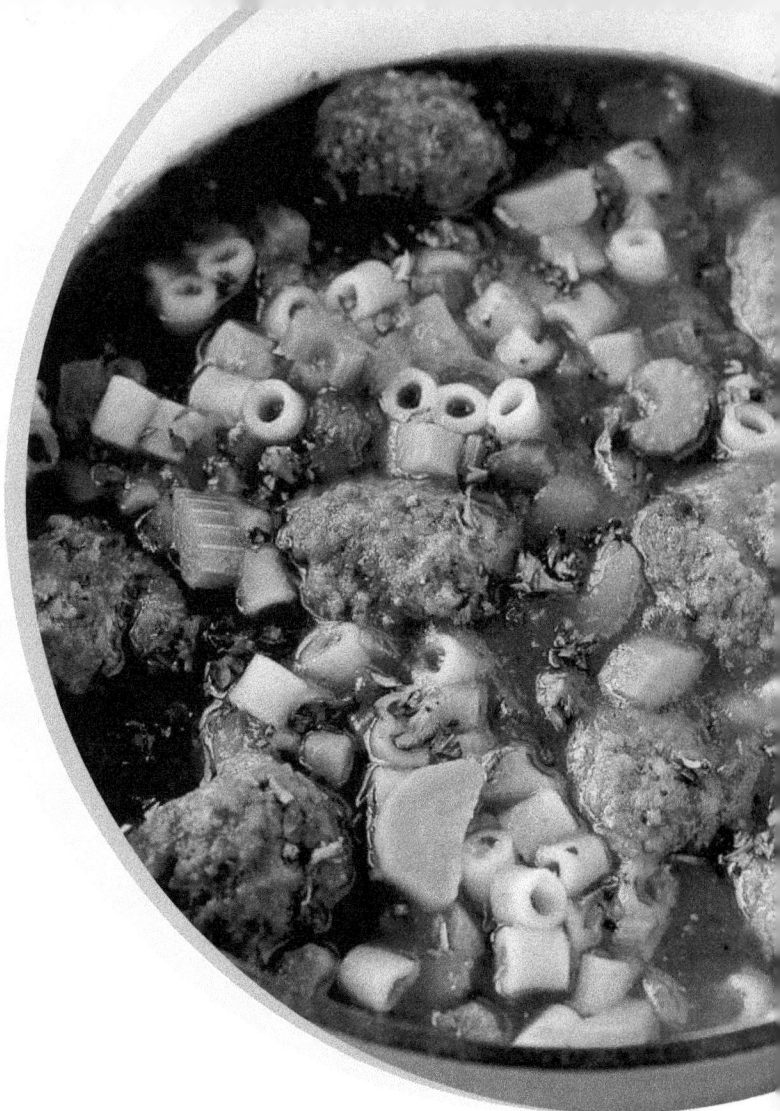

Carbohydrates: 4g

76 | VEGETABLE STEW

Preparation Time: 15 minutes

Cooking Time: 15 minutes

Servings: 8

INGREDIENTS:

- 1 teaspoon olive oil
- 1 sweet onion, chopped
- 1 teaspoon minced garlic
- 2 zucchinis, chopped
- 1 red bell pepper, diced
- 2 carrots, chopped
- 2 cups low-sodium vegetable stock
- 2 large tomatoes, chopped
- 2 cups broccoli florets
- 1 teaspoon ground coriander
- ½ teaspoon ground cumin
- Pinch cayenne pepper
- Freshly ground black pepper
- 2 tablespoons chopped fresh cilantro

DIRECTIONS:

1. Cook garlic and onion in a saucepan until softened.
2. Put zucchini, bell pepper, and carrots, and sauté for 5 minutes.
3. Mix vegetable stock, tomatoes, broccoli, coriander, cumin, and cayenne pepper.
4. Let it boil and simmer to medium-low until the vegetables are tender, often stirring about 5 minutes.
5. Add pepper and serve hot, topped with the cilantro.

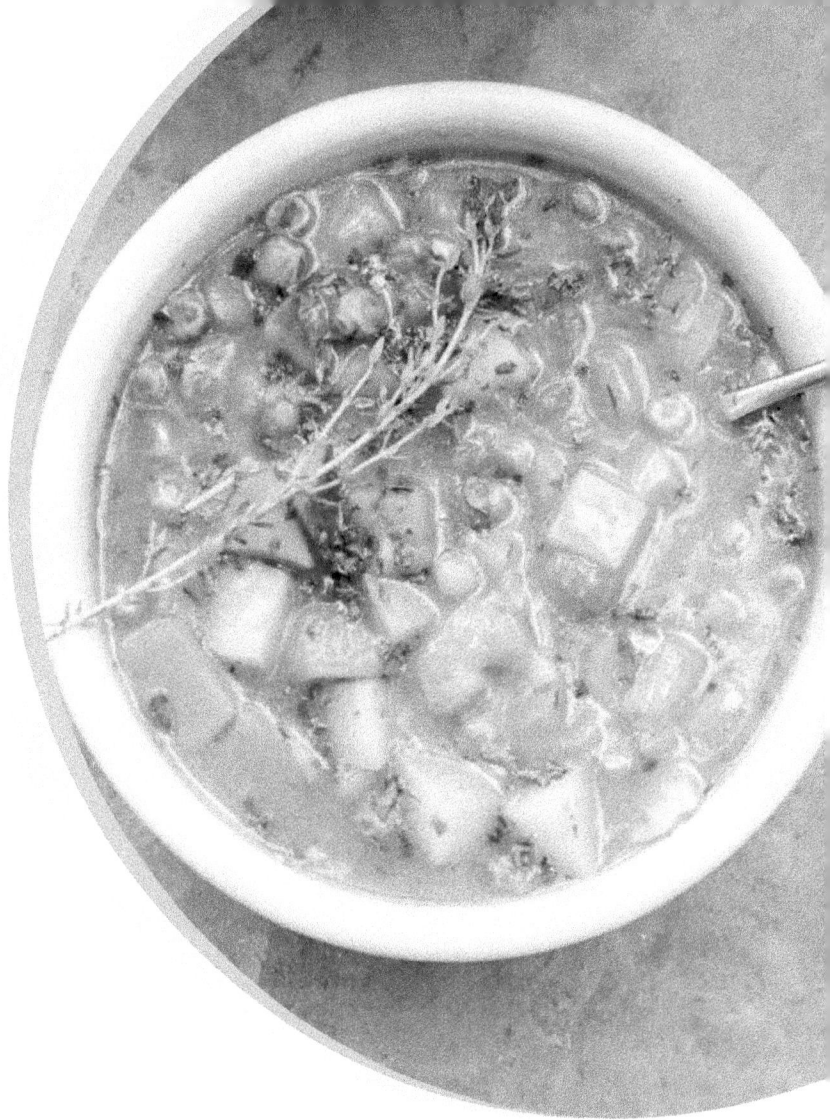

Calories: 45
Fat: 1g
Carbohydrates: 5g
Protein: 1g
Sodium: 194mg
Phosphorus: 21mg
Potassium: 184mg

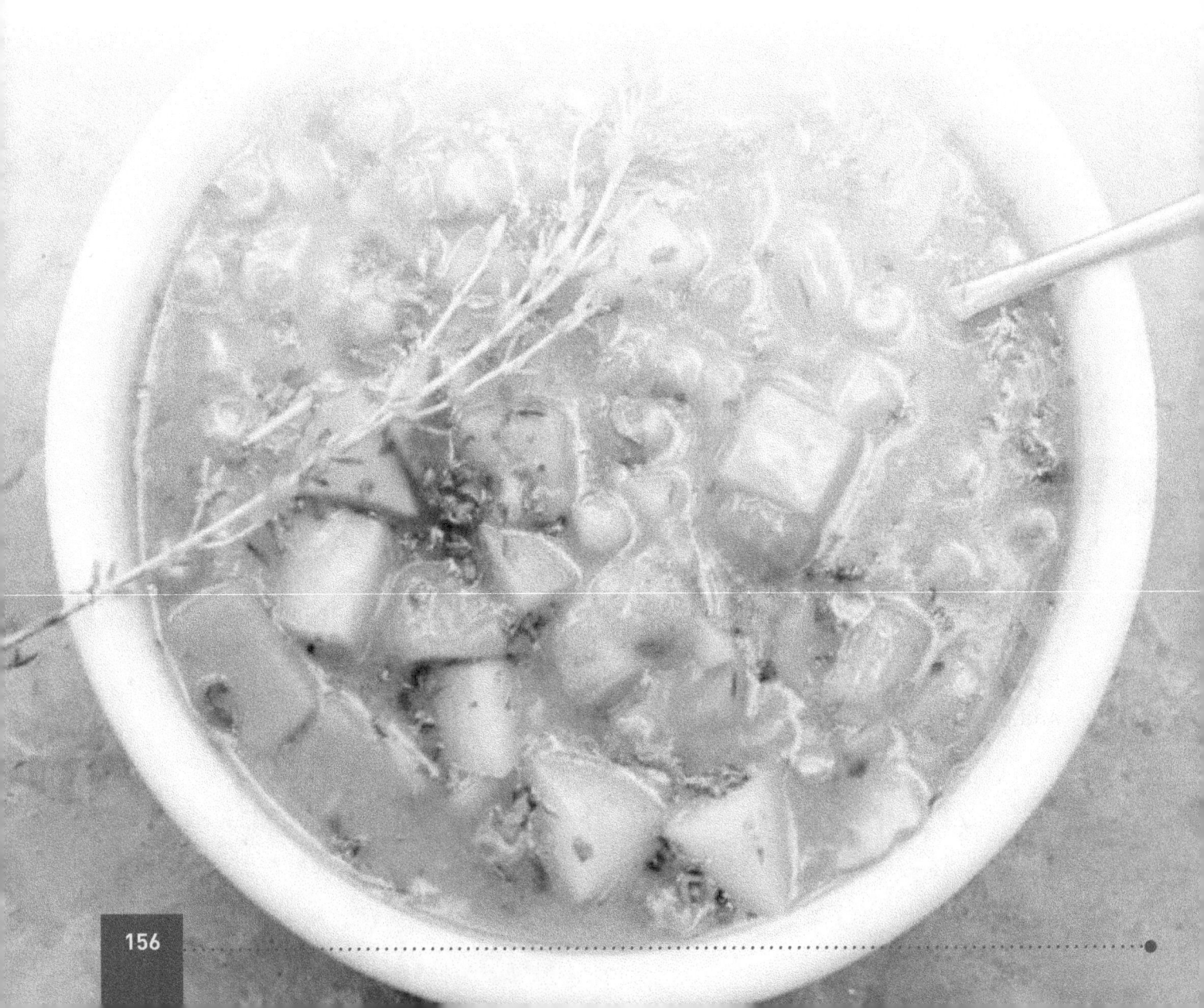

77 SAUSAGE & EGG SOUP

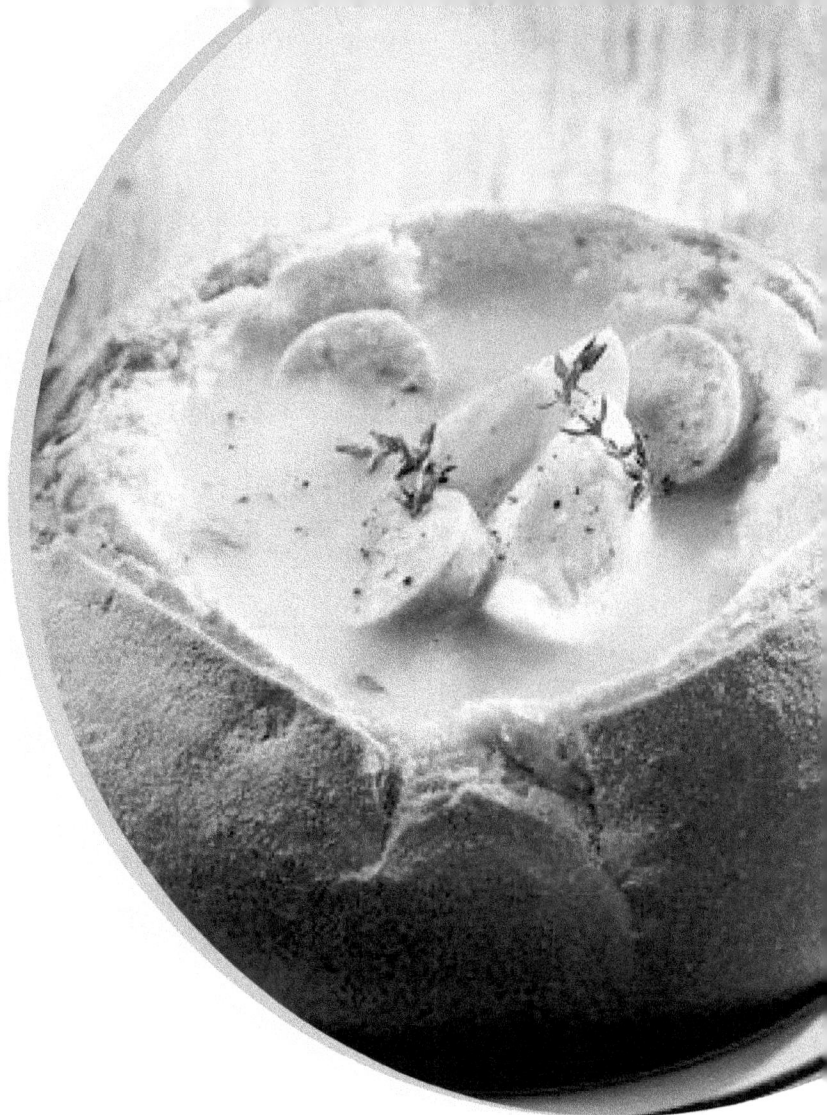

Preparation Time: 15 minutes

Cooking Time: 30 minutes

Servings: 4

INGREDIENTS:

- 1/2 lb. ground beef
- Black pepper
- 1/2 teaspoon ground sage
- 1/2 teaspoon garlic powder
- 1/2 teaspoon dried basil
- 4 slices bread (one day old), cubed
- 2 tablespoons olive oil
-
  1 tablespoon herb seasoning blend
- 2 garlic cloves, minced
- 3 cups low-sodium chicken broth
- 1 cup of water
- 4 tablespoons fresh parsley
- 4 eggs
- 2 tablespoons Parmesan cheese, grated

DIRECTIONS:

1. Preheat your oven to 375 degrees F.
2. Mix the first five ingredients to make the sausage—Toss bread cubes in oil and seasoning blend.
3. Bake in the oven for 8 minutes. Set aside.
4. Cook the sausage in a pan over medium heat.

5. Cook the garlic in the sausage drippings for 2 minutes.
6. Stir in the broth, water, and parsley and let it boil. Simmer for 10 minutes.
7. Pour into serving bowls and top with baked bread, egg, and sausage.

NUTRITION:

Calories: 196
Fat: 11g
Carbohydrates: 17g
Protein: 7g
Sodium: 148mg
Potassium: 537mg
Phosphorus: 125mg

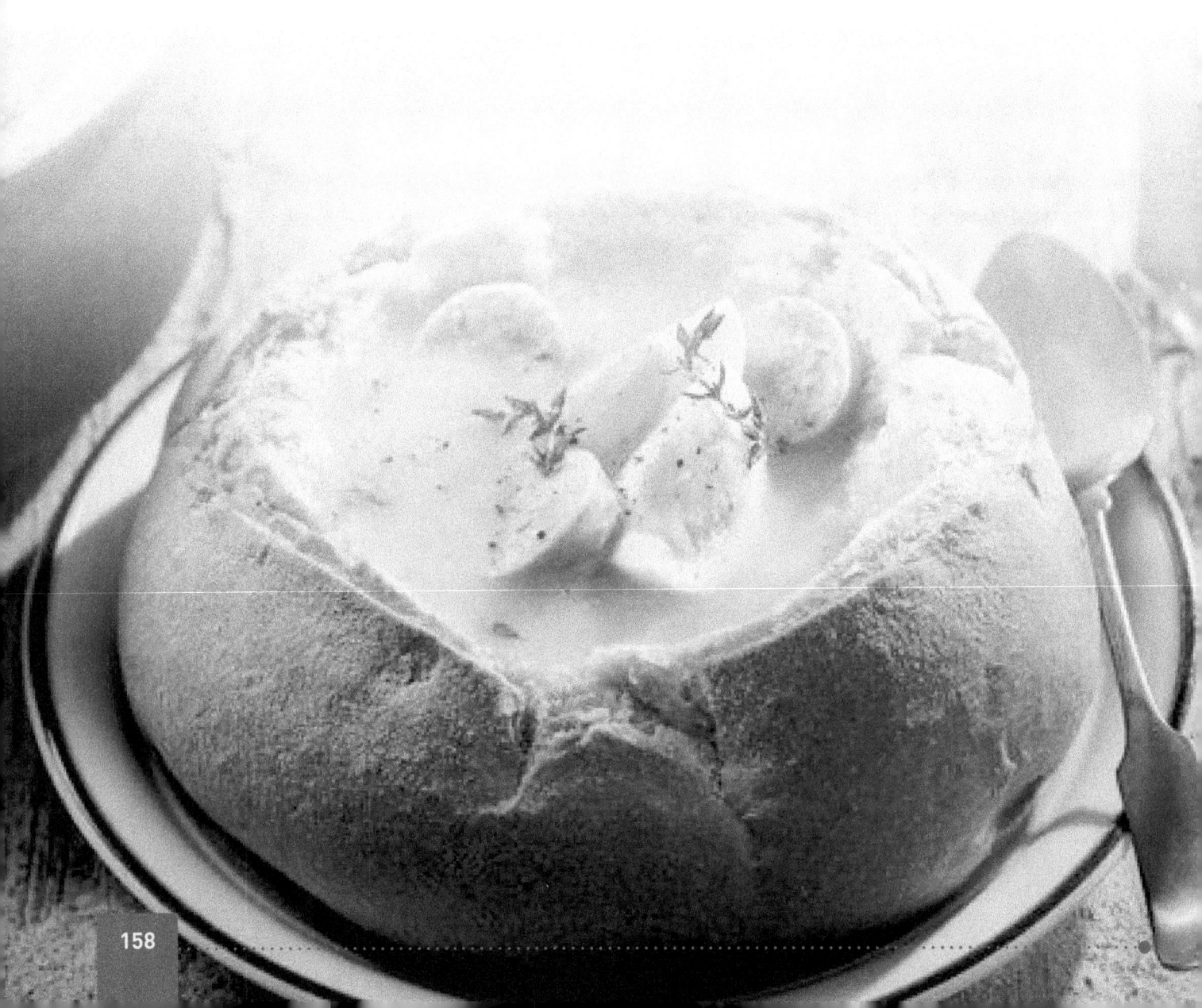

78 SEAFOOD CHOWDER WITH CORN

Preparation Time: 15 minutes

Cooking Time: 20 minutes

Servings: 10

INGREDIENTS:

- 1 tablespoon butter (unsalted)
- 1 cup onion, chopped
- ½ cup red bell pepper, chopped
- ½ cup green bell pepper, chopped
- ¼ cup celery, chopped
- 1 tablespoon all-purpose white flour
- 14 oz. low-sodium chicken broth
- 2 cups non-dairy creamer
- 6 oz. almond milk
- 10 oz. crab flakes
- 2 cups corn kernels
- ½ teaspoon paprika
- Black pepper to taste

DIRECTIONS:

1. Melt the butter in a pan. Cook the onion, bell peppers, and celery for 4 minutes. Stir in the flour and cook for 2 minutes.
2. Add the broth and bring to a boil.
3. Add the rest of the ingredients.
4. Stir occasionally and cook for 5 minutes.

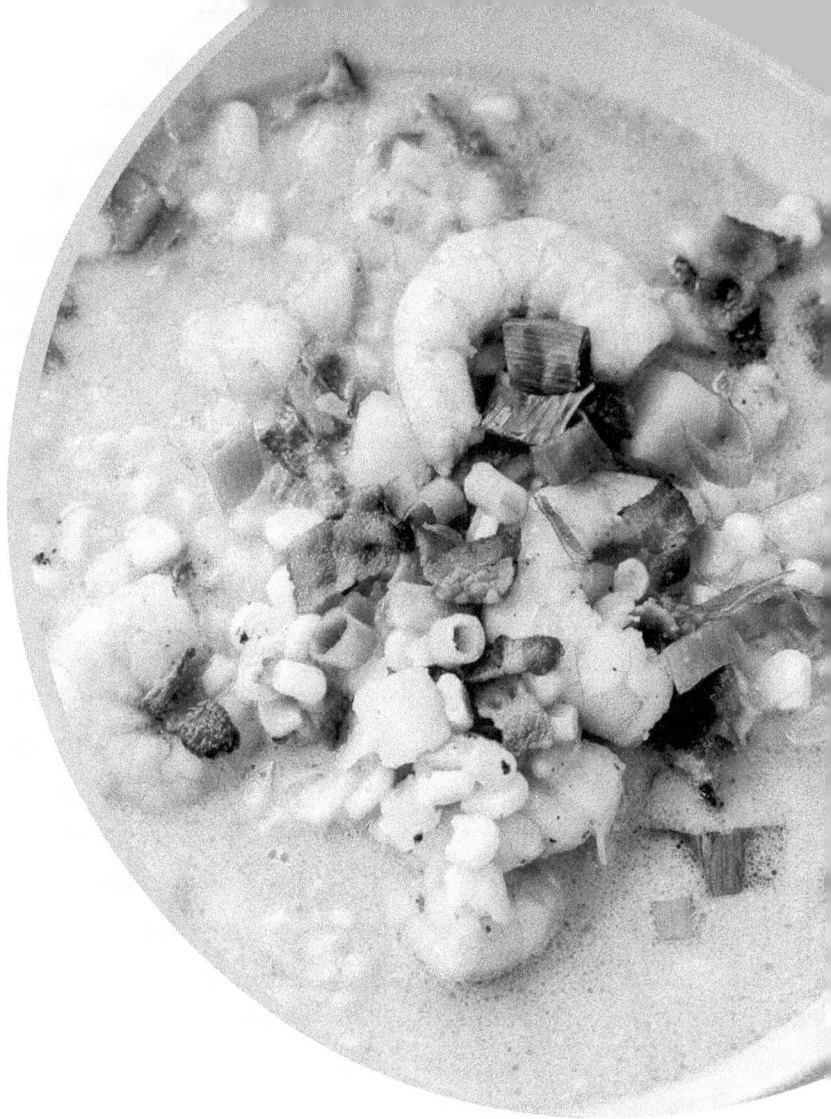

Calories: 156
Fat: 11g
Carbohydrates: 17g
Protein: 7g
Sodium: 128mg
Potassium: 527mg
Phosphorus: 125mg

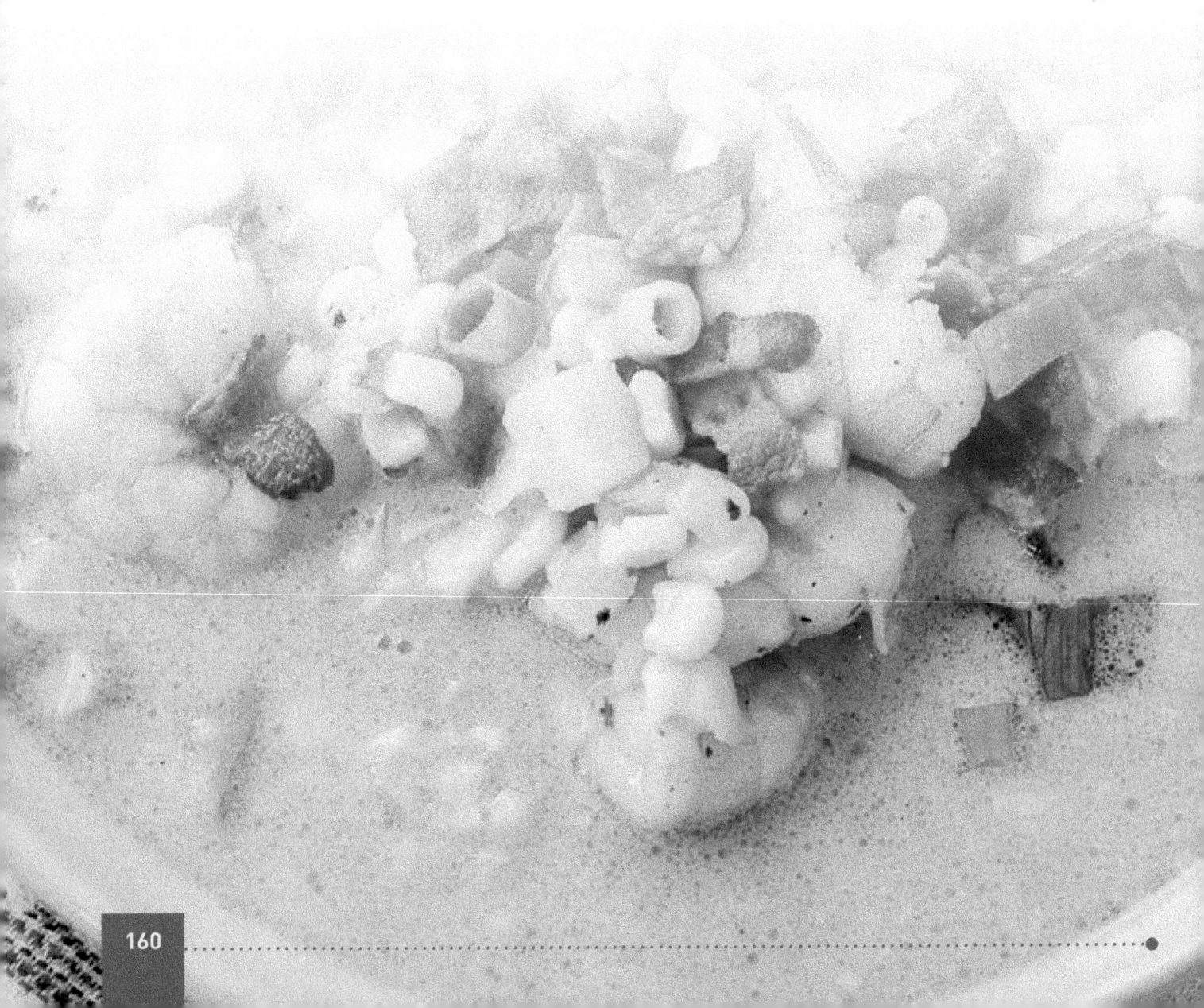

79 LAMB STEW

Preparation Time: 30 minutes

Cooking Time: 1 hour and 40 minutes

Servings: 6

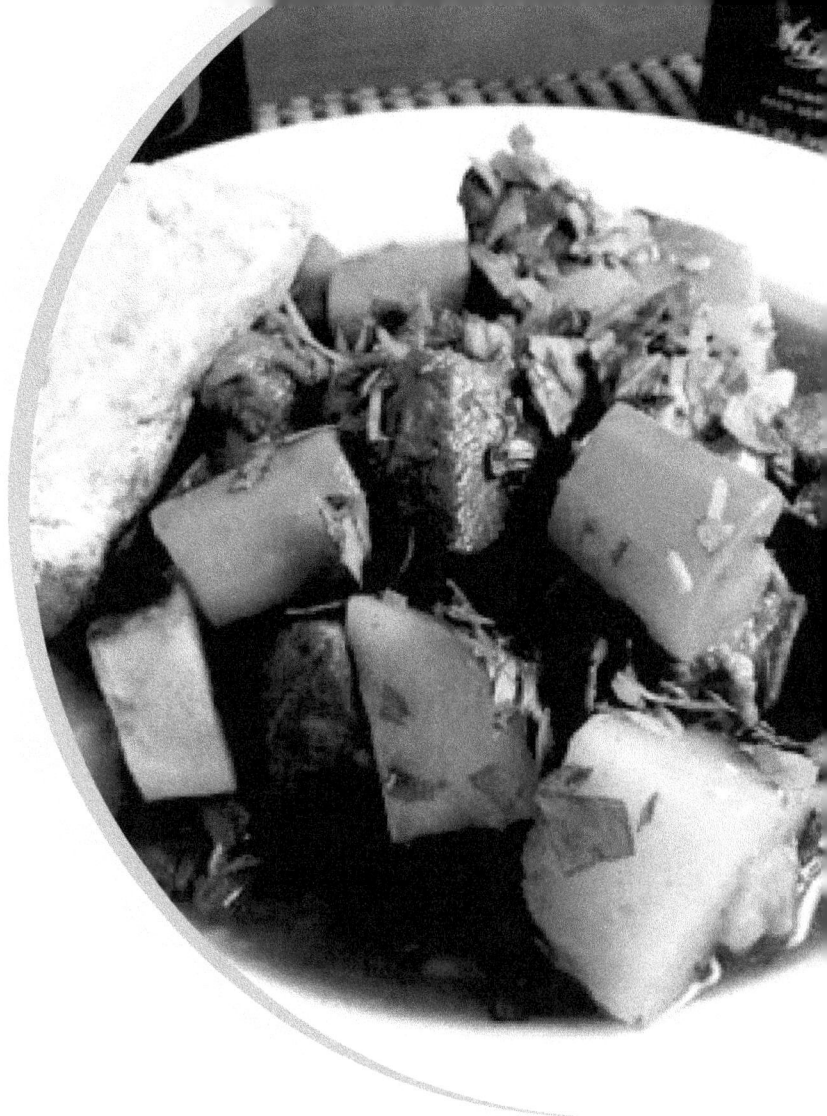

INGREDIENTS:

- 1 lb. boneless lamb shoulder, trimmed and cubes
- Black pepper to taste
- 1/4 cup all-purpose flour
- 1 tablespoon olive oil
- 1 onion, chopped
- 3 garlic cloves, chopped
- 1/2 cup tomato sauce
- 2 cups low-sodium beef broth
- 1 teaspoon dried thyme
- 2 parsnips, sliced
- 2 carrots, sliced
- 1 cup frozen peas

DIRECTIONS:

1. Season the lamb with pepper. Coat it evenly with flour.
2. Pour oil into a pot over medium heat.
3. Cook the lamb and then set aside.
4. Add onion to the pot. Cook for 2 minutes.
5. Add garlic and sauté for 30 seconds.
6. Pour in the broth to deglaze the pot.
7. Add the tomato sauce and thyme.
8. Put the lamb back in the pot.
9. Let it boil and then simmer for 1 hour.
10. Add parsnips and carrots—Cook for 30 minutes.
11. Put green peas and cook for 5 minutes.

Calories: 156;
Fat: 11g;
Carbohydrates: 17g;
Protein: 7g
Sodium: 148mg
Potassium: 567mg
Phosphorus: 115mg

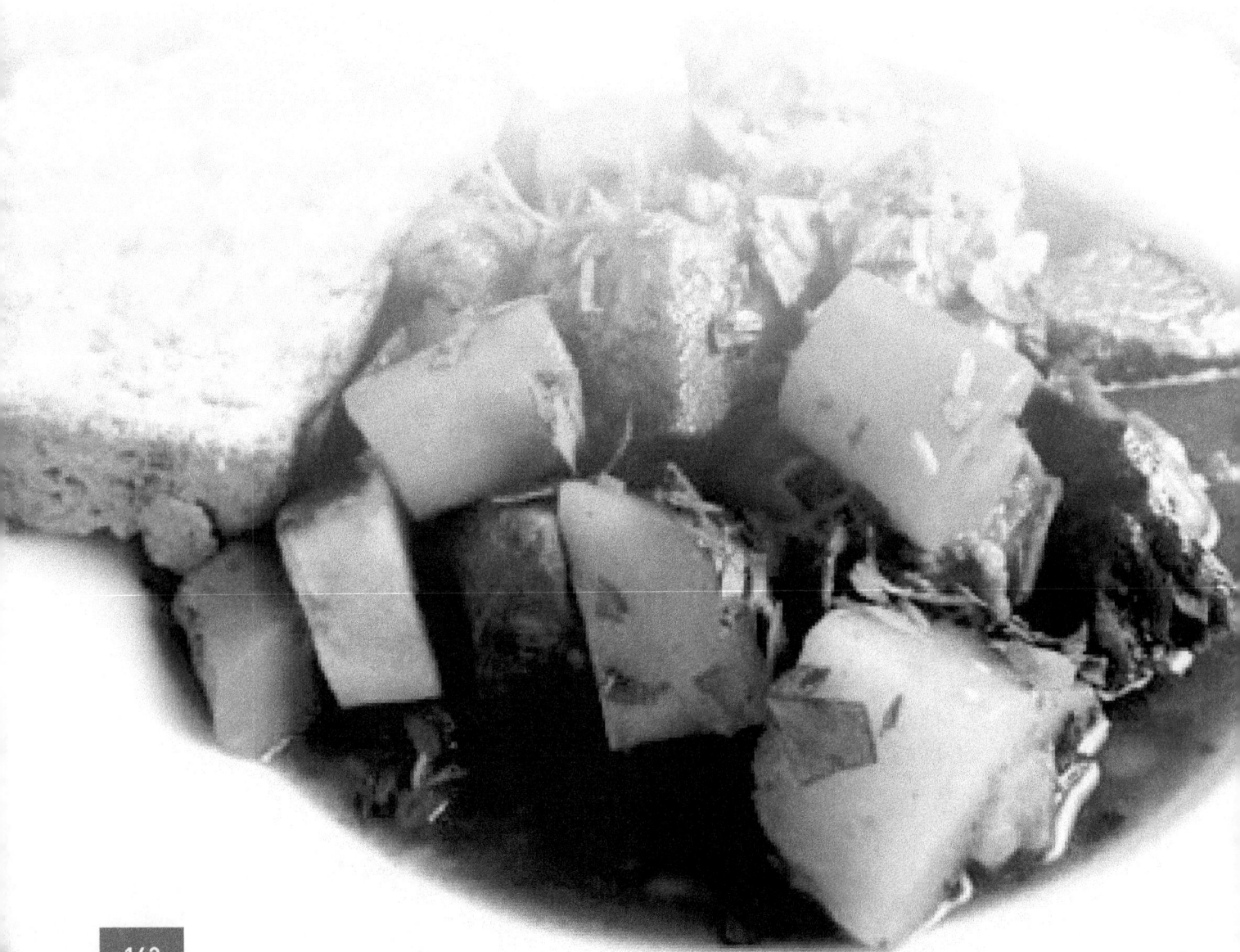

80 SPRING VEGGIE SOUP

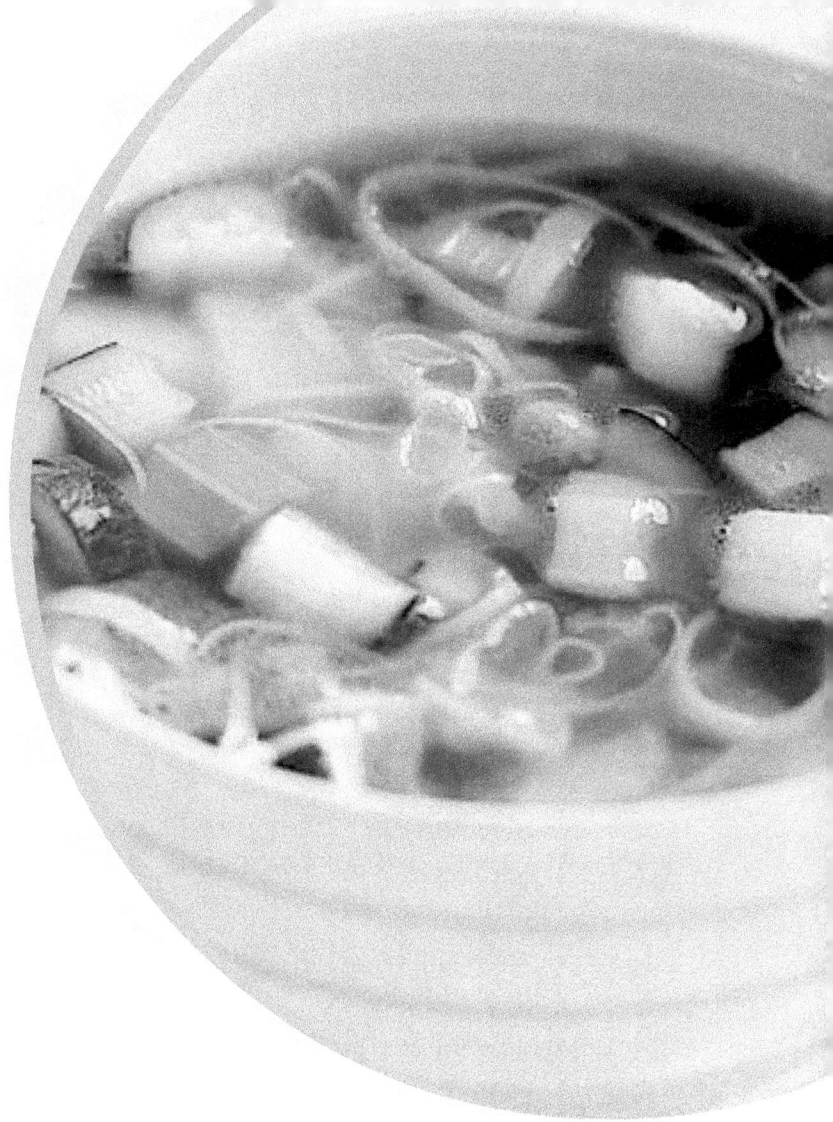

Preparation Time: 20 minutes

Cooking Time: 45 minutes

Servings: 5

INGREDIENTS:

- 2 tablespoons olive oil
- 1/2 cup onion, diced
- 1/2 cup mushrooms, sliced
- 1/8 cup celery, chopped
- 1 tomato, diced
- 1/2 cup carrots, diced
- 1 cup green beans, trimmed
- 1/2 cup frozen corn
- 1 teaspoon garlic powder
- 1 teaspoon dried oregano leaves
- 4 cups low-sodium vegetable broth

DIRECTIONS:

1. In a pot, pour the olive oil and cook the onion and celery for 2 minutes.
2. Add the rest of the ingredients.
3. Bring to a boil.
4. Reduce heat and simmer for 45 minutes.

NUTRITION:

Calories: 136
Fat: 11g
Carbohydrates: 17g
Protein: 7g

Sodium: 138mg
Potassium: 527mg
Phosphorus: 125mg

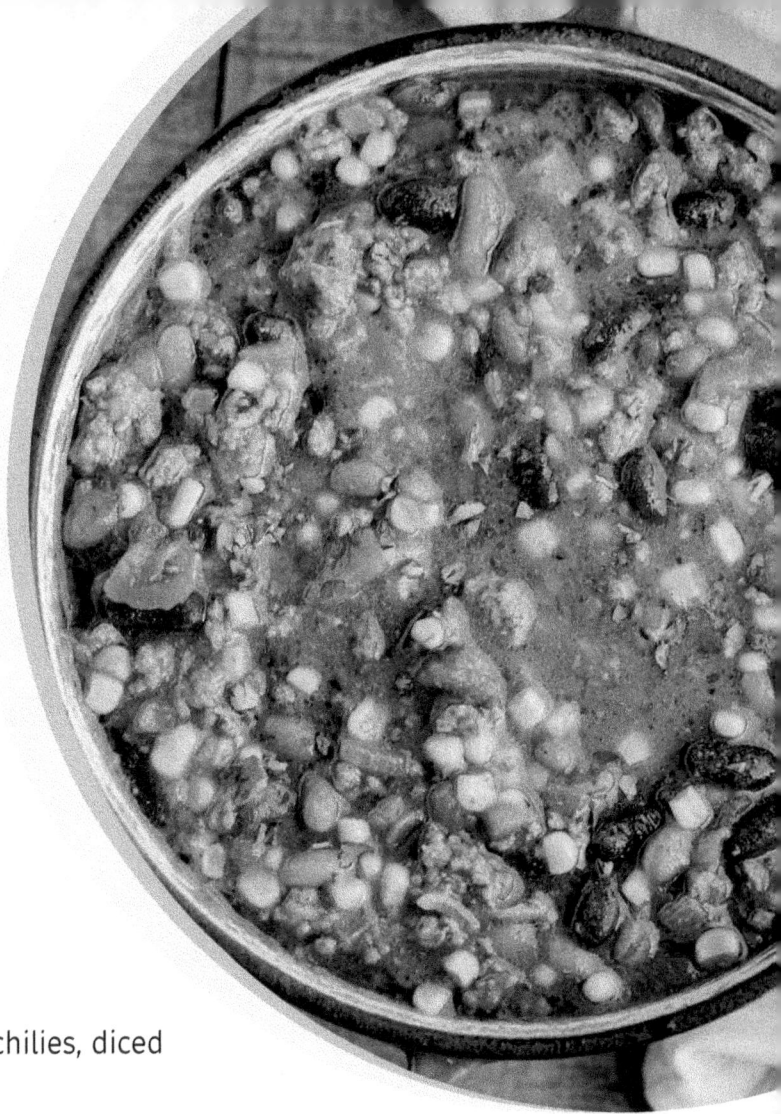

81 | TACO SOUP

Preparation Time: 30 minutes

Cooking Time: 7 hours

Servings: 10

INGREDIENTS:

1. 1 lb. chicken breast (boneless, skinless)
2. 15 oz. canned red kidney beans
3. 15 oz. low-sodium white corn, rinsed and drained
4. 15 oz. canned yellow hominy, rinsed and drained
5. 1 cup canned tomatoes with green chilies, diced
6. 1/2 cup onion, chopped
7. 1/2 cup green bell peppers, chopped
8. 1 clove garlic, chopped
9. 1 jalapeno, chopped
10. 1 tablespoon low-sodium taco seasoning
11. 2 cups low-sodium chicken broth

DIRECTIONS:

1. Put the chicken in the slow cooker.
2. Top with the rest of the ingredients. Cook on high for 1 hour.
3. Cook in low for 6 hours.
4. Shred chicken and serve with the soup.

NUTRITION:

Calories: 86
Fat: 18g
Carbohydrates: 17g
Protein: 7g

Sodium: 248mg
Potassium: 517mg
Phosphorus: 125mg

82 CURRIED CARROT AND BEET SOUP

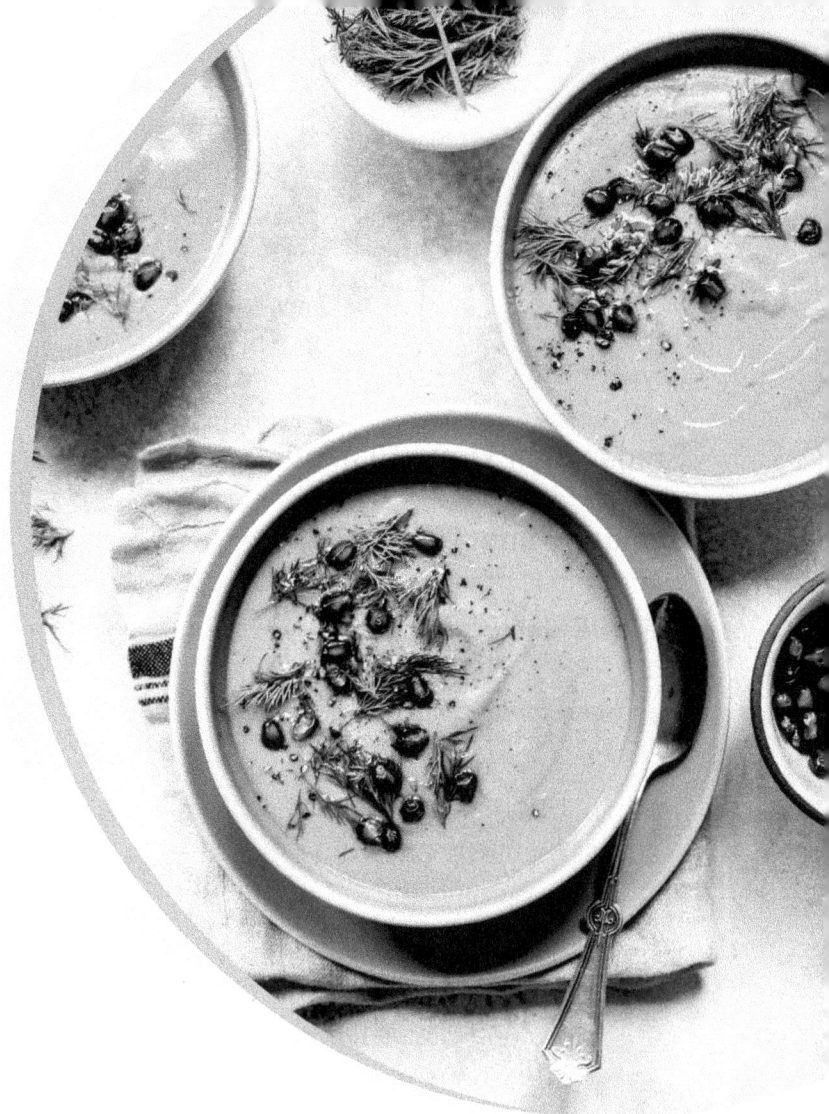

Preparation Time: 10 minutes

Cooking Time: 50 minutes

Servings: 4

INGREDIENTS:

- 1 large red beet
- 5 carrots, chopped
- 1 tablespoon curry powder
- 3 cups Homemade Rice Milk or unsweetened store-bought rice milk
- Freshly ground black pepper
- Yogurt, for serving

DIRECTIONS:

1. Preheat the oven to 400°F.
2. Cover beet in aluminum foil and roast for 45 minutes, until the vegetable is tender when pierced with a fork. Remove from the oven and let cool.
3. In a saucepan, add the carrots and cover with water. Bring to a boil, reduce the heat, cover, and simmer for 10 minutes until tender.
4. Transfer the carrots and beet to a food processor and process until smooth. Add the curry powder and rice milk. Season it with pepper. Serve topped with a dollop of yogurt.

NUTRITION:

Calories: 186
Fat: 11g
Carbohydrates: 17g
Protein: 7g

Sodium: 248mg
Potassium: 357mg
Phosphorus: 225mg

83 ASPARAGUS LEMON SOUP

Preparation Time: 10 minutes

Cooking Time: 25 minutes

Servings: 4

INGREDIENTS:

- 1-pound asparagus
- 2 tablespoons extra-virgin olive oil
- ½ sweet onion, chopped
- 4 cups low-sodium chicken stock
- ½ cup Homemade Rice Milk or unsweetened store-bought rice milk
- Freshly ground black pepper
- Juice of 1 lemon

DIRECTIONS:

1. Cut the asparagus tips from the spears and set aside.
2. Heat the olive oil in a small stockpot. Add the onion and cook, frequently stirring for 3 to 5 minutes, until it softens.
3. Add the stock and asparagus stalks and bring to a boil. Reduce the heat and simmer until the asparagus is tender about 15 minutes.
4. Put to a blender or food processor and carefully purée until smooth. Return to the pot, add the asparagus tips, and simmer until tender, about 5 minutes.
5. Add the rice milk, pepper, and lemon juice, and stir until heated through. Serve.

NUTRITION:

Calories: 86
Fat: 11g
Carbohydrates: 17g

Protein: 7g
Sodium: 128mg

Potassium: 257mg
Phosphorus: 155mg

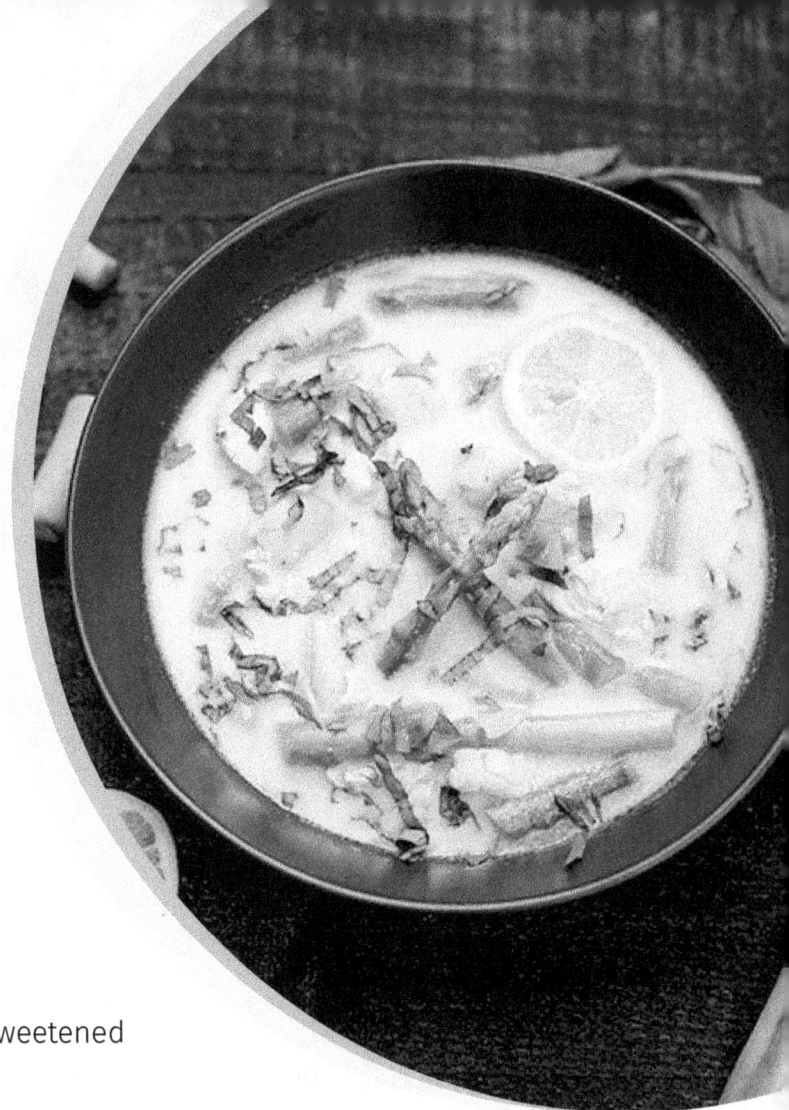

84 CAULIFLOWER AND CHIVE SOUP

Preparation Time: 10 minutes

Cooking Time: 20 minutes

Servings: 4

INGREDIENTS:

- 2 tablespoons extra-virgin olive oil
- ½ sweet onion, chopped
- 2 garlic cloves, minced
- 2 cups Simple Chicken Broth or low-sodium store-bought chicken stock
- 1 cauliflower head, broken into florets
- Freshly ground black pepper
- 4 tablespoons (¼ cups) finely chopped chives

DIRECTIONS:

1. Heat the olive oil. Add and cook the onion, frequently stirring, until it softens for 3 to 5 minutes.
2. Add the garlic and stir until fragrant.
3. Add the broth and cauliflower and bring to a boil. Reduce the heat and simmer until the cauliflower is tender about 15 minutes.
4. Transfer the soup in batches to a blender or food processor and purée until smooth or use an immersion blender.
5. Return the soup to the pot, and season with pepper. Before serving, top each bowl with 1 tablespoon of chives.

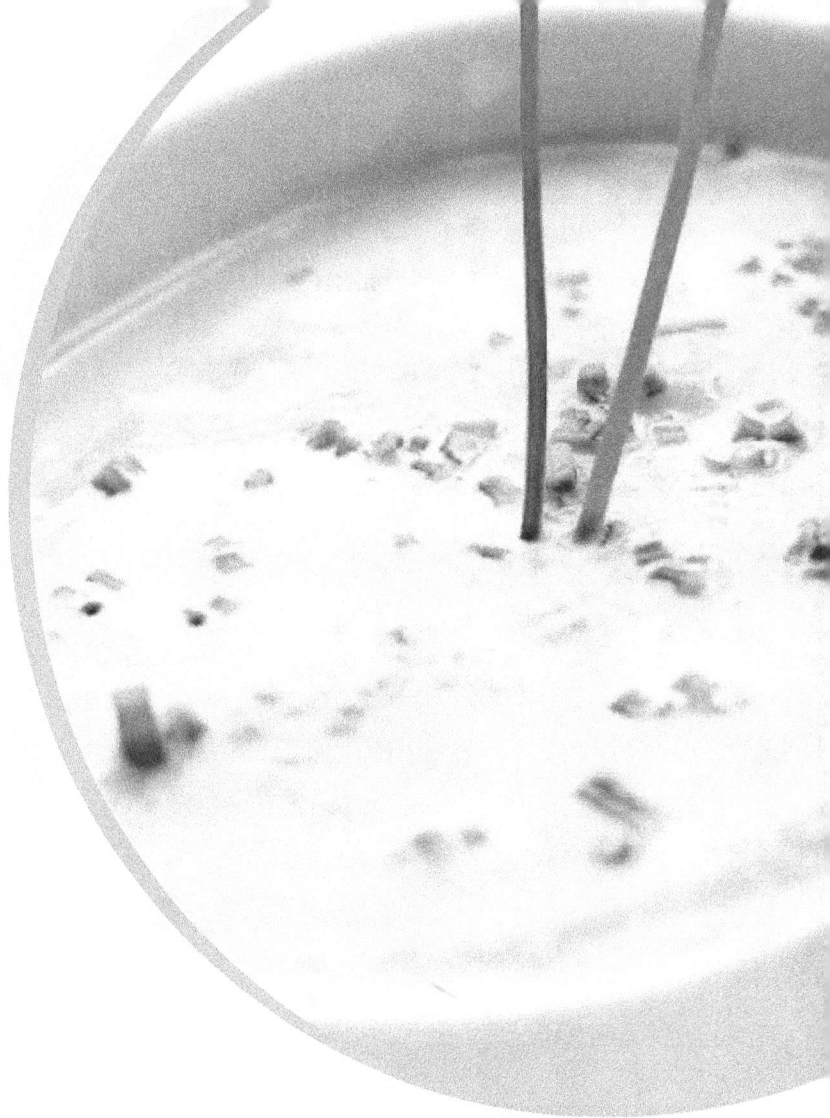

Calories: 156
Fat: 11g
Carbohydrates: 17g
Protein: 7g
Sodium: 248mg
Potassium: 527mg
Phosphorus: 125mg

85 SIMPLE CHICKEN AND RICE SOUP

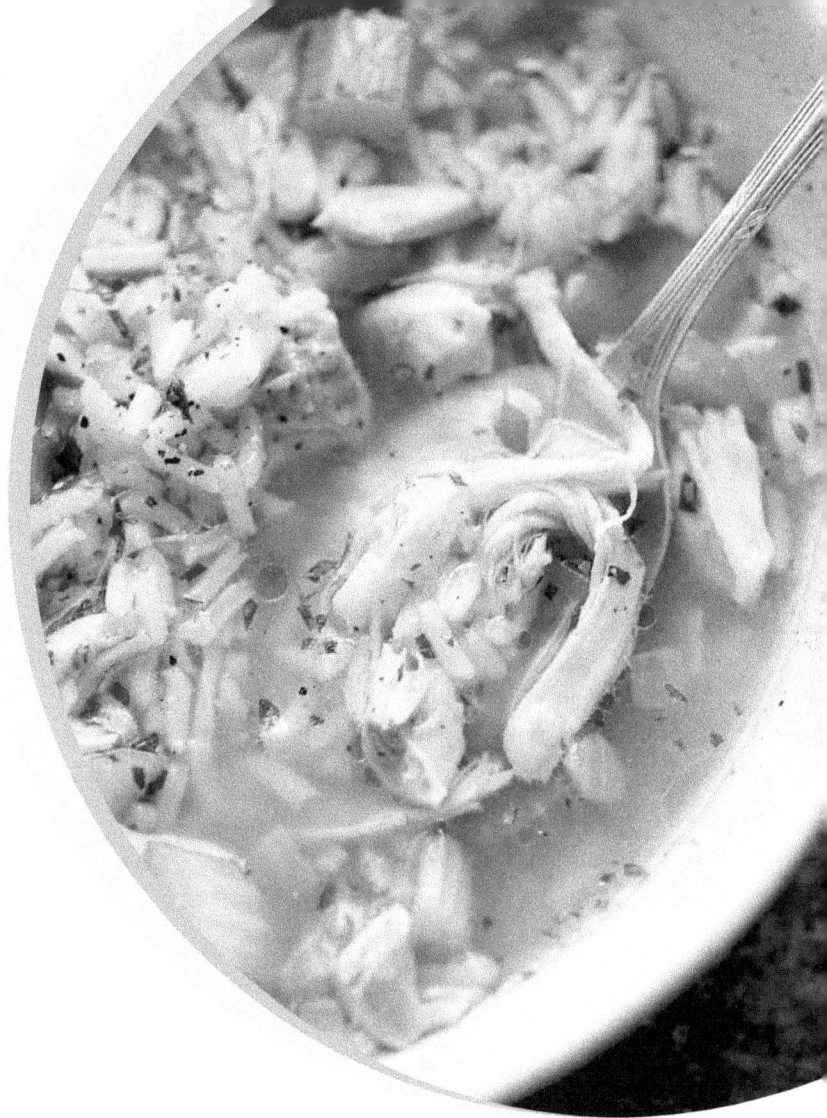

Preparation Time: 10 minutes

Cooking Time: 15 minutes

Servings: 4

INGREDIENTS:

- 1 tablespoon extra-virgin olive oil
- ½ sweet onion, chopped
- 2 celery stalks, chopped
- 2 carrots, chopped
- 8 ounces chicken breast, diced
- 4 cups Simple Chicken Broth or low-sodium store-bought chicken stock
- ¼ teaspoon dried thyme leaves
- 1 cup cooked rice
- Juice of 1 lime
- Freshly ground black pepper
- 2 tablespoons chopped parsley leaves, for garnish

DIRECTIONS:

1. Heat the olive oil over medium-high heat. Add the onion, celery, carrots, and cook, often stirring, for about 5 minutes, until the onion begins to soften.
2. Add the chicken breast and continue stirring until the meat is just browned but not cooked through. Add the broth and thyme and bring to a boil.
3. Simmer for 10 minutes, until the chicken is cooked through and the vegetables are tender.
4. Add the rice and lime juice. Season it with pepper. Serve and garnished with parsley leaves.

NUTRITION:

Calories: 176
Fat: 11g
Carbohydrates: 17g
Protein: 7g
Sodium: 128mg
Potassium: 357mg
Phosphorus: 225mg

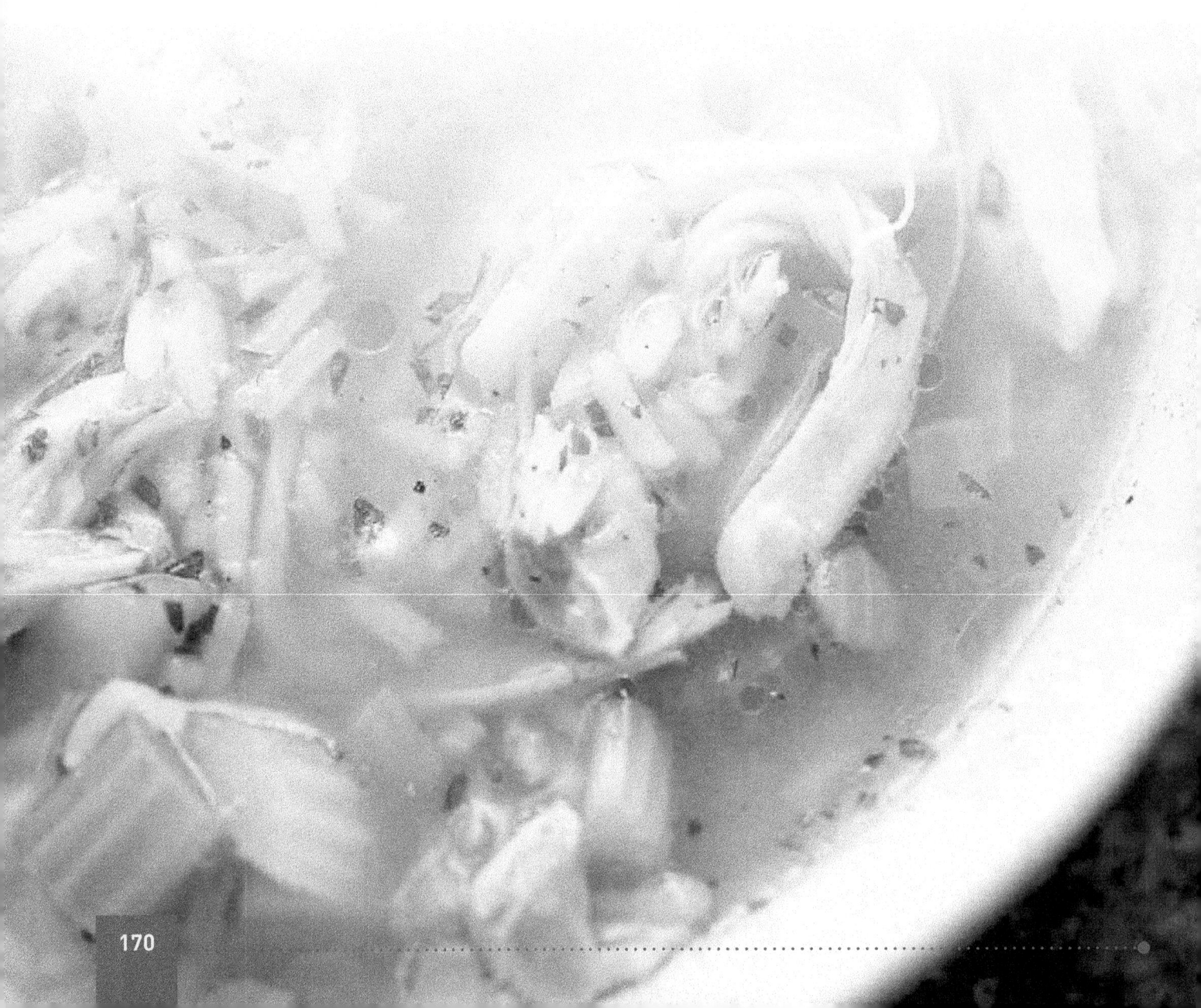

86 TURKEY, WILD RICE, AND MUSHROOM SOUP

Preparation Time: 15 minutes

Cooking Time: 2-3 hours

Servings: 6

INGREDIENTS:

- ½ cup onion, chopped
- ½ cup red bell pepper, chopped
- ½ cup carrots, chopped
- 2 garlic cloves, minced
- 2 cup cooked turkey, shredded
- 5 cup chicken broth (see recipe)
- ½ cup quick-cooking wild rice, uncooked
- 1 tbsp olive oil
- 1 cup mushrooms, sliced
- 2 bay leaves
- ¼ tsp Mrs. Dash® Original salt-free herb seasoning blend
- 1 tsp dried thyme
- ½ tsp low sodium salt
- ¼ tsp black pepper

DIRECTIONS:

1. Cook rice in a saucepan with 1-2 cups of broth. Set aside.
2. Heat the oil in a skillet and sauté the onion, bell pepper, carrots, and garlic until soft. Add to a 4 to 6-quart slow cooker.
3. Add remaining ingredients to the slow cooker except for the rice and mushrooms.
4. Cook for 2-3 hours on low with cover.

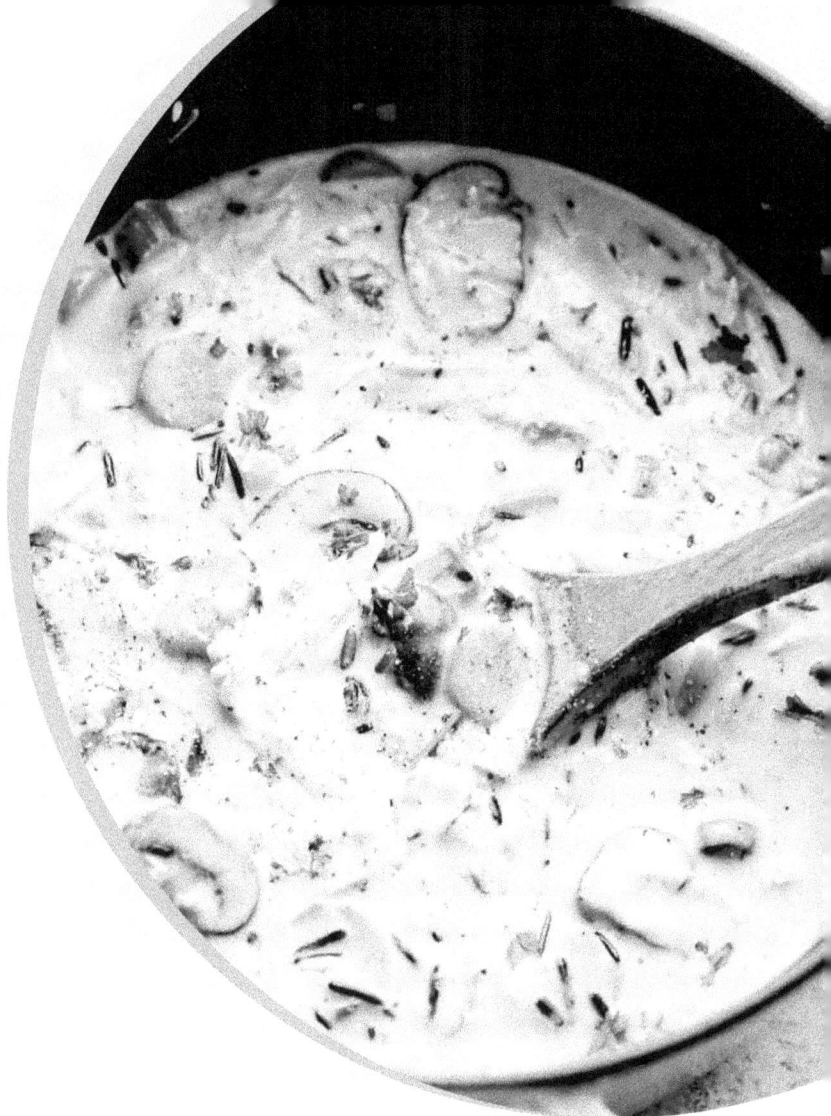

5. Put the mushrooms and rice. Cook for another 15 minutes.
6. Remove the bay leaves and serve.

NUTRITION:

Calories: 136
Fat: 11g
Carbohydrates: 15g
Protein: 5g
Sodium: 128mg
Potassium: 537mg
Phosphorus: 145mg

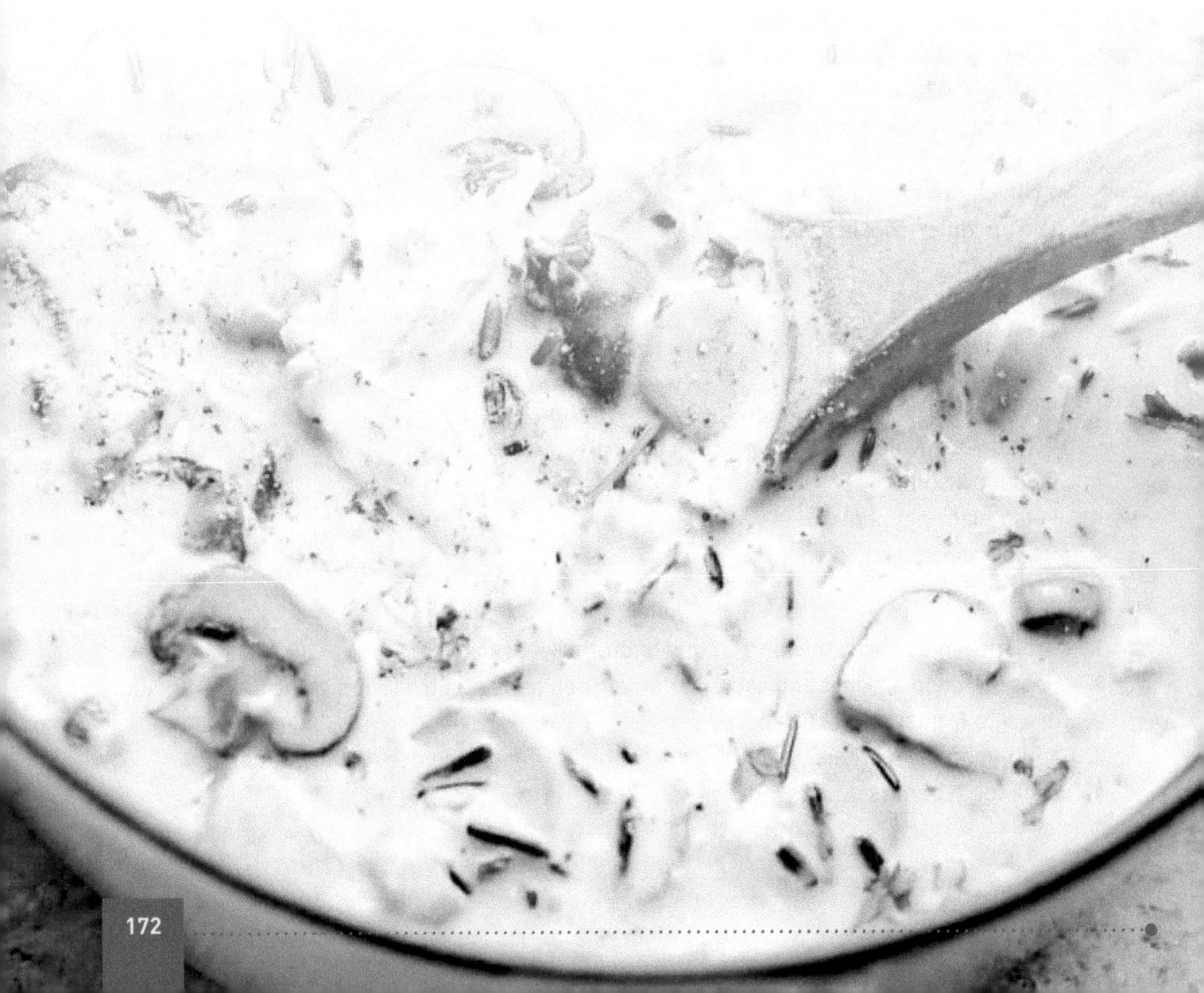

87 TURKEY BURGER SOUP

Preparation Time: 10minutes

Cooking Time: 25 minutes

Servings: 4

INGREDIENTS:

- 2 tablespoons extra-virgin olive oil
- 1-pound ground turkey breast
- ½ sweet onion, chopped
- 3 garlic cloves, minced
- Freshly ground black pepper
- 1 (16-ounce) can low-sodium diced tomatoes, drained
- 4 cups Simple Chicken Broth or low-sodium store-bought chicken stock
- 1 cup sliced carrots
- 1 cup sliced celery
- 1 tablespoon chopped fresh basil
- 1 tablespoon chopped fresh oregano
- 1 tablespoon chopped fresh thyme

DIRECTIONS:

1. Prepare the olive oil. Add the turkey, onion, and garlic in a medium stockpot.
2. Cook, stirring until the turkey is browned. Season it with pepper.
3. Add the drained tomatoes, broth, carrots, celery, basil, oregano, and thyme.
4. Reduce the heat to low, and simmer for 20 minutes. Serve.

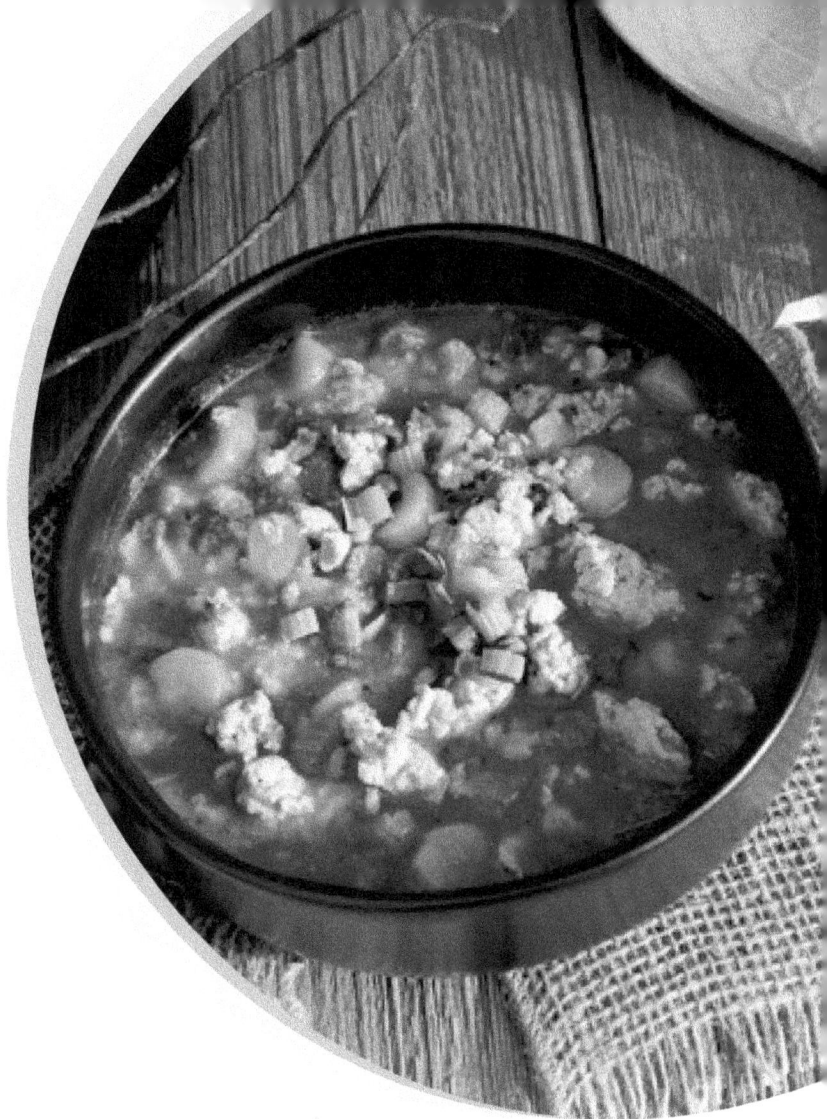

Calories: 186
Fat: 11g
Carbohydrates: 17g
Protein: 7g
Sodium: 128mg
Potassium: 257mg
Phosphorus: 115mg

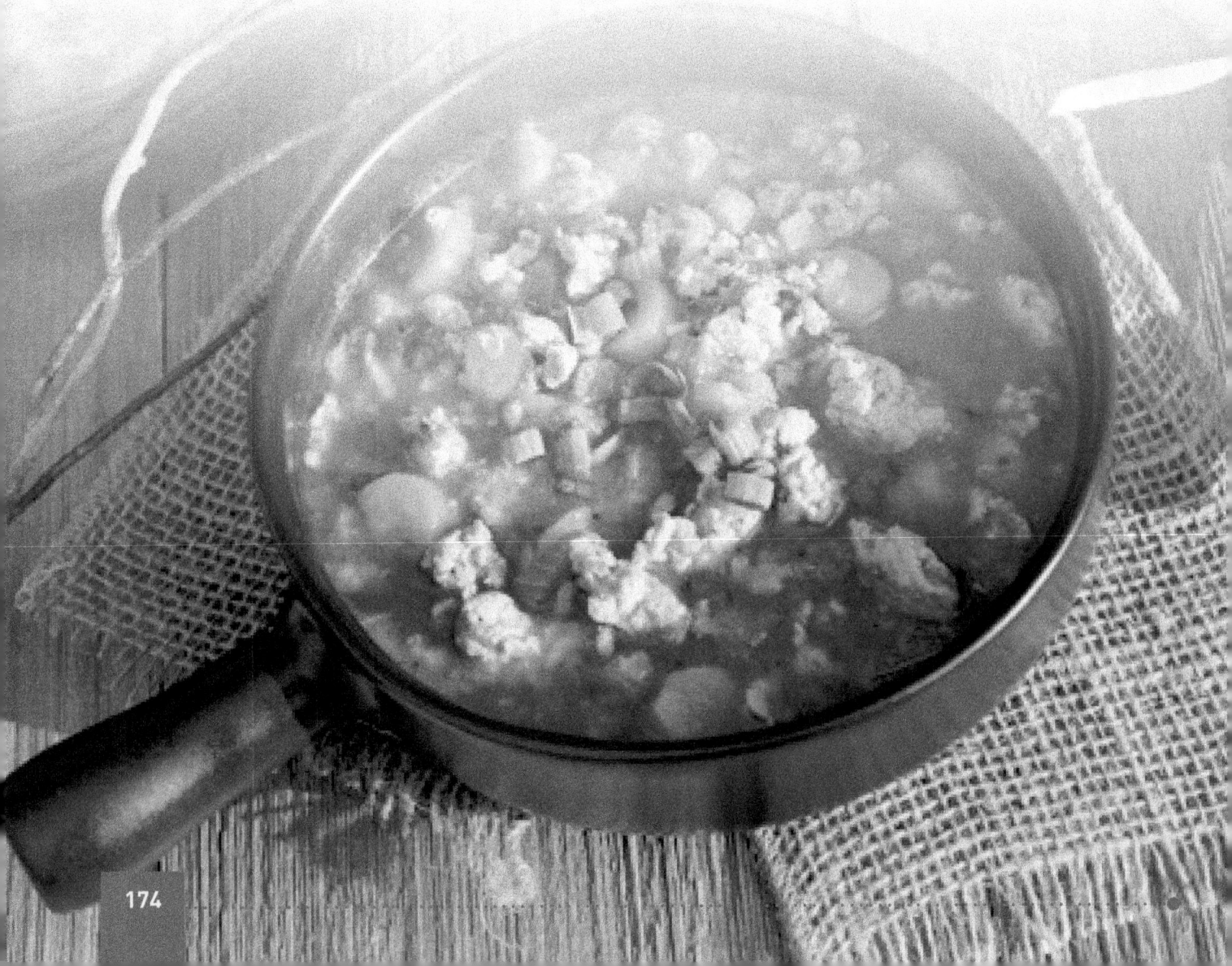

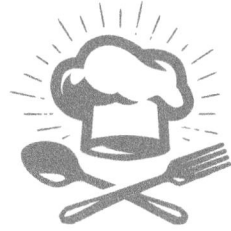

CHAPTER 16

VEGETABLE RECIPES

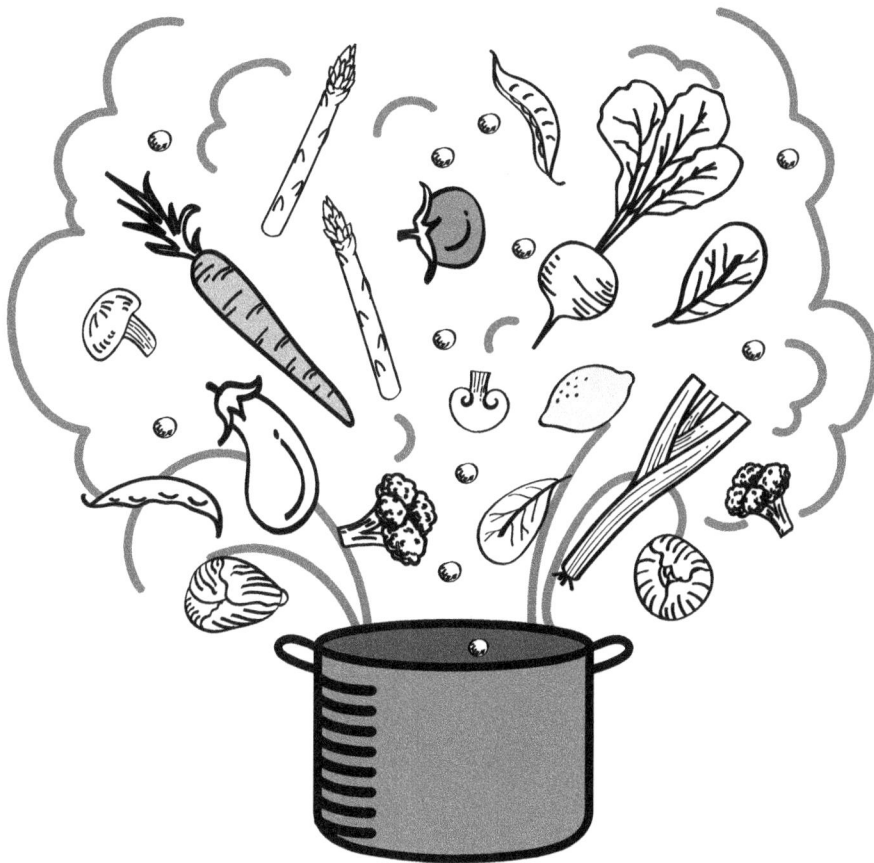

88 SPICY MUSHROOM STIR-FRY

Preparation Time: 10 minutes

Cooking Time: 10 minutes

Servings: 4

INGREDIENTS:

- 1 cup low-sodium vegetable broth
- 2 tablespoons cornstarch
- 1 teaspoon low-sodium soy sauce
- 1/2 teaspoon ground ginger
- 1/8 teaspoon cayenne pepper
- 2 tablespoons olive oil
- 2 (8-ounce) packages sliced button mushrooms
- 1 red bell pepper, chopped
- 1 jalapeño pepper, minced
- 3 cups brown rice that has been cooked in unsalted water
- 2 tablespoons sesame oil

DIRECTIONS:

1. In a small bowl, whisk together the broth, cornstarch, soy sauce, ginger, and cayenne pepper and set aside.
2. Heat the olive oil in a wok or heavy skillet over high heat.
3. Add the mushrooms and peppers and stir-fry for 3 to 5 minutes or until the vegetables are tender-crisp.
4. Stir the broth mixture and add it to the wok; stir-fry for 3 to 5 minutes longer or until the vegetables are tender and the sauce has thickened.
5. Serve the stir-fry over the hot cooked brown rice and drizzle with the sesame oil.

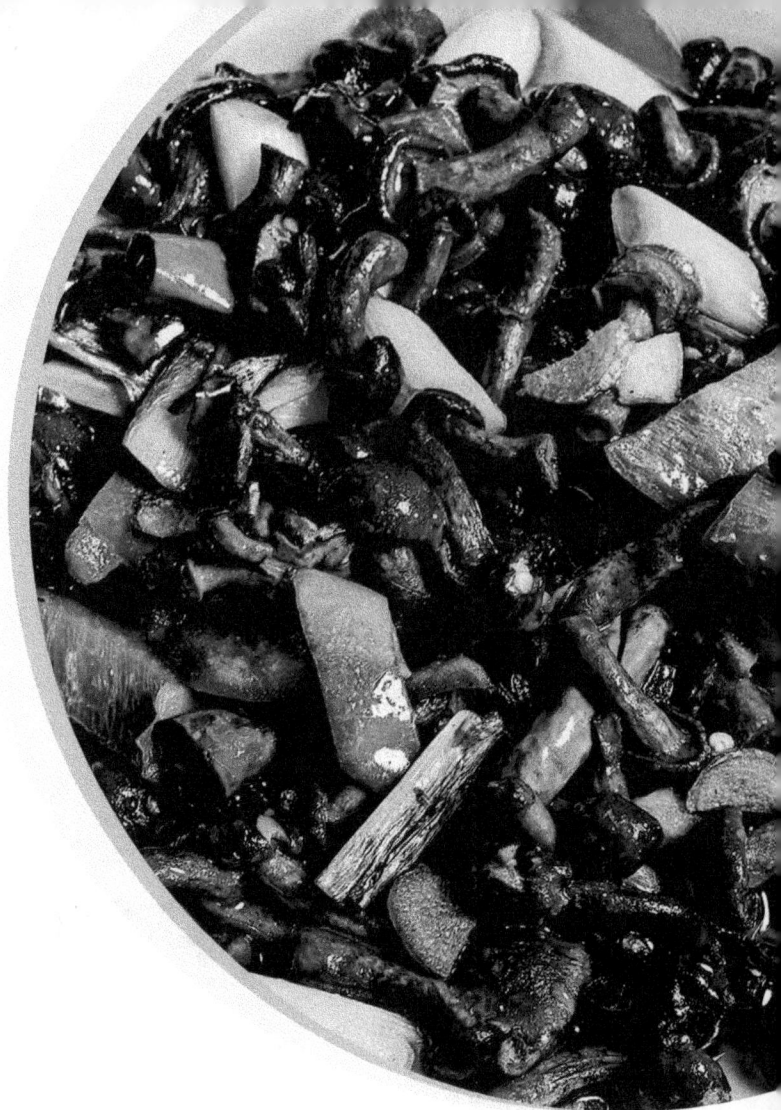

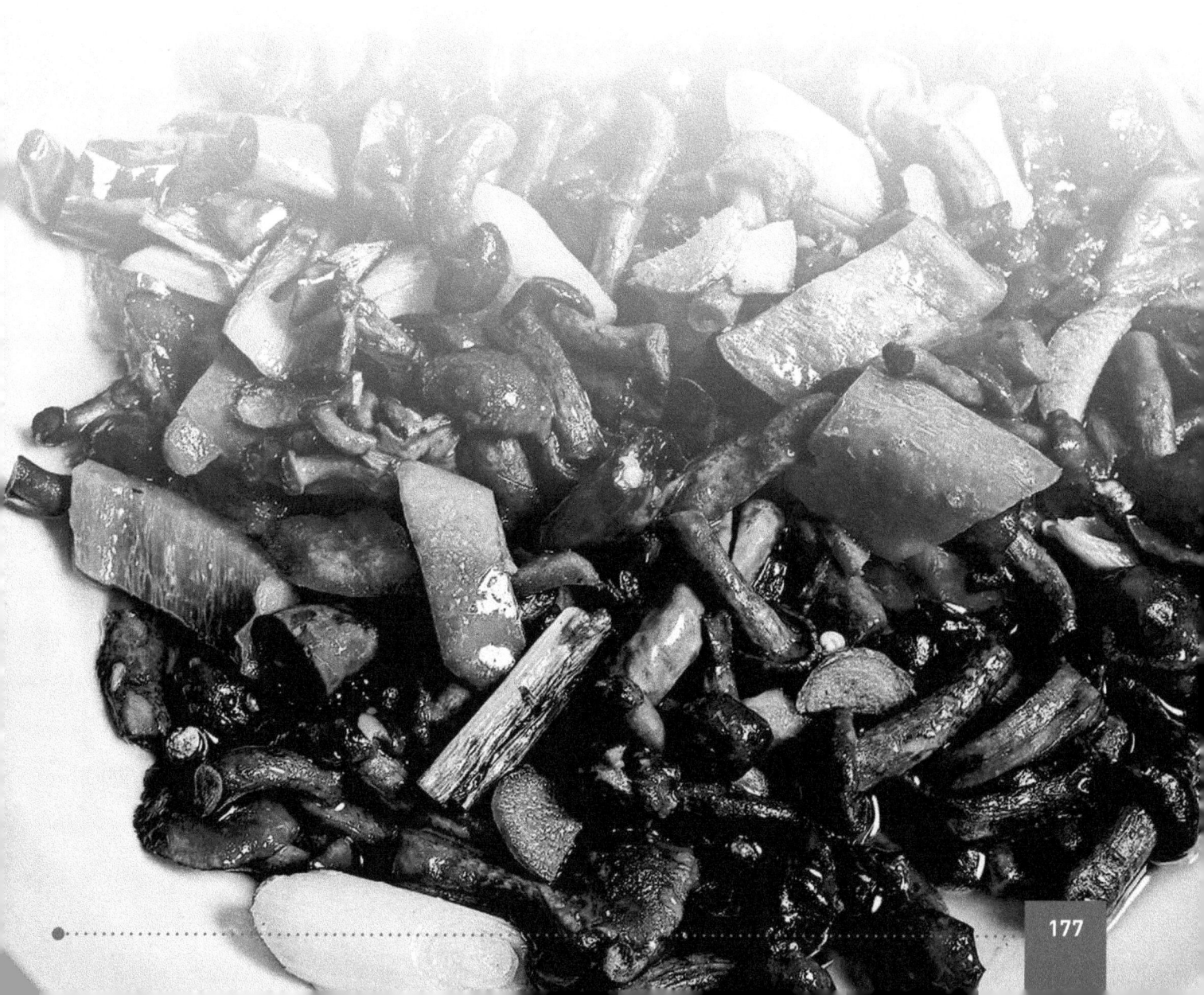

89 CURRIED VEGGIES AND RICE

Preparation Time: 12 minutes

Cooking Time: 18 minutes

Servings: 4

INGREDIENTS:

- 1/4 cup olive oil
- 1 cup long-grain white basmati rice
- 4 garlic cloves, minced
- 2 1/2 teaspoons curry powder
- 1/2 cup sliced shiitake mushrooms
- 1 red bell pepper, chopped
- 1 cup frozen, shelled edamame
- 2 cups low-sodium vegetable broth
- 1/8 teaspoon freshly ground black pepper

DIRECTIONS:

1. Heat the olive oil on medium heat.
2. Add the rice, garlic, curry powder, mushrooms, bell pepper, and edamame; cook, stirring, for 2 minutes.
3. Add the broth and black pepper and bring to a boil.
4. Reduce the heat to low, partially cover the pot, and simmer for 15 to 18 minutes or until the rice is tender. Stir and serve.

NUTRITION:

Calories: 347
Fat: 16g
Carbohydrates: 44g
Protein: 8g

Sodium: 114mg
Phosphorus: 131mg
Potassium: 334mg

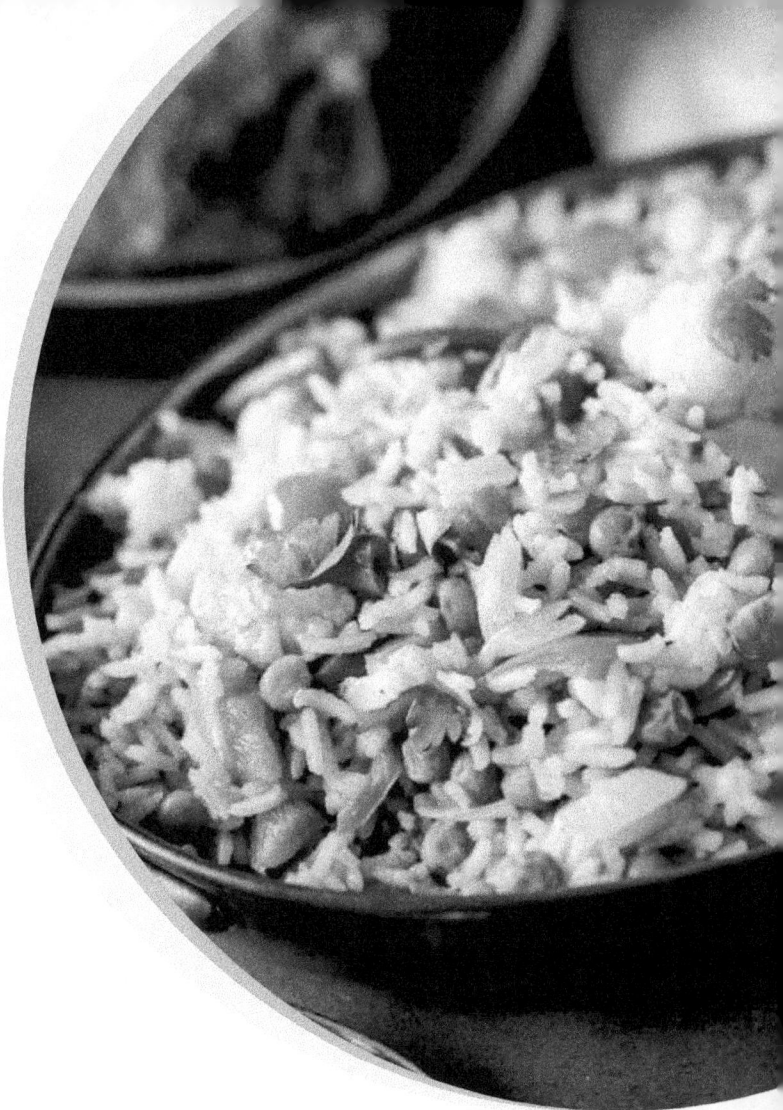

90 | SPICY VEGGIE PANCAKES

Preparation Time: 10 minutes

Cooking Time: 10 minutes

Servings: 4

INGREDIENTS:

- 3 tablespoons olive oil, divided
- 2 small onions, finely chopped
- 1 jalapeño pepper, minced
- 3/4 cup carrot, grated
- 3/4 cup cabbage, finely chopped
- 11/2 cups quick-cooking oats
- 3/4 cup cooked brown rice
- 3/4 cup of water
- ½ cup whole-wheat flour
- 1 large egg
- 1 large egg white
- 1 teaspoon baking soda
- 1/4 teaspoon cayenne pepper

DIRECTIONS:

1. In a skillet, heat 2 teaspoons oil over medium heat.
2. Sauté the onion, jalapeño, carrot, and cabbage for 4 minutes.
3. While the veggies are cooking, combine the oats, rice, water, flour, egg, egg white, baking soda, and cayenne pepper in a medium bowl until well mixed.
4. Add the cooked vegetables to the mixture and stir to combine.
5. Heat the remaining oil in a large skillet over medium heat.
6. Drop the mixture into the skillet, about 1/3 cup per pancake. Cook for 4 minutes, or until bubbles form on the pancakes' surface and the edges look cooked, then carefully flip them over.
7. Repeat with the remaining mixture and serve.

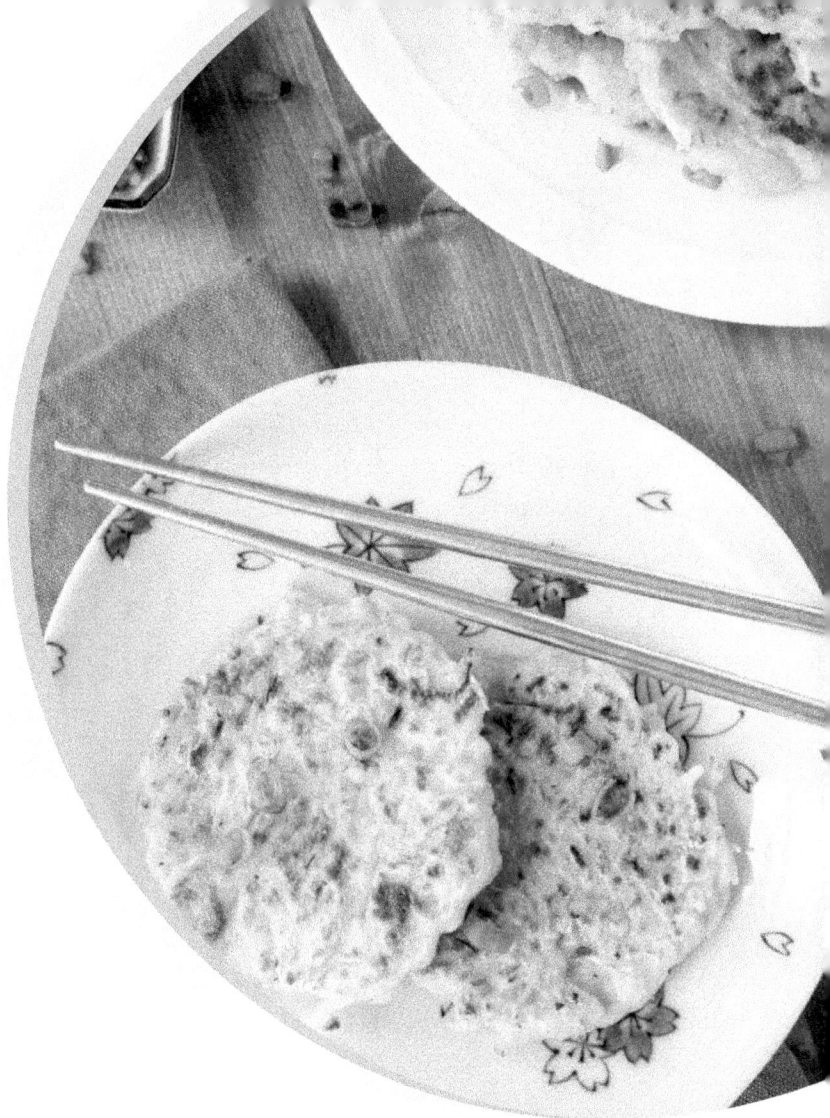

Calories: 323
Fat: 11g
Carbohydrates: 48g
Protein: 10g
Sodium: 366mg
Potassium: 381mg
Phosphorus: 263mg

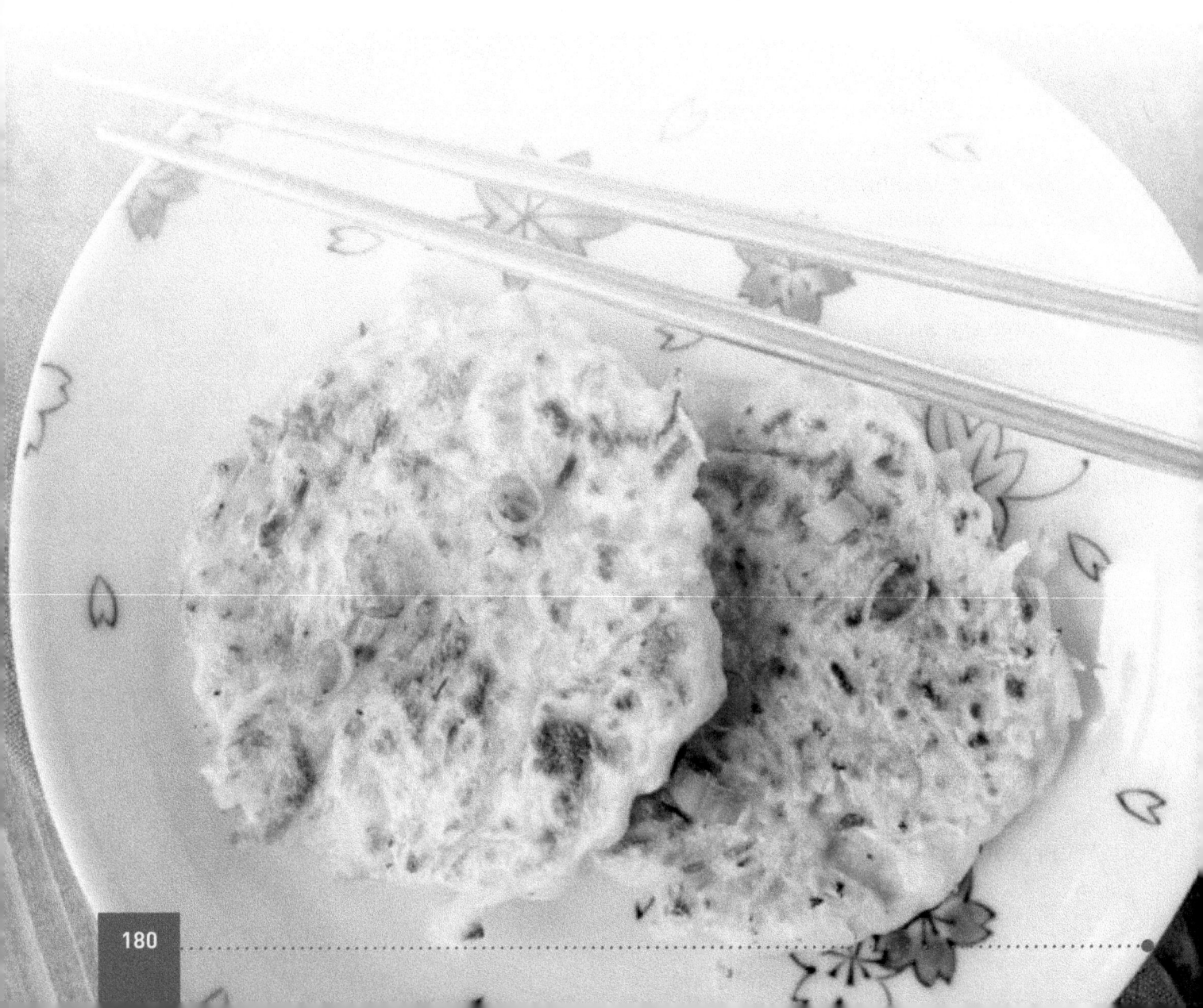

91 EGG AND VEGGIE FAJITAS

Preparation Time: 15 minutes

Cooking Time: 10 minutes

Servings: 4

INGREDIENTS:

- 3 large eggs
- 3 egg whites
- 2 teaspoons chili powder
- 1 tablespoon unsalted butter
- 1 onion, chopped
- 2 garlic cloves, minced
- 1 jalapeño pepper, minced
- 1 red bell pepper, chopped
-
  1 cup frozen corn, thawed and drained
- 8 (6-inch) corn tortillas

DIRECTIONS:

1. Whisk the eggs, egg whites, and chili powder in a small bowl until well combined. Set aside.
2. Prepare a large skillet and melt the butter on medium heat.
3. Sauté the onion, garlic, jalapeño, bell pepper, and corn until the vegetables are tender, 3 to 4 minutes.
4. Add the beaten egg mixture to the skillet. Cook, occasionally stirring, until the eggs form large curds and are set, 3 to 5 minutes.
5. Meanwhile, soften the corn tortillas as directed on the package.
6. Divide the egg mixture evenly among the softened corn tortillas. Roll the tortillas up and serve.

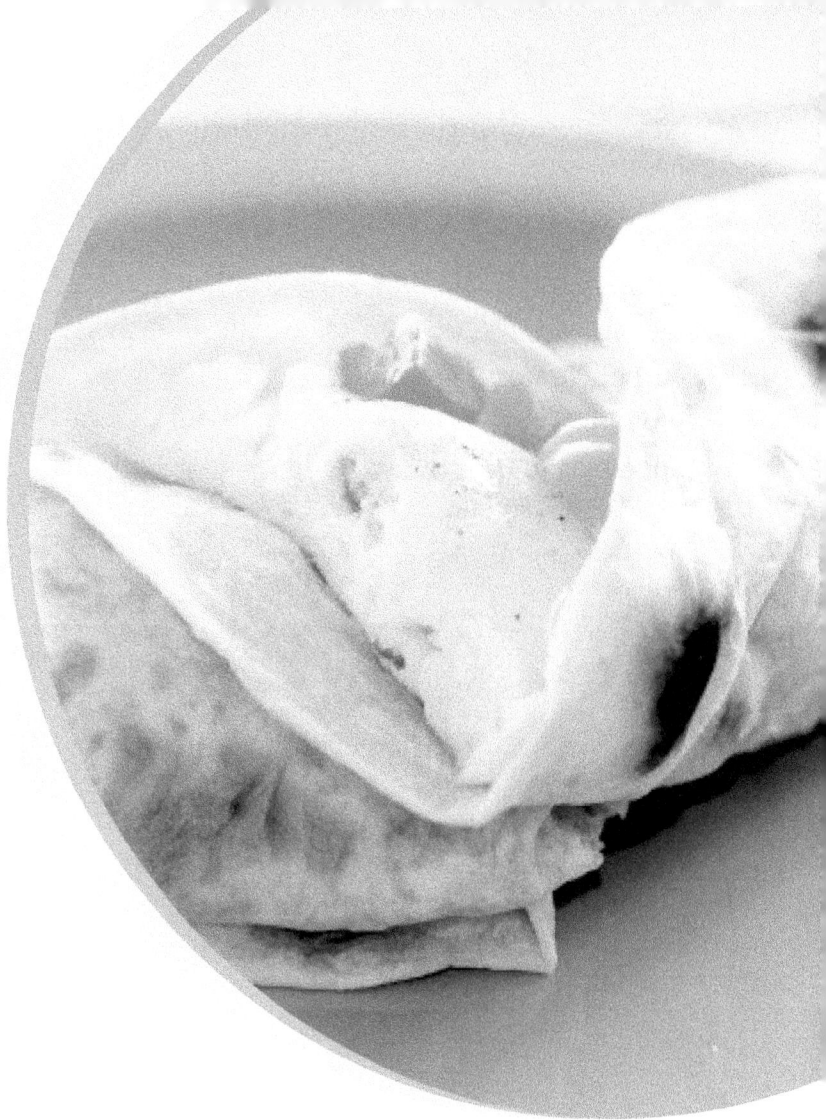

Calories: 316
Fat 14g
Carbohydrates: 35g
Protein: 14g
Sodium: 167mg
Potassium: 408mg
Phosphorus: 287mg

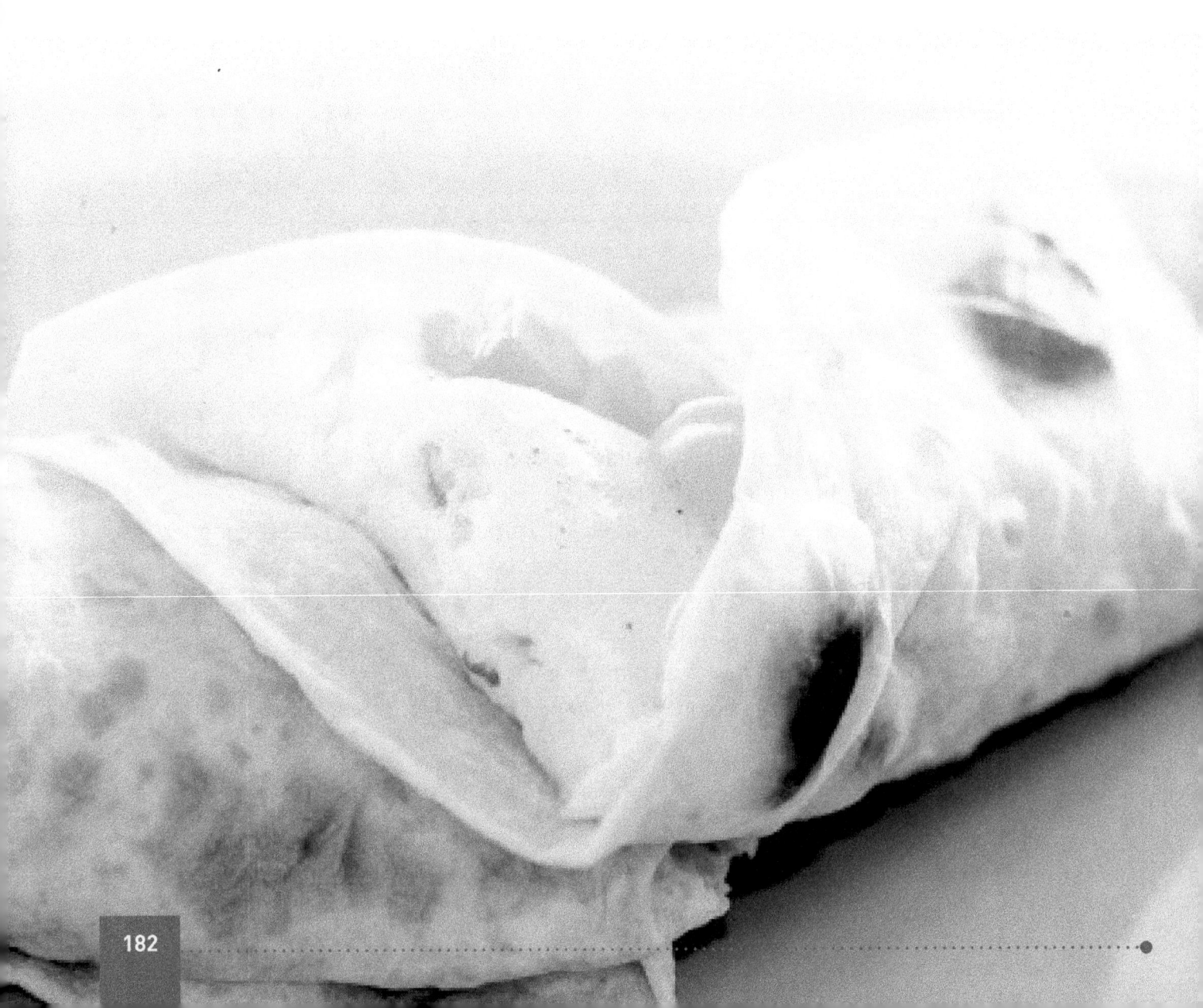

92 VEGETABLE BIRYANI

Preparation Time: 10 minutes

Cooking Time: 15 minutes

Servings: 4

INGREDIENTS:

- 2 tablespoons olive oil
- 1 onion, diced
- 4 garlic cloves, minced
- 1 tbsp. peeled and grated fresh ginger root
- 1 cup carrot, grated
- 2 cups chopped cauliflower
- 1 cup thawed frozen baby peas
- 2 teaspoons curry powder
- 1 cup low-sodium vegetable broth
- 3 cups of frozen cooked brown rice

DIRECTIONS:

1. Get a skillet and heat the olive oil on medium heat.
2. Add onion, garlic, and ginger root. Sauté, frequently stirring, until tender-crisp, 2 minutes.
3. Add the carrot, cauliflower, peas, and curry powder and cook for 2 minutes longer.
4. Put vegetable broth. Cover the skillet partially, and simmer on low for 6 to 7 minutes or until the vegetables are tender.
5. Meanwhile, heat the rice as directed on the package.
6. Stir the rice into the vegetable mixture and serve.

NUTRITION:

Calories: 378
Fat 16g
Carbohydrates: 53g

Protein: 8g
Sodium: 113mg

Potassium: 510mg
Phosphorus: 236mg

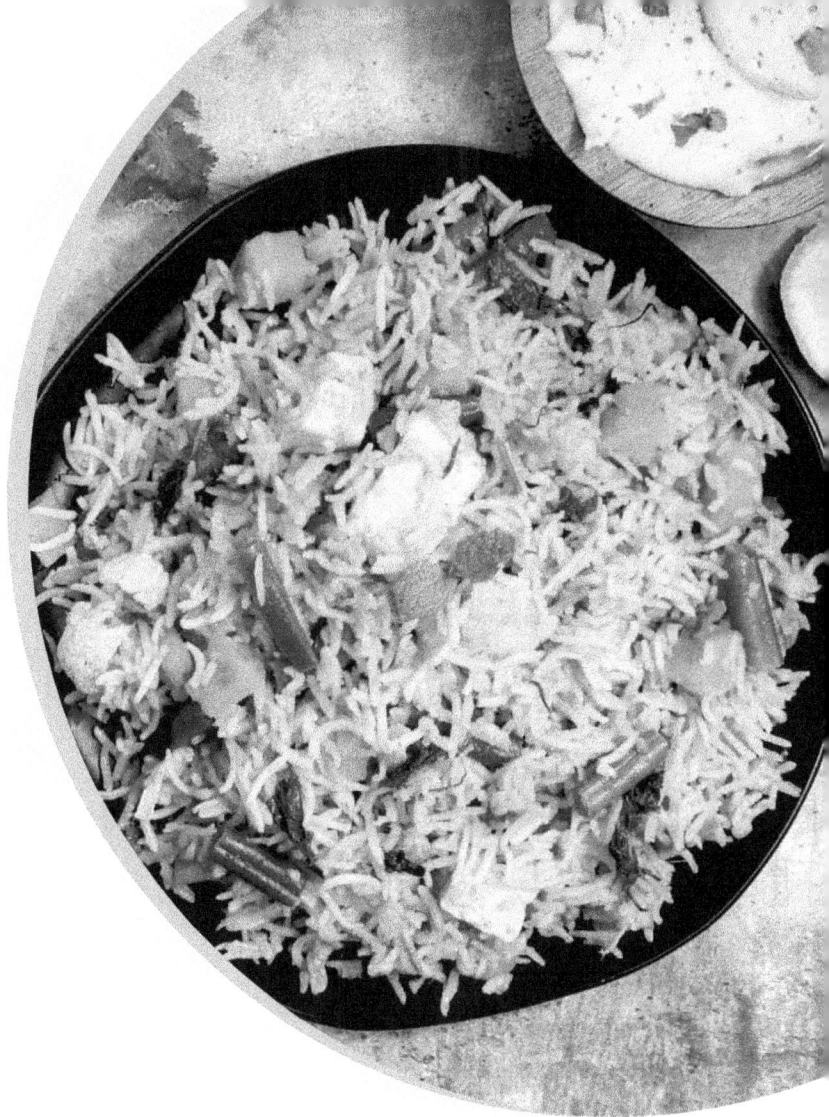

93 | PESTO PASTA SALAD

Preparation Time: 15 minutes

Cooking Time: 15 minutes

Servings: 4

INGREDIENTS:

- 1 cup fresh basil leaves
- ½ cup packed fresh flat-leaf parsley leaves
- ½ cup arugula, chopped
- 2 tablespoons Parmesan cheese, grated
- ¼ cup extra-virgin olive oil
- 3 tablespoons mayonnaise
- 2 tablespoons water
- 12 ounces whole-wheat rotini pasta
- 1 red bell pepper, chopped
- 1 medium yellow summer squash, sliced
- 1 cup frozen baby peas

DIRECTIONS:

1. Boil water in a large pot.
2. Meanwhile, combine the basil, parsley, arugula, cheese, and olive oil in a blender or food processor. Process until the herbs are finely chopped. Add the mayonnaise and water, then process again. Set aside.
3. Prepare the pasta to the pot of boiling water; cook according to package directions, about 8 to 9 minutes. Drain well, reserving ¼ cup of the cooking liquid.
4. Combine the pesto, pasta, bell pepper, squash, and peas in a large bowl and toss gently, adding enough reserved pasta cooking liquid to make a sauce on the salad. Serve immediately or cover and chill, then serve.
5. Store covered in the refrigerator for up to 3 days.

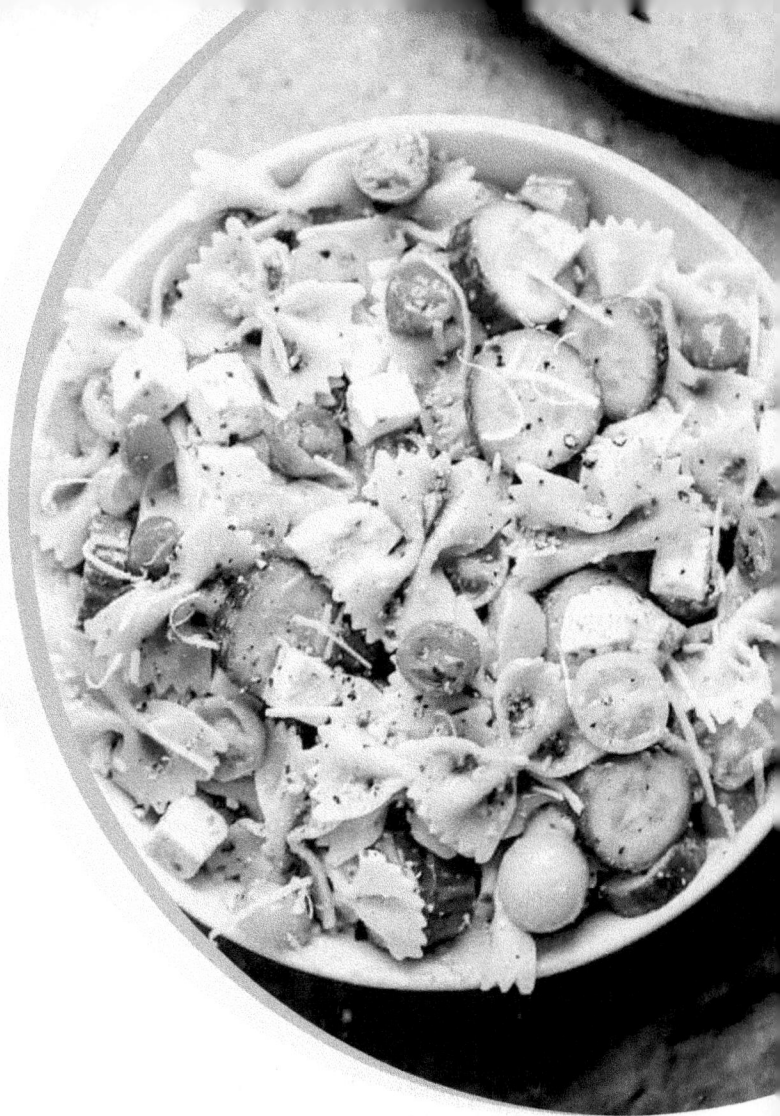

Calories: 378
Fat: 24g
Carbohydrates: 35g
Protein: 9g
Sodium: 163mg
Potassium: 472mg
Phosphorus: 213mg

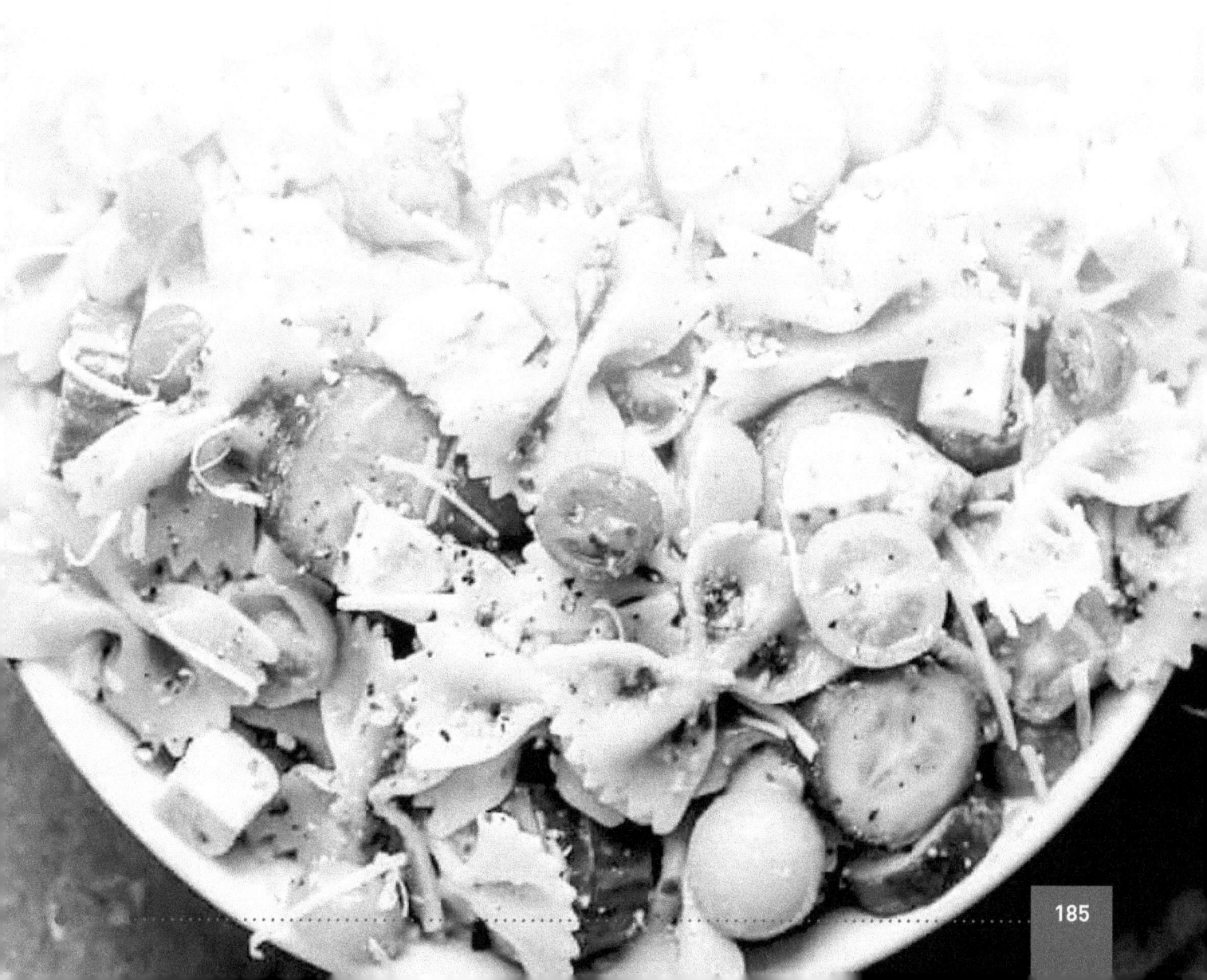

94 BARLEY BLUEBERRY AVOCADO SALAD

Preparation Time: 15 minutes

Cooking Time: 15 minutes

Servings: 4

INGREDIENTS:

- 1 cup quick-cooking barley
- 3 cups low-sodium vegetable broth
- 3 tablespoons extra-virgin olive oil
- 2 tablespoons freshly squeezed lemon juice
- 1 teaspoon yellow mustard
- 1 teaspoon honey
- ½ avocado, peeled and chopped
- 2 cups blueberries
- ¼ cup crumbled feta cheese

DIRECTIONS:

1. Combine the barley and vegetable broth in a medium saucepan and bring to a simmer.
2. Reduce the heat to low, partially cover the pan, and simmer for 10 to 12 minutes or until the barley is tender.
3. Meanwhile, whisk together the olive oil, lemon juice, mustard, and honey in a serving bowl until blended.
4. Drain the barley if necessary and add to the bowl; toss to combine.
5. Add the avocado, blueberries, and feta and toss gently. Serve.

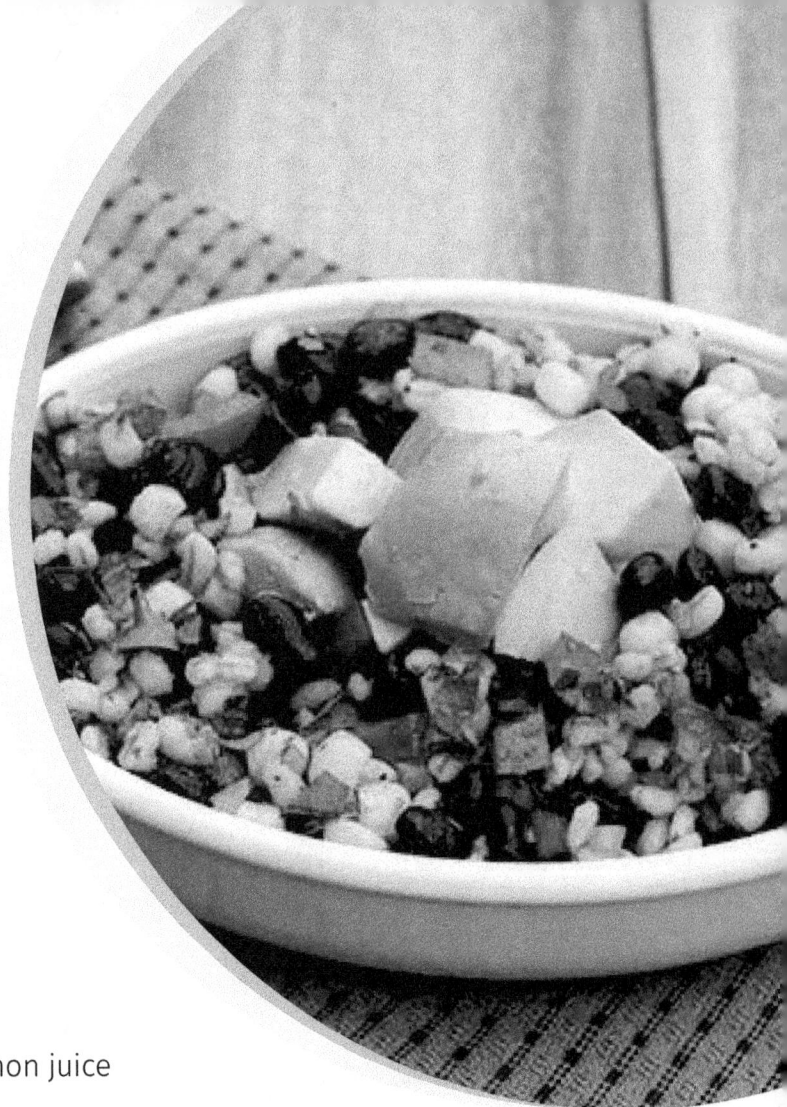

Calories: 345

Fat 16g

Carbohydrates: 44g

Protein: 7g

Sodium: 259mg

Potassium: 301mg

Phosphorus: 152mg

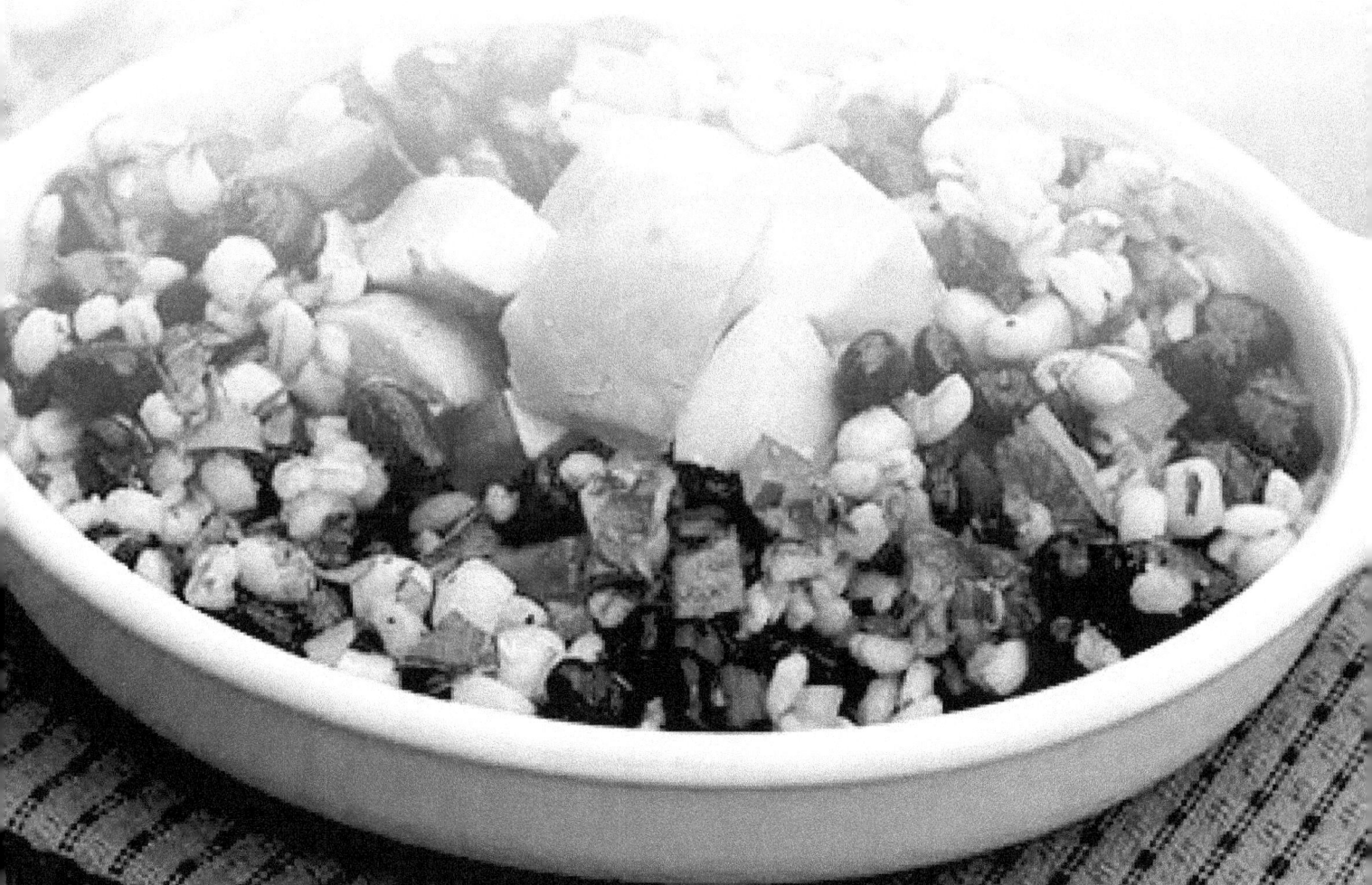

95 PASTA WITH CREAMY BROCCOLI SAUCE

Preparation Time: 15 minutes

Cooking Time: 15 minutes

Servings: 4

INGREDIENTS:

1. 2 tablespoons olive oil
2. 1-pound broccoli florets
3. 3 garlic cloves, halved
4. 1 cup low-sodium vegetable broth
5. ½ pound whole-wheat spaghetti pasta
6. 4 ounces cream cheese
7. 1 teaspoon dried basil leaves
8. ½ cup grated Parmesan cheese

DIRECTIONS:

1. Prepare a large pot of water to a boil.
2. Put olive oil in a large skillet. Sauté the broccoli and garlic for 3 minutes.
3. Add the broth to the skillet and bring to a simmer. Reduce the heat to low, partially cover the skillet, and simmer until the broccoli is tender about 5 to 6 minutes.
4. Cook the pasta according to package directions. Drain when al dente, reserving 1 cup pasta water.
5. When the broccoli is tender, add the cream cheese and basil—purée using an immersion blender.
6. Put mixture into a food processor, about half at a time, and purée until smooth and transfer the sauce back into the skillet.
7. Add the cooked pasta to the broccoli sauce. Toss, adding enough pasta water until the sauce coats the pasta completely. Sprinkle with the Parmesan and serve.

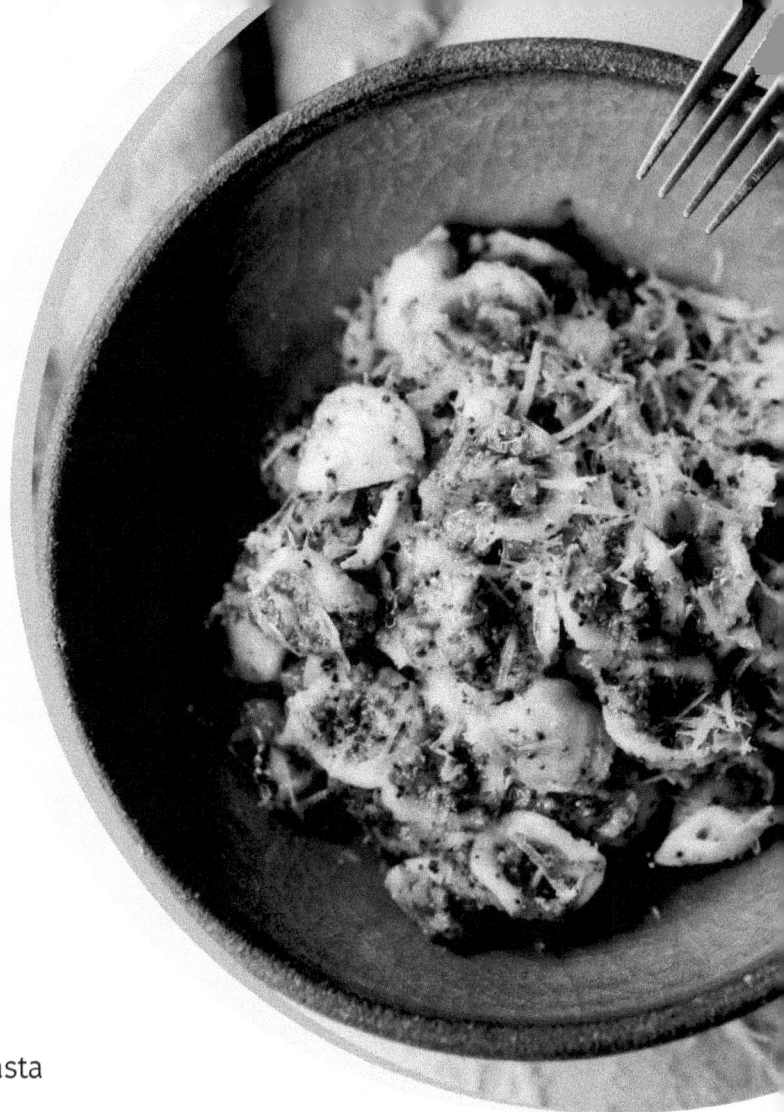

Calories: 302

Fat 14g

Carbohydrates: 36g

Protein: 11g

Sodium: 260mg

Potassium: 375mg

Phosphorus: 223mg

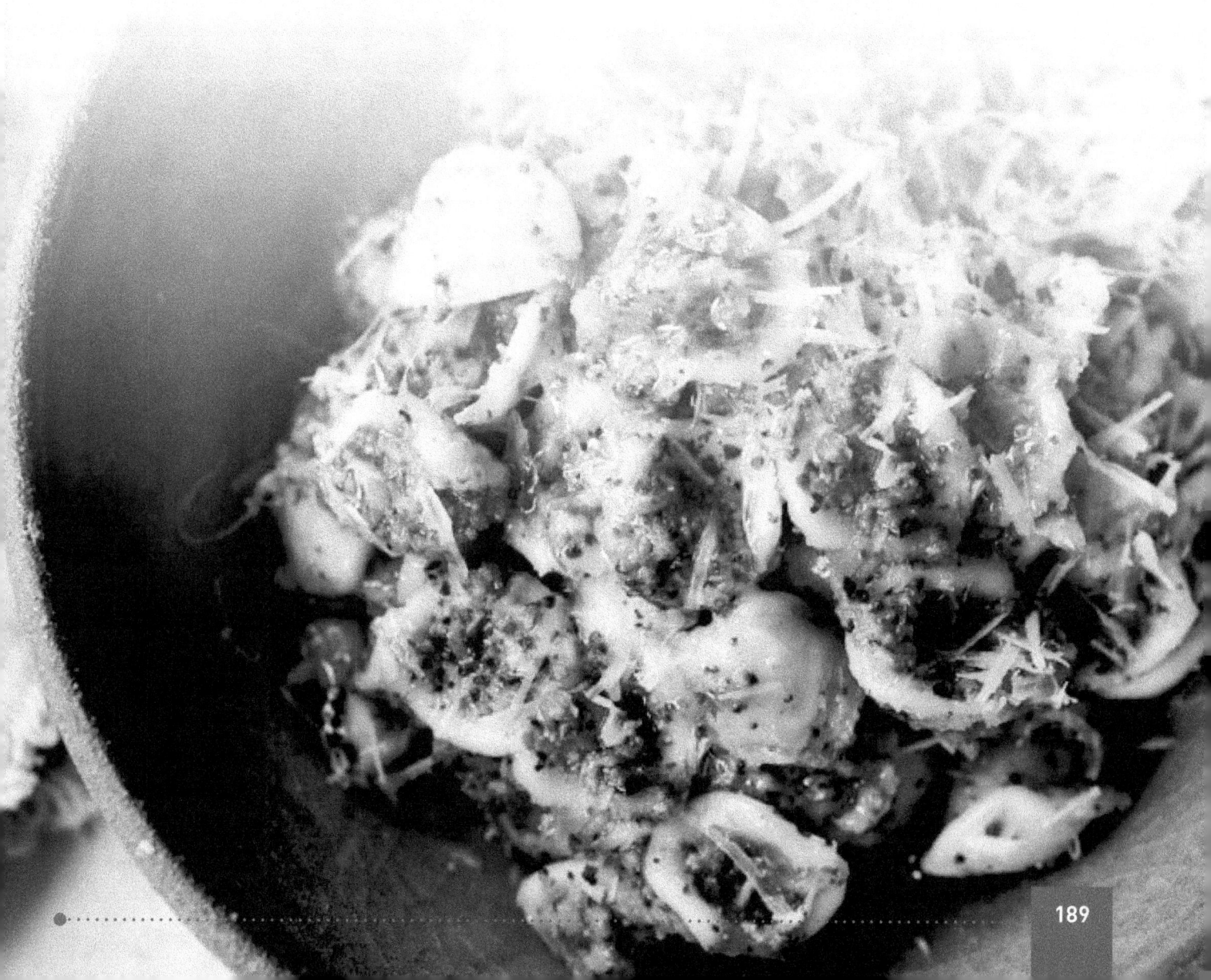

96 ASPARAGUS FRIED RICE

Preparation Time: 10 minutes

Cooking Time: 10 minutes

Servings: 1

INGREDIENTS:

- 3 large eggs, beaten
- ½ teaspoon ground ginger
- 2 teaspoons low-sodium soy sauce
- 2 tablespoons olive oil
- 1 onion, diced
- 4 garlic cloves, minced
- 1 cup sliced cremini mushrooms
- 1 (10-ounce) package frozen brown rice, thawed
- 8 ounces fresh asparagus, about 15 spears, cut into 1-inch pieces
- 1 teaspoon sesame oil

DIRECTIONS:

1. Whisk the eggs, ginger, and soy sauce in a small bowl and set aside.
2. Heat the olive oil in a medium skillet or wok over medium heat.
3. Add the onion and garlic and sauté for 2 minutes until tender crisp.
4. Add the mushrooms and rice; stir-fry for 3 minutes longer.
5. Put asparagus and cook for 2 minutes.6.
6. Pour in the egg mixture. Stir the eggs until cooked through, 2 to 3 minutes, and stir into the rice mixture.
7. Sprinkle the fried rice with the sesame oil and serve.

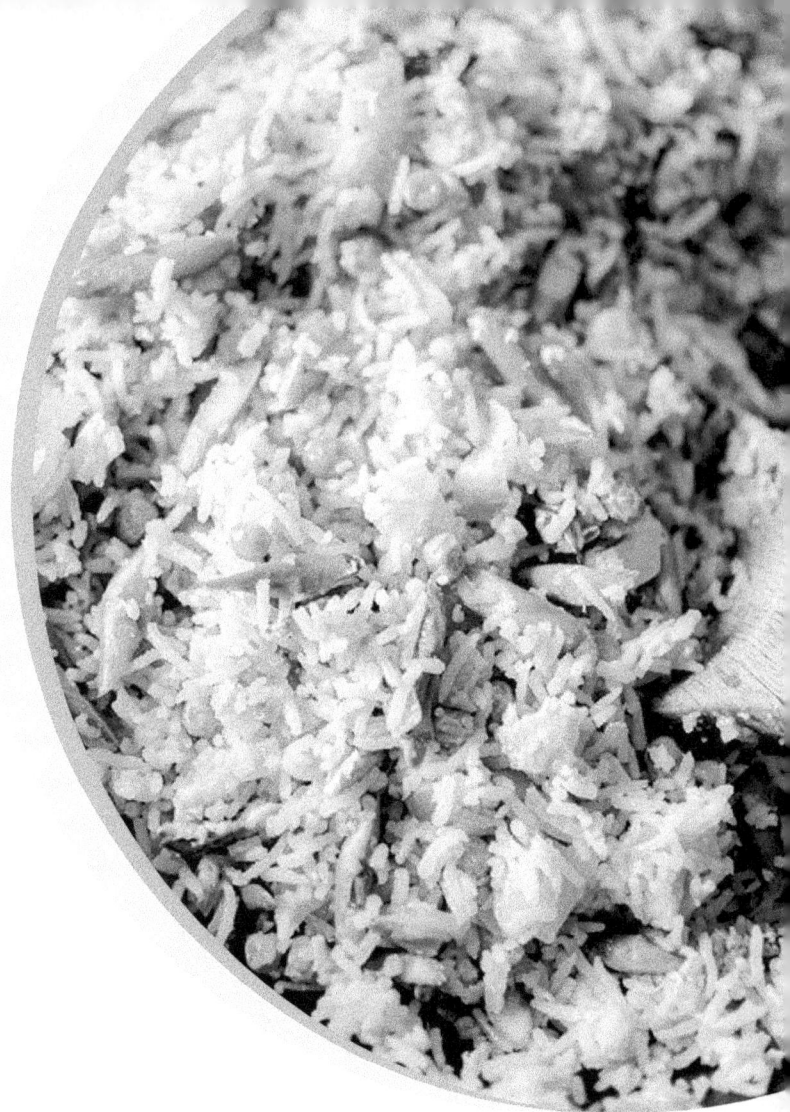

Calories: 247

Fat: 13g

Carbohydrates: 25g

Protein: 9g

Sodium: 149mg

Potassium: 367mg

Phosphorus: 206mg

VEGETARIAN TACO SALAD

Preparation Time: 15 minutes

Cooking Time: 15 minutes

Servings: 2

INGREDIENTS:

- 1½ cups canned low-sodium or no-salt-added pinto beans, rinsed and drained
- 1 (10-ounce) package frozen brown rice, thawed
- 1 red bell pepper, chopped
- 3 scallions, white and green parts, chopped
- 1 jalapeño pepper, minced
- 1 cup frozen corn, thawed and drained
- 1 tablespoon chili powder
- 1 cup chopped romaine lettuce
- 2 cups chopped butter lettuce
- ½ cup Powerhouse Salsa
- ½ cup grated pepper Jack cheese

DIRECTIONS:

1. In a medium bowl, combine the beans, rice, bell pepper, scallions, jalapeño, and corn.
2. Sprinkle with the chili powder and stir gently.
3. Stir in the romaine and butter lettuce.
4. Serve topped with Powerhouse Salsa and cheese.

NUTRITION:

Calories: 254

Fat: 7g

Carbohydrates: 39g

Protein: 11g

Sodium: 440mg

Potassium: 599mg

Phosphorus: 240mg

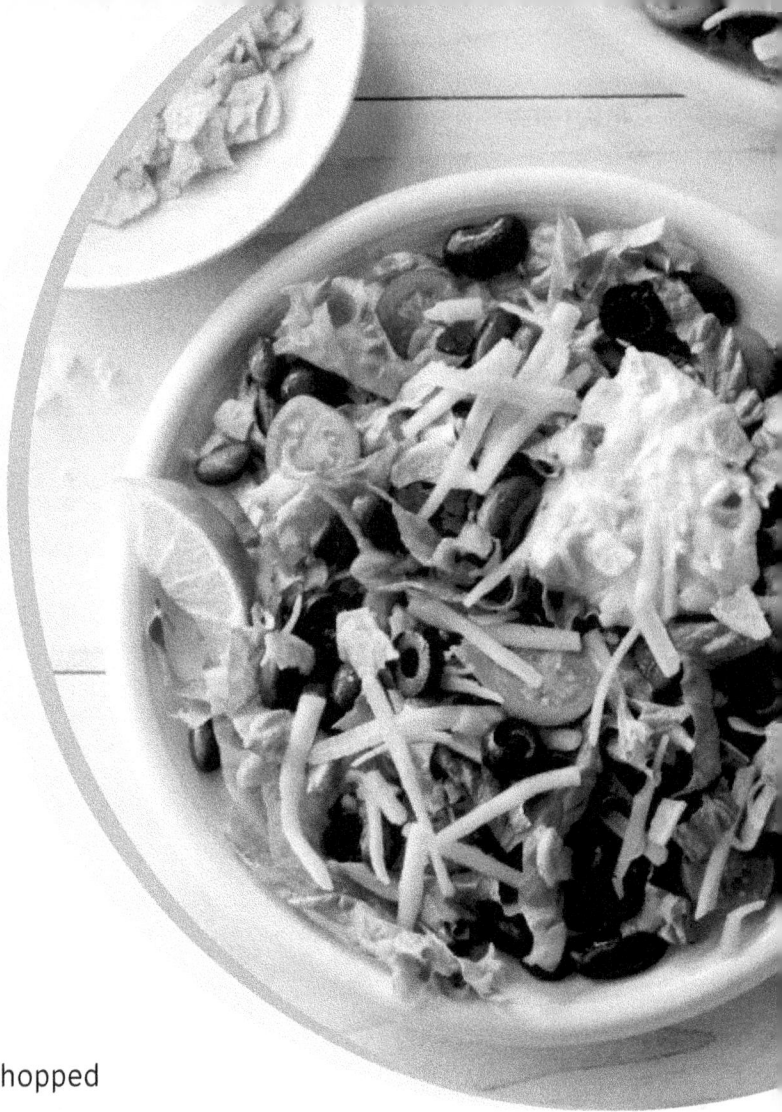

98 SAUTÉED GREEN BEANS

Preparation Time: 10 minutes

Cooking Time: 15 minutes

Servings: 4

INGREDIENTS:

- 2 cup frozen green beans
- ½ cup red bell pepper
- 4 tsp margarine
- ¼ cup onion
- 1 tsp dried dill weed
- 1 tsp dried parsley
- ¼ tsp black pepper

DIRECTIONS:

1. Cook green beans in a large pan of boiling water until tender, then drain.
2. 2.While the beans are cooking, melt the margarine in a skillet and fry the other vegetables.
3. Add the beans to sautéed vegetables.
4. Sprinkle with freshly ground pepper and serve with meat and fish dishes.

NUTRITION:

Calories 67
Carbs 8g
Protein 4g
Sodium 5mg
Potassium 179mg
Phosphorous 32mg

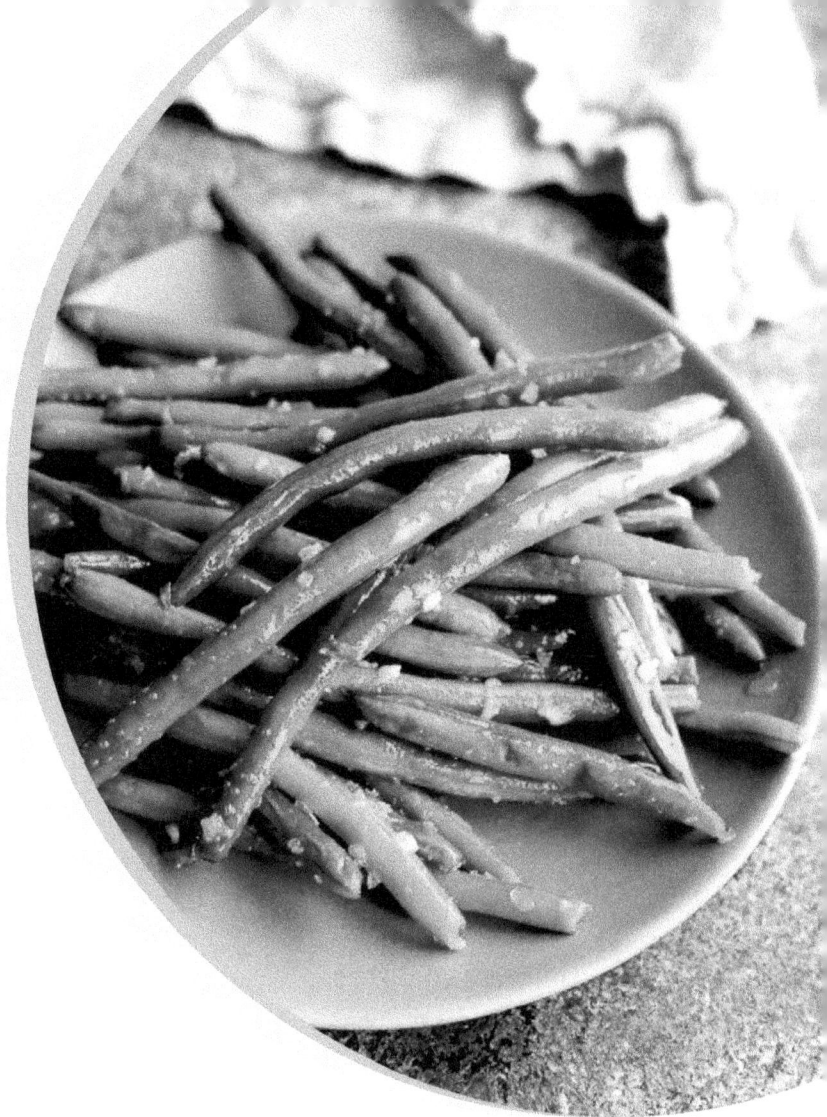

GARLICKY PENNE PASTA WITH ASPARAGUS

Preparation Time: 10 minutes

Cooking Time: 10 minutes

Servings: 4

INGREDIENTS:

- 2 tbsp butter
- 1lb asparagus, cut into 2-inch pieces
- 2 tsp lemon juice
- 4 cup whole wheat penne pasta, cooked
- ¼ cup shredded Parmesan cheese
- ¼ tsp Tabasco® hot sauce

DIRECTIONS:

1. Add olive oil and butter in a skillet over medium heat.
2. Fry garlic and red pepper flakes for 2-3 minutes.
3. Add asparagus, Tabasco sauce, lemon juice, and black pepper to skillet and cook for a further 6 minutes.
4. Add hot pasta and cheese. Toss and serve.

NUTRITION:

Calories 387

Carbs 49g

Protein 13g

Sodium 93

Potassium 258mg

Phosphorous 252mg

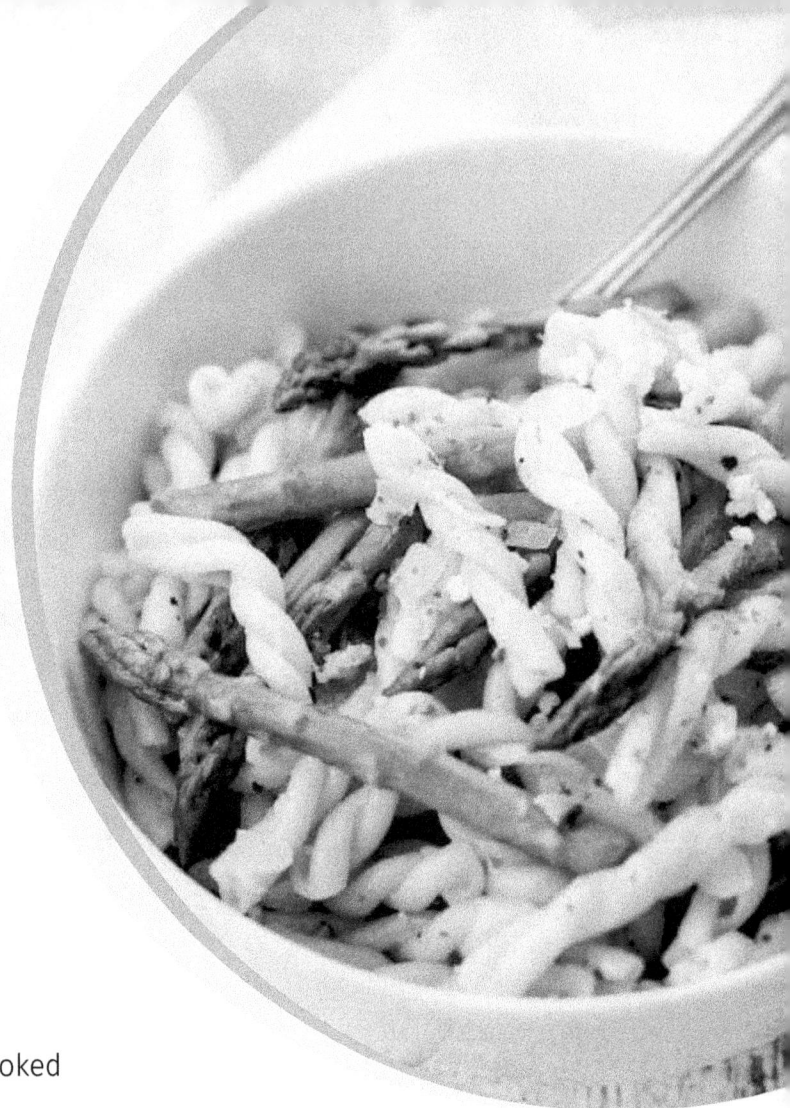

100 GARLIC MASHED POTATOES

Preparation Time: 5 minutes

Cooking Time: 20 minutes

Servings: 4

INGREDIENTS:

- 2 medium potatoes, peeled and sliced
- ¼ cup butter
- ¼ cup 1% low-fat milk
- 2 garlic cloves

DIRECTIONS:

1. Double-boil or soak the potatoes to reduce potassium if you are on a low potassium diet.
2. Boil potatoes and garlic until soft. Drain.
3. Beat the potatoes and garlic with butter and milk until smooth.

NUTRITION:

Calories 168

Carbs 29g

Protein 5g

Sodium 59

Potassium 161g

Phosphorous 57mg

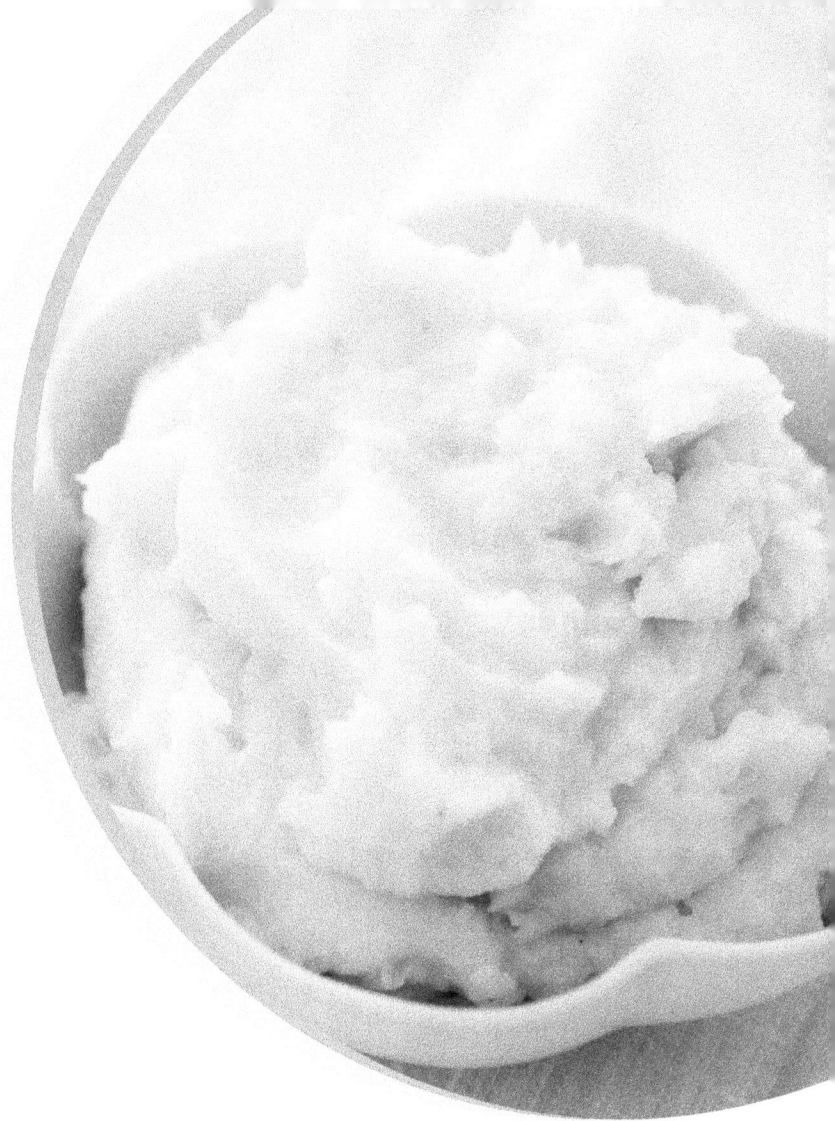

101 GINGER GLAZED CARROTS

Preparation Time: 10 minutes

Cooking Time: 20 minutes

Servings: 4

INGREDIENTS:

- 2 cups carrots, sliced into 1-inch pieces
- ¼ cup apple juice
- 2 tbsp margarine, melted
- ¼ cup boiling water
- 1 tbsp sugar
- 1 tsp cornstarch
- ¼ tsp salt
- ¼ tsp ground ginger

DIRECTIONS:

1. Cook carrots until tender.
2. Mix sugar, cornstarch, salt, ginger, apple juice, and margarine together
3. Pour mixture over carrots and cook for 10 minutes until thickened.

NUTRITION:

Calories 101

Fat 3

Carbs 14g

Protein 1g

Sodium 87

Potassium 202g

Phosphorous 26mg

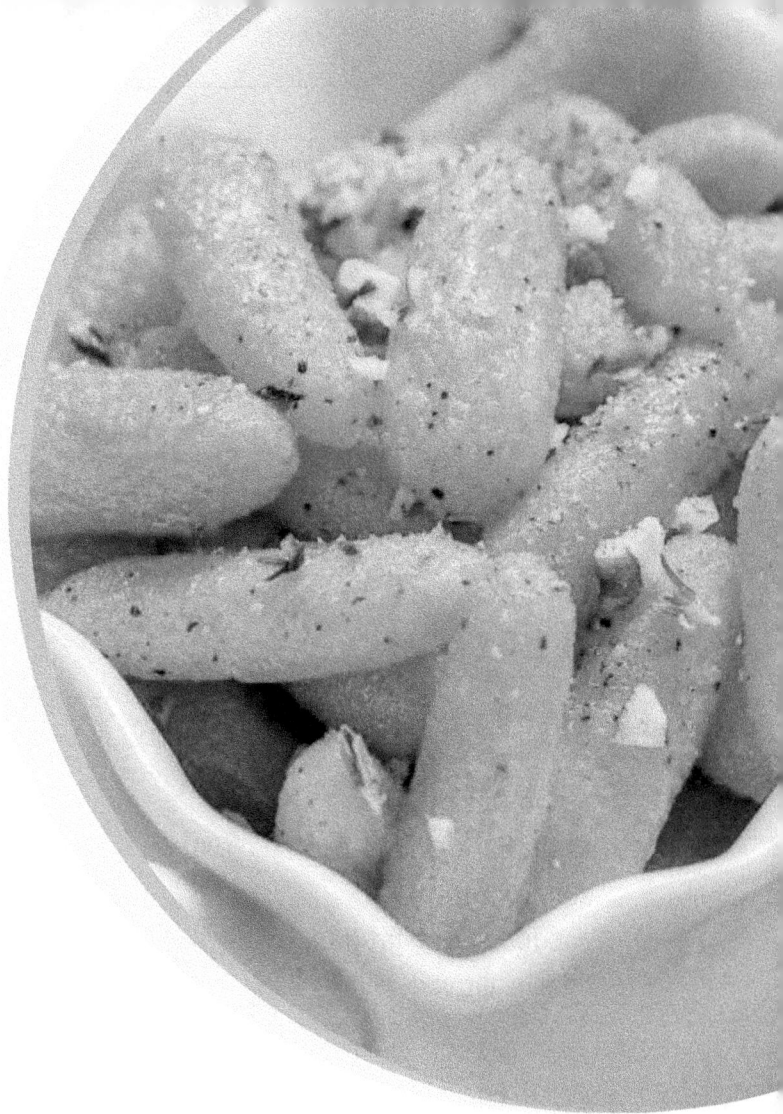

102 CARROT-APPLE CASSEROLE

Preparation Time: 15 minutes

Cooking Time: 50 minutes

Servings: 8

INGREDIENTS:

- 6 large carrots, peeled and sliced
- 4 large apples, peeled and sliced
- 3 tbsp butter
- ½ cup apple juice
- 5 tbsp all-purpose flour
- 2 tbsp brown sugar
- ½ tsp ground nutmeg

DIRECTIONS:

1. Preheat oven to 350° F.
2. Let the carrots boil for 5 minutes or until tender. Drain.
3. Arrange the carrots and apples in a large casserole dish.
4. Mix the flour, brown sugar, and nutmeg in a small bowl.
5. Rub in butter to make a crumb topping.
6. Sprinkle the crumb over the carrots and apples, then drizzle with juice.
7. Bake until bubbling and golden brown.

NUTRITION:

Calories 245
Fat 6g
Carbs 49g
Protein 1g

Sodium 91mg
Potassium 169mg
Phosphorous 17mg

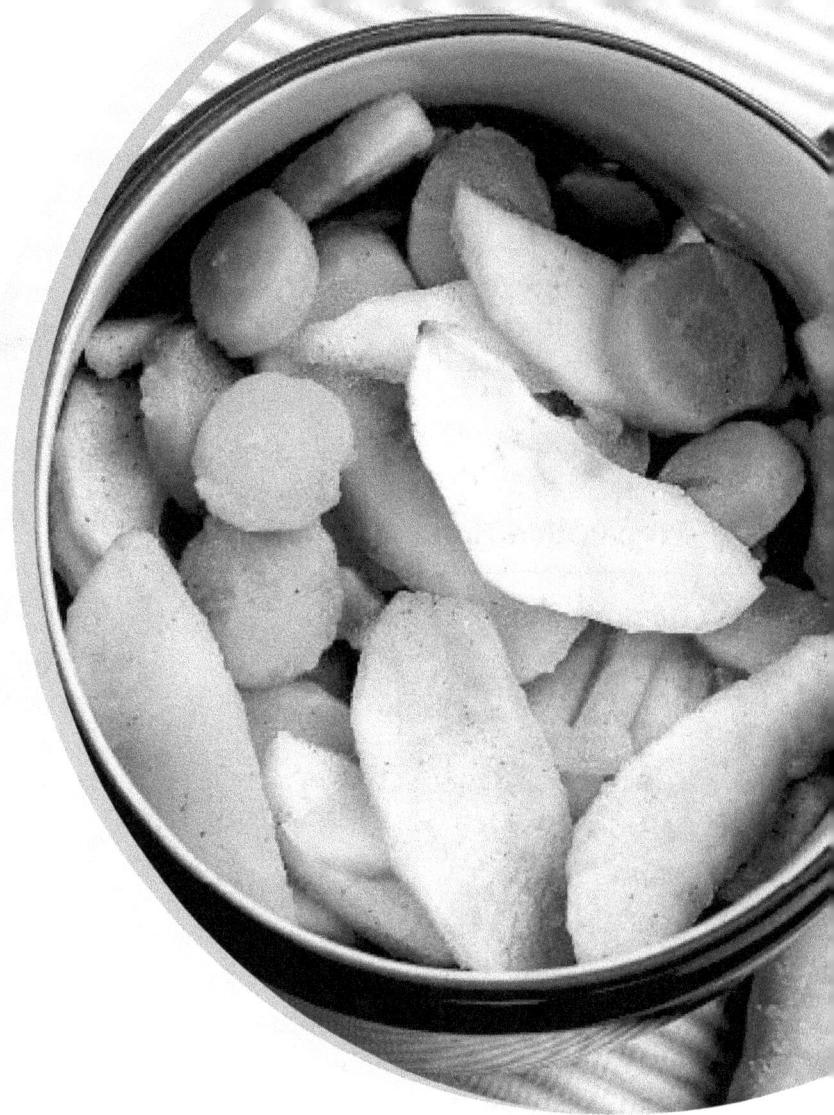

103 CREAMY SHELLS WITH PEAS AND BACON

Preparation Time: 15 minutes

Cooking Time: 15 minutes

Servings: 4

INGREDIENTS:

- 1 cup part-skim ricotta cheese
- ½ cup grated Parmesan cheese
- 3 slices bacon, cut into strips
- 1 cup onion, chopped
- ¾ cup of frozen green peas
- 1 tbsp olive oil
- ¼ tsp black pepper
- 3 garlic cloves, minced
- 3 cup cooked whole-wheat small shell pasta
- 1 tbsp lemon juice
- 2 tbsp unsalted butter

DIRECTIONS:

1. Place ricotta, Parmesan cheese, butter, and pepper in a large bowl.
2. Cook bacon in a skillet until crisp. Set aside.
3. Add the garlic and onion to the same skillet and fry until soft. Add to bowl with ricotta.
4. Cook the peas and add to the ricotta.
5. Add half a cup of the reserved cooking water and lemon juice to the ricotta mixture and mix well.
6. Add the pasta, bacon, and peas to the bowl and mix well.
7. Put freshly ground black pepper and serve.

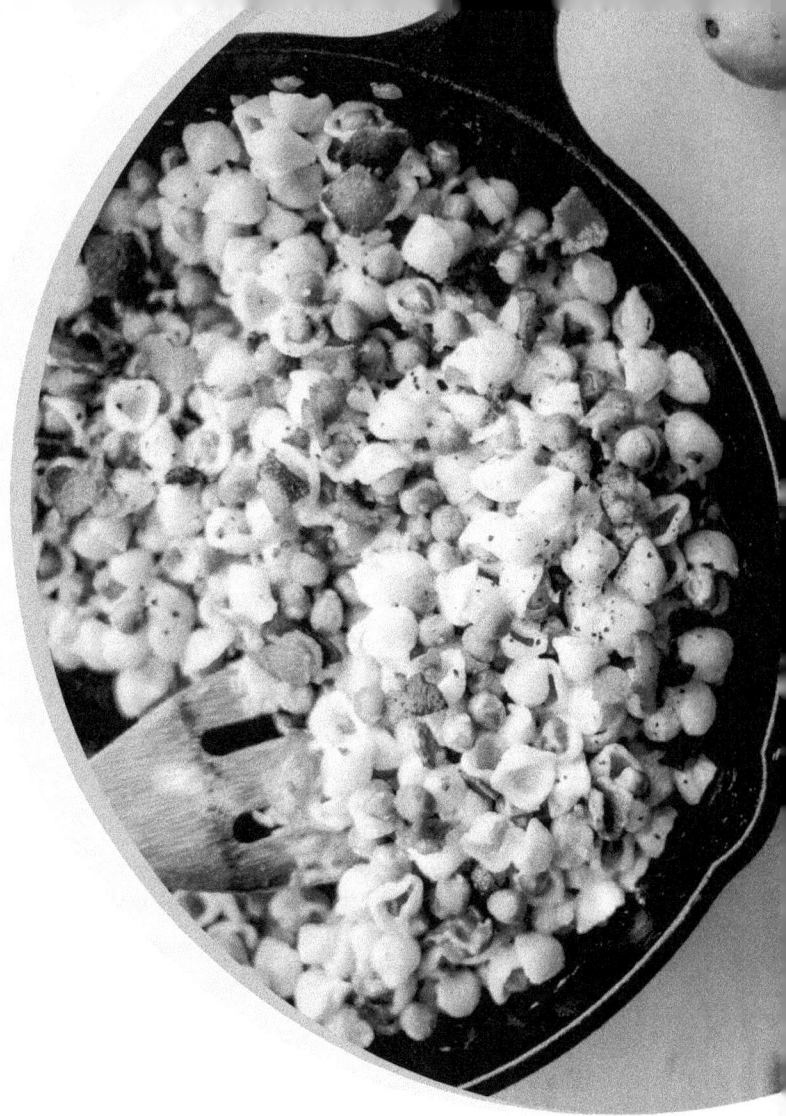

Calories 429

Fat 14g

Carbs 27g

Protein 13g

Sodium 244mg

Potassium 172mg

Phosphorous 203mg

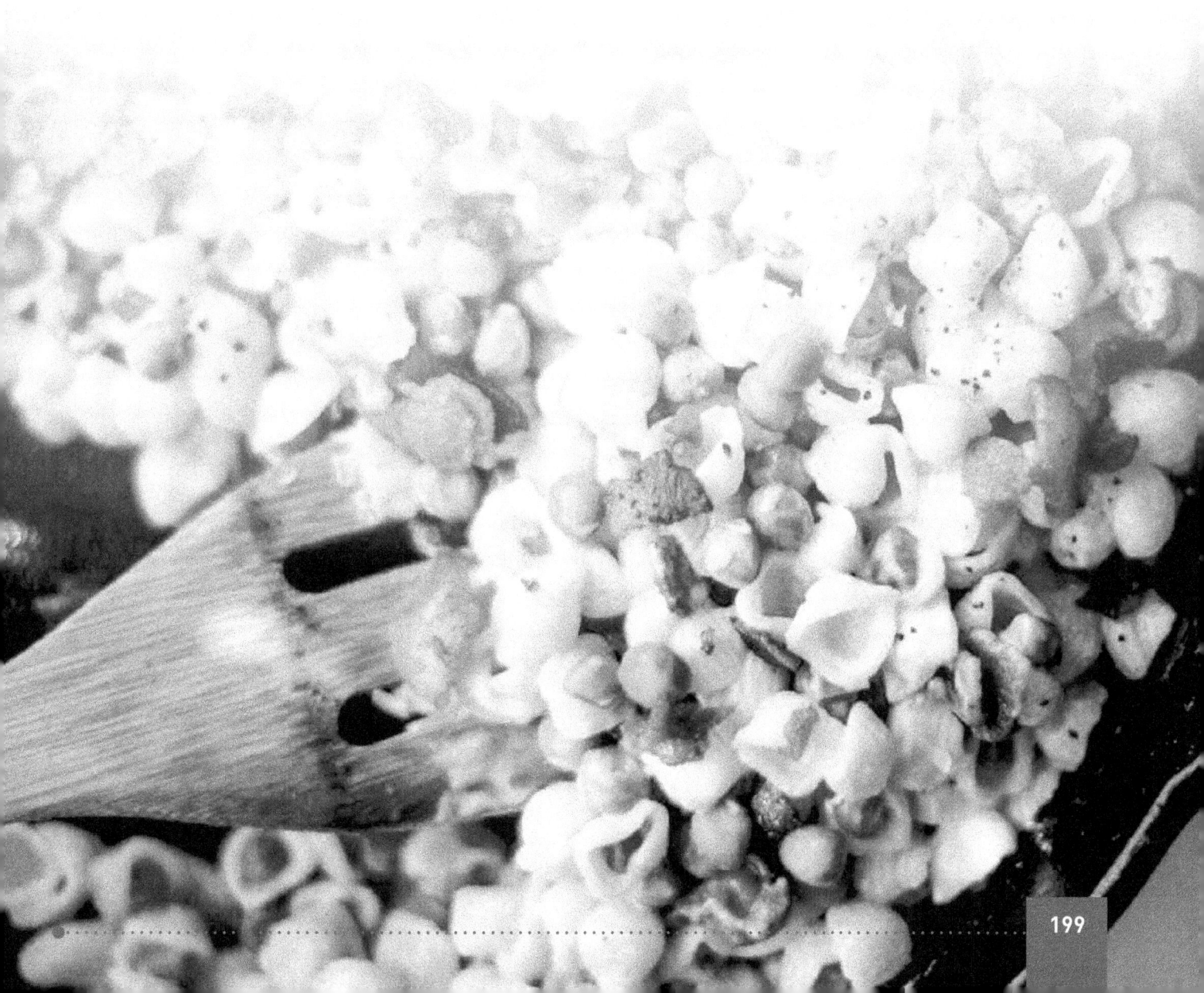

104 DOUBLE-BOILED STEWED POTATOES

Preparation Time: 20 minutes

Cooking Time: 30 minutes

Servings: 4

INGREDIENTS:

- 2 cup potatoes, diced into ½ inch cubes
- ½ cup hot water
- ½ cup liquid non-dairy creamer
- ¼ tsp garlic powder
- ¼ tsp black pepper
- 2 tbsp margarine
- 2 tsp all-purpose white flour

DIRECTIONS:

1. Soak or double boil the potatoes if you are on a low potassium diet.
2. Boil potatoes for 15 minutes.
3. Drain potatoes and return to pan. Add half a cup of hot water, the creamer, garlic powder, pepper, and margarine. Heat to a boil.
4. Mix the flour with a tablespoon of water and then stir this into the potatoes. Cook for 3 minutes until the mixture has thickened and the flour has cooked.

NUTRITION:

Calories 184
Carbs 25g
Protein 2g
Potassium 161mg
Phosphorous 65mg

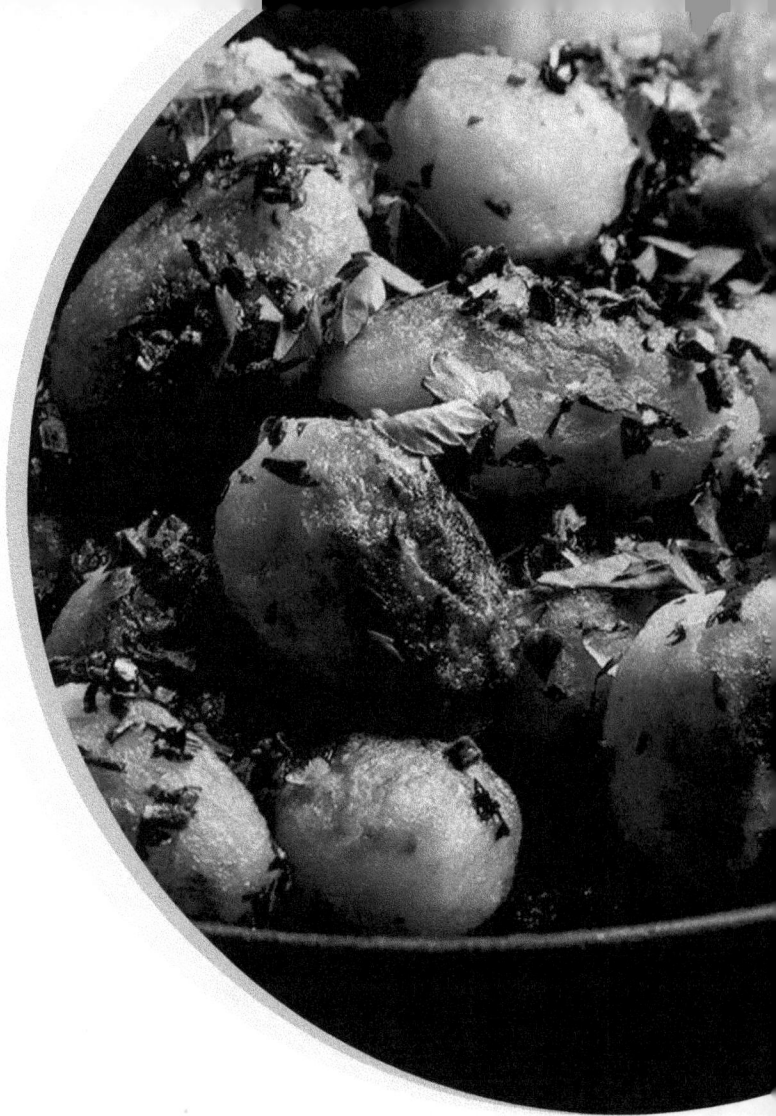

105 DOUBLE-BOILED COUNTRY STYLE FRIED POTATOES

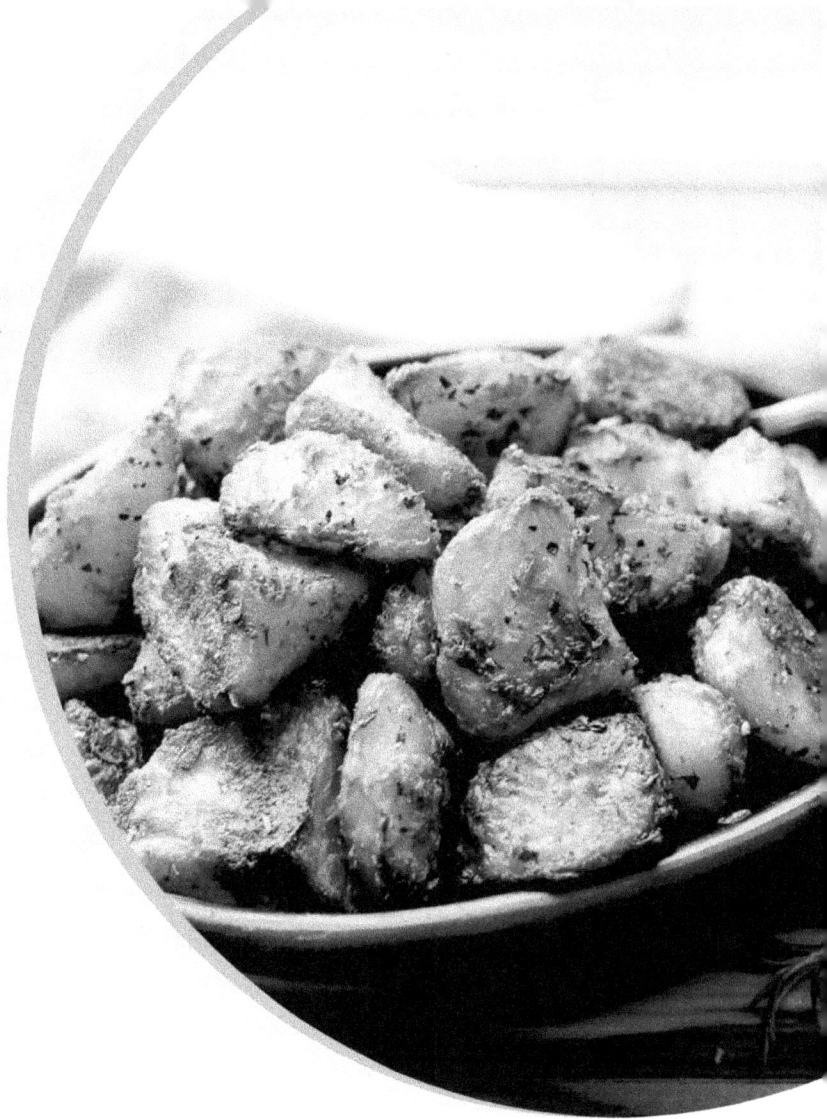

Preparation Time: 20 minutes

Cooking Time: 20 minutes

Servings: 4

INGREDIENTS:

- 2 medium potatoes, cut into large chips
- ½ cup canola oil
- ¼ tsp ground cumin
- ¼ tsp paprika
- ¼ tsp white pepper
- 3 tbsp ketchup

DIRECTIONS:

1. Soak or double boil the potatoes if you are on a low potassium diet.
2. Heat oil over medium heat in a skillet.
3. Fry the potatoes for around 10 minutes until golden brown.
4. Drain potatoes, then sprinkle with cumin, pepper, and paprika.
5. Serve with ketchup or mayo.

NUTRITION:

Calories 156
Fat 0.1g
Carbs 21g
Protein 2g
Sodium 3mg
Potassium 296mg
Phosphorous 34mg

106 BROCCOLI-ONION LATKES

Preparation Time: 15 minutes

Cooking Time: 20 minutes

Servings: 4

INGREDIENTS:

- 3 cups broccoli florets, diced
- ½ cup onion, chopped
- 2 large eggs, beaten
- 2 tbsp all-purpose white flour
- 2 tbsp olive oil

DIRECTIONS:

1. Cook the broccoli for around 5 minutes until tender. Drain.
2. Mix the flour into the eggs.
3. Combine the onion, broccoli, and egg mixture and stir through.
4. Prepare olive oil in a skillet on medium-high heat.
5. Drop a spoon of the mixture onto the pan to make 4 latkes.
6. Cook each side until golden brown.
7. Drain on a paper towel and serve.

NUTRITION:

Calories 140
Fat
Carbs 7g
Protein 6g
Sodium 58mg
Potassium 276mg
Phosphorous 101mg

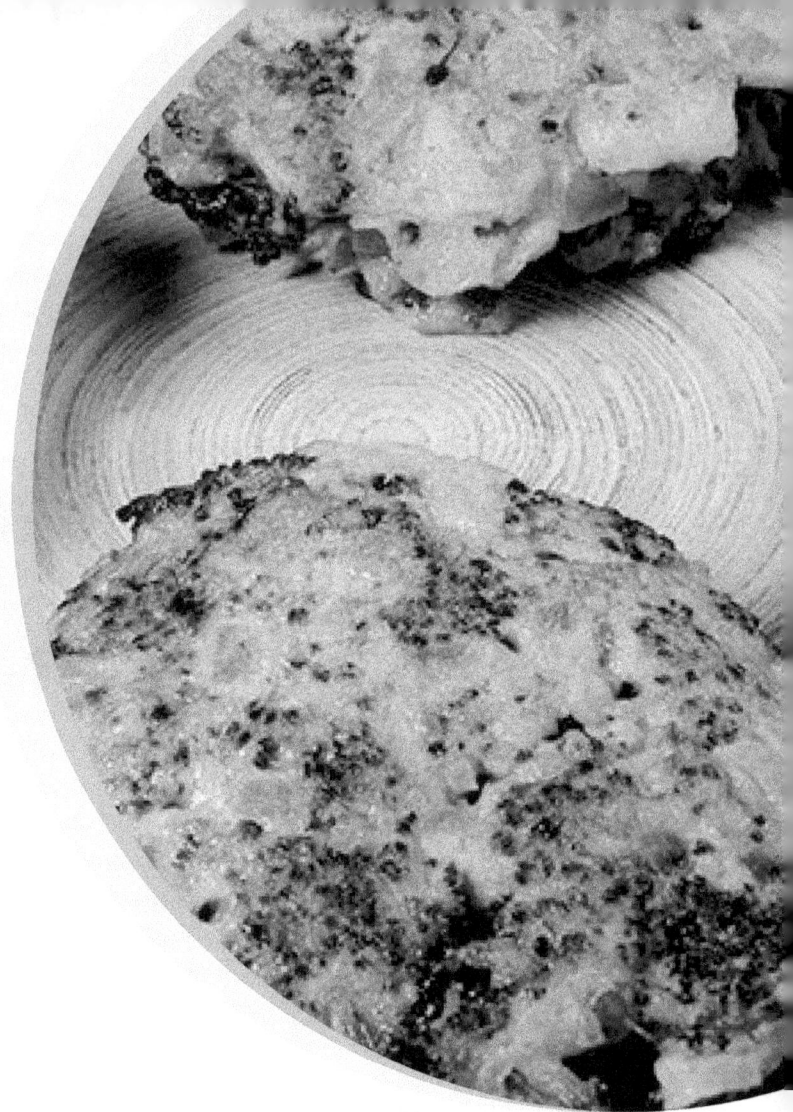

107 CRANBERRY CABBAGE

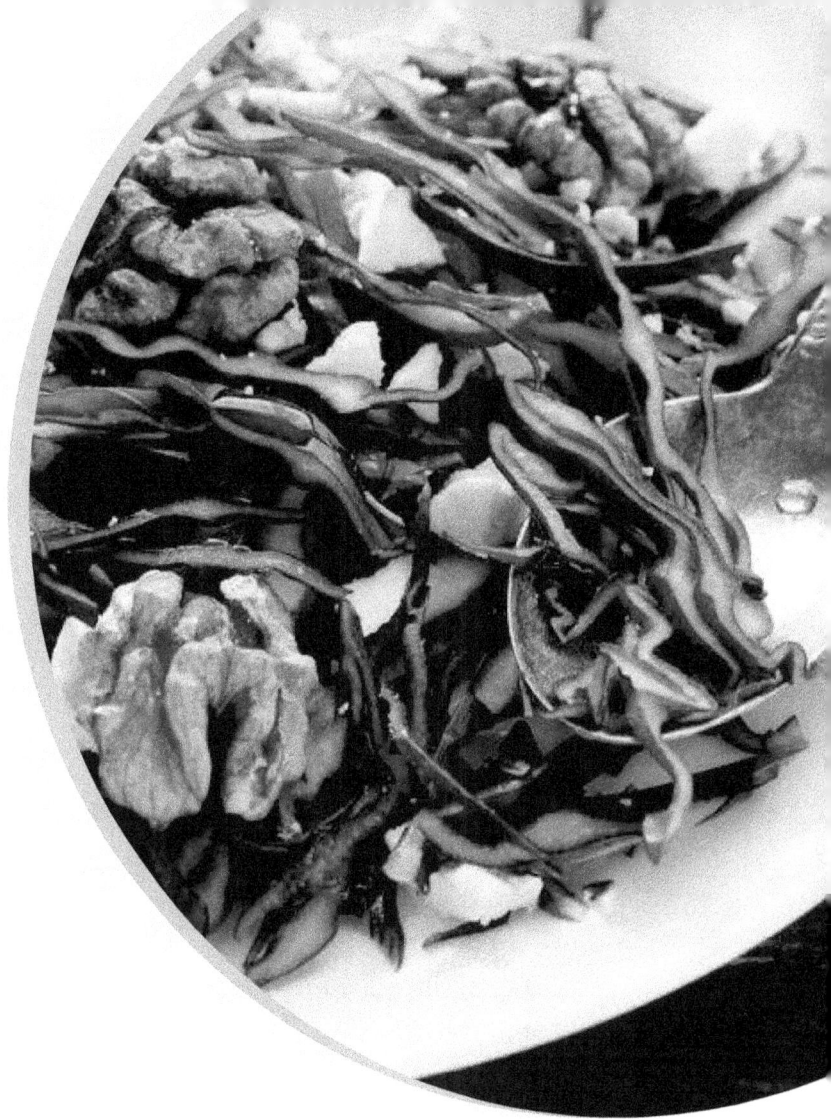

Preparation Time: 10 minutes

Cooking Time: 20 minutes

Servings: 8

INGREDIENTS:

- 10 ounces canned whole-berry cranberry sauce
- 1 tablespoon fresh lemon juice
- 1 medium head red cabbage
- 1/4 teaspoon ground cloves

DIRECTIONS:

1. Place the cranberry sauce, lemon juice, and cloves in a large pan and bring to the boil.
2. Add the cabbage and reduce it to a simmer.
3. Cook until the cabbage is tender, occasionally stirring to make sure the sauce does not stick.
4. Delicious served with beef, lamb, or pork.

NUTRITION:

Calories 73
Fat 0g
Carbs 18g
Protein 1g
Sodium 32mg
Potassium 138mg
Phosphorous 18mg

108 CAULIFLOWER RICE

Preparation Time: 5 minutes

Cooking Time: 10 minutes

Servings: 1

INGREDIENTS:

- 1 small head cauliflower cut into florets
- 1 tbsp butter
- ¼ tsp black pepper
- ¼ tsp garlic powder
- ¼ tsp salt-free herb seasoning blend

DIRECTIONS:

1. Blitz cauliflower pieces in a food processor until it has a grain-like consistency.
2. Melt butter in a saucepan and add spices.
3. Add the cauliflower rice grains and cook over low-medium heat for approximately 10 minutes.
4. Use a fork to fluff the rice before serving.
5. Serve as an alternative to rice with curries, stews, and starch to accompany meat and fish dishes.

NUTRITION:

Calories 47
Fat
Carbs 4g
Protein 1g

Sodium 300mg
Potassium 206mg
Phosphorous 31mg

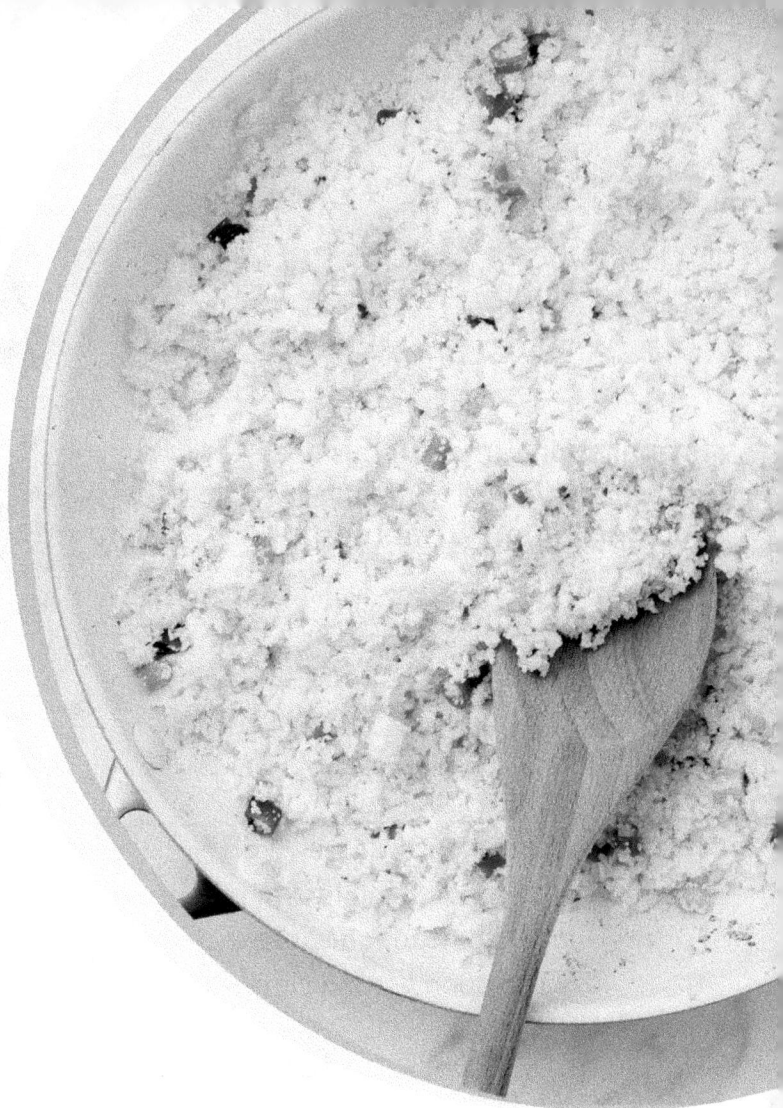

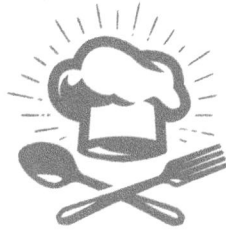

CHAPTER 17

SMOOTHIES AND DRINKS RECIPES

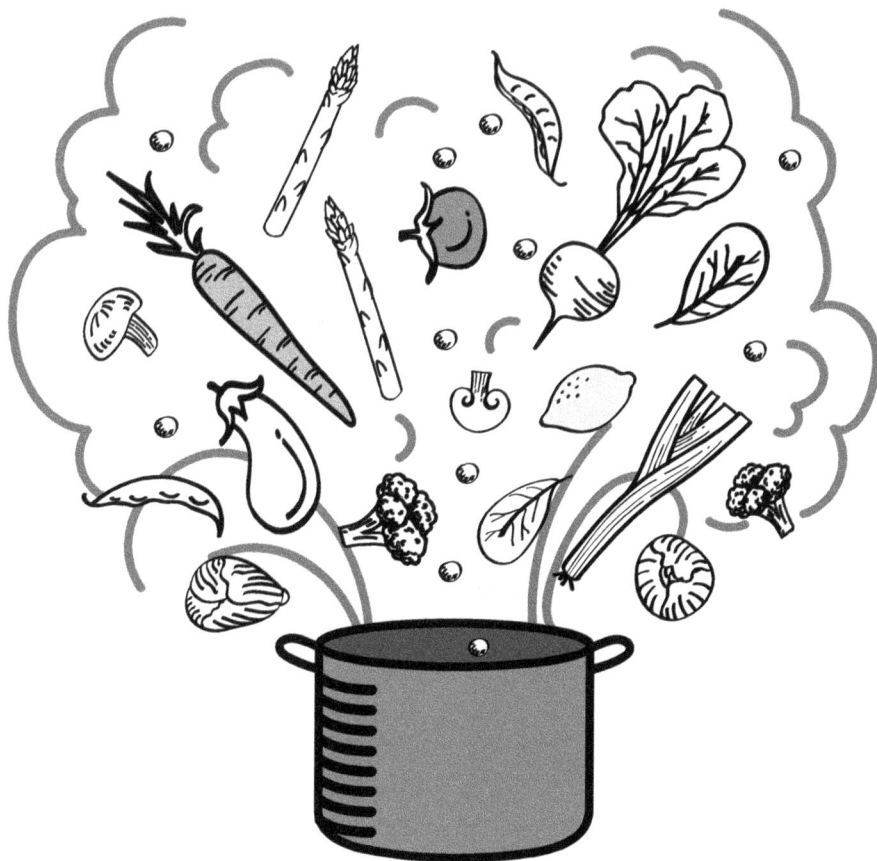

109 BLACKBERRY SAGE COCKTAIL

Preparation Time: 5 minutes

Cooking Time: 10 minutes

Servings: 6

INGREDIENTS:

- Sage Simple Syrup
- 1 cup water
- 1 cup0granulated sugar
- 8 fresh sage leaves, plus more for garnish
- 1-pint fresh blackberries, muddled and strained (juices reserved)
- Juice of 1/2 a lemon
- 8 oz St. Germain Liqueur
- 16 oz vodka
- seltzer water

DIRECTIONS:

1. Place water and sugar in a small saucepan.
2. Simmer until sugar dissolves for 7 to 10 minutes.
3. Remove from heat. Add sage leaves, and cover, allowing the mixture for about 2 hours.
4. Combine fresh blackberry juice, lemon juice, sage simple syrup, cocktail pitcher.
5. Mix and refrigerate covered until well chilled.
6. Serve in cocktail glasses filled with ice and garnish with fresh sage leaves and top with a splash of seltzer water.

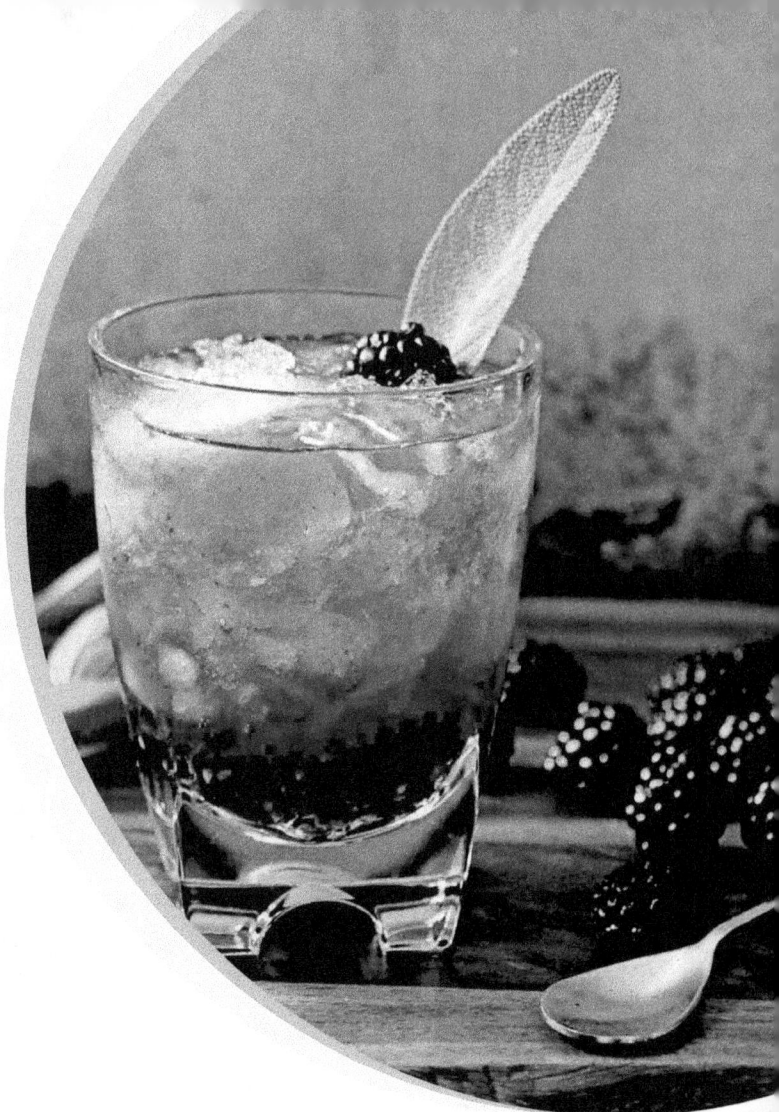

Calories: 68
Fat: 1g
Carbs: 15g
Protein: 3g
Sodium: 3mg
Potassium: 133mg
Phosphorus: 38mg

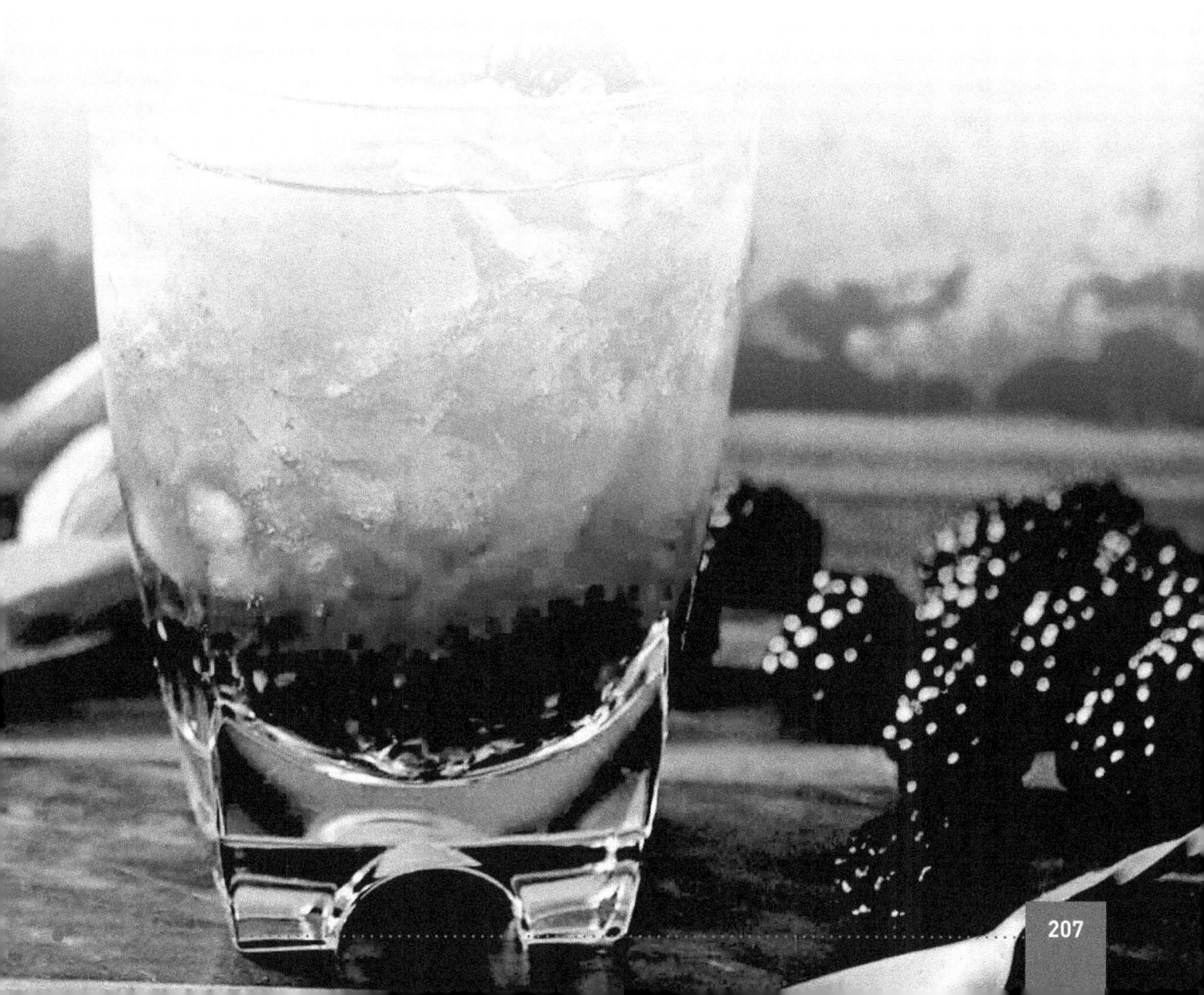

110 APPLE-CINNAMON DRINK

Preparation Time: 10 minutes

Cooking Time: 20 minutes

Servings: 4

INGREDIENTS:

- 13 fresh apples
- 750ml-1L cold water
- 3-4 tablespoons cinnamon
- 1-2 tablespoons sugar (brown or caster)

DIRECTIONS:

1. Peel, chop and cook 13 fresh apples.
2. Once they were half-cooked, add water leaving for 2 minutes
3. Add a lot of cinnamon (3-4 tablespoons, but you can add as much as you please, really) and 1-2 tablespoons sugar.
4. Keep cooking for another 5 minutes.
5. Drain and put into the new container back in the pan and bring it to the boil.
6. Add more cinnamon and a bit of water to thin it out a bit.
7. Pour into a cup and enjoy.

NUTRITION:

Calories: 130
Fat: 0g
Carbs: 32g
Protein: 0g

Sodium: 20mg
Potassium: 0mg
Phosphorus: 0mg

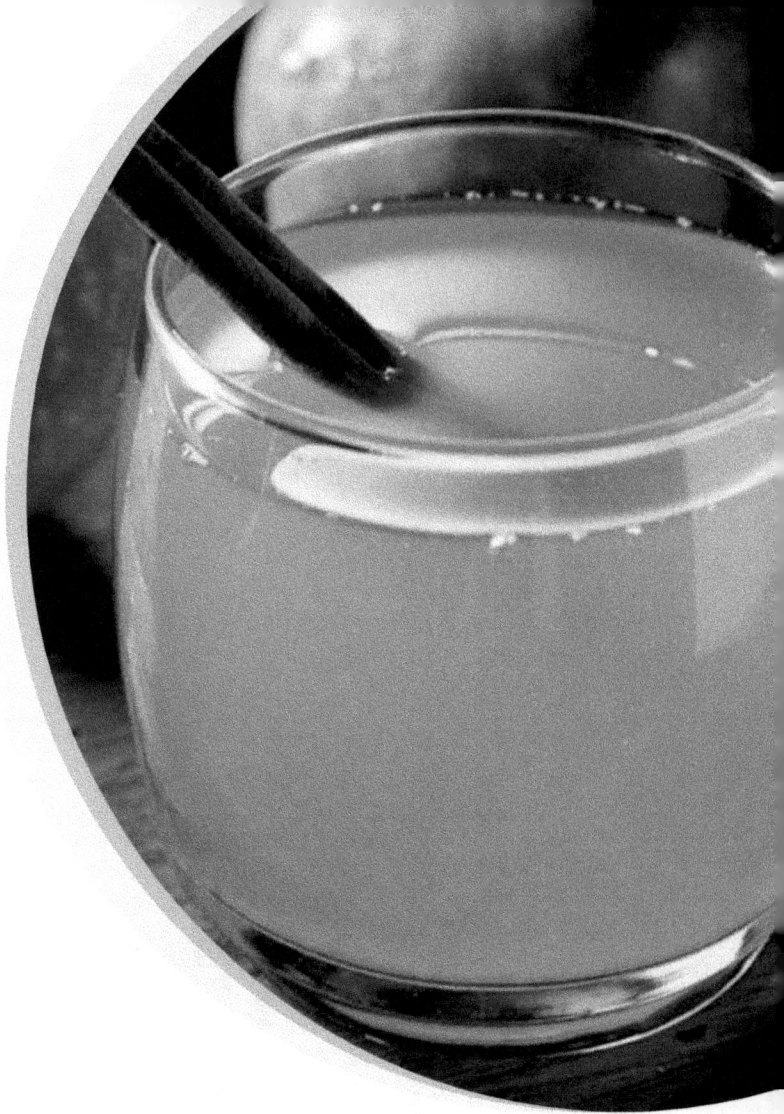

111 DETOXIFYING BEET JUICE

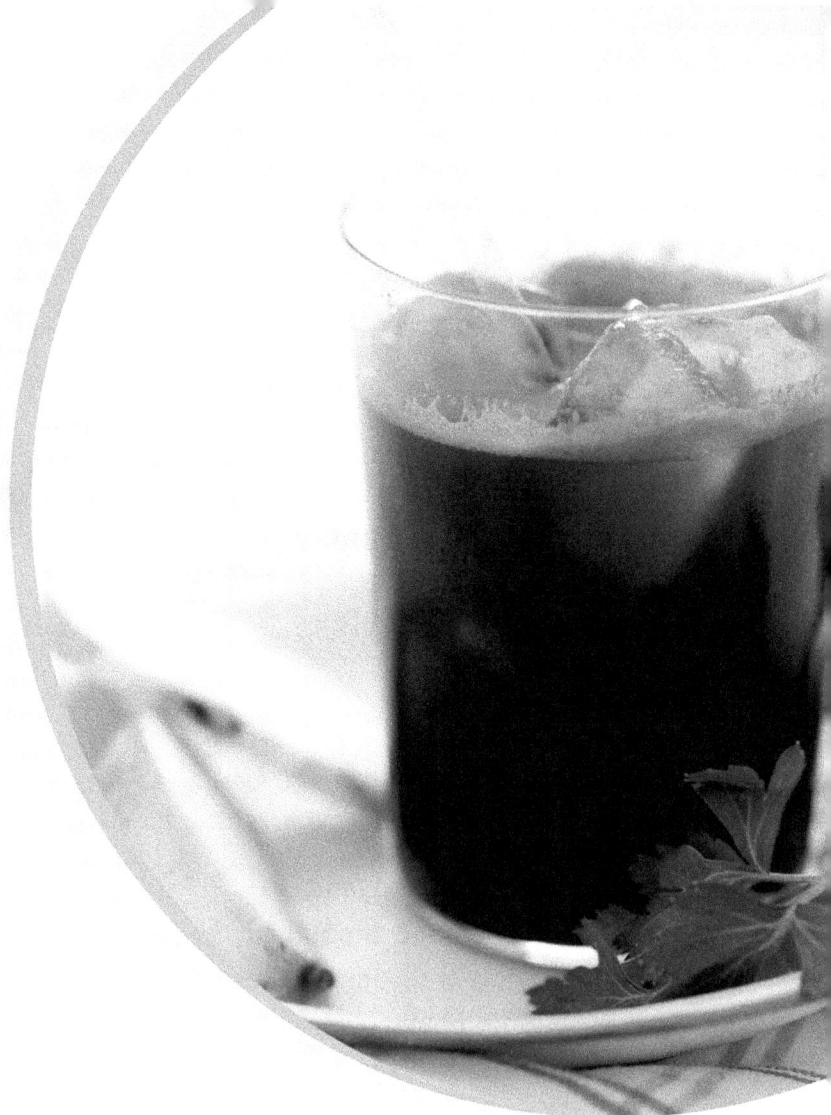

Preparation Time: 10 minutes

Cooking Time: 10 minutes

Servings: 4

INGREDIENTS:

- 1-pound beets, washed with ends cut off
- 2 pounds carrots, washed with ends cut off
- 1 bunch celery, washed and broken into ribs
- 2 lemons, peel cut off and quartered
- 1 lime, peel cut off and quartered
- 1 bunch flat-leaf parsley, washed
- 1 Fuji or Honeycrisp red apple, chopped (optional, for extra sweetness)

DIRECTIONS:

1. Wash produce and chop so pieces will fit into the feeder tube of your juicer.
2. Feed the vegetable pieces through the juicer, alternating harder and softer textured pieces to aid in the juicing process.
3. Serve immediately or store in the refrigerator in a highly sealed container.
4. The juice is best when served within 48 hours of making.

NUTRITION:

Calories: 58
Fat: 0g
Carbs: 13g
Protein: 2g

Sodium: 106mg
Potassium: 442mg
Phosphorus: 54mg

112 HONEY CINNAMON LATTE

Preparation Time: 5 minutes

Cooking Time: 5 minutes

Servings: 2

INGREDIENTS:

- 1-½ cups of organic, unsweetened almond milk
- 1 scoop of organic vanilla protein powder
- 1 teaspoon of organic cinnamon
- ½ teaspoon of pure, local honey
- 1-2 shots of espresso

DIRECTIONS:

1. Heat almond milk in the microwave until hot to the touch.
2. Add honey and stir until completely melted.
3. Using a whisk, add cinnamon, and protein powder and thoroughly combine.
4. Pour into a manual milk and froth concoction until foamy and creamy.
5. Pour espresso shots into a mug and add in milk mixture.

NUTRITION:

Calories: 115
Fat: 3g
Carbs: 26g
Protein: 3g
Sodium: 125mg
Potassium: 10.9mg
Phosphorus: 0.1mg

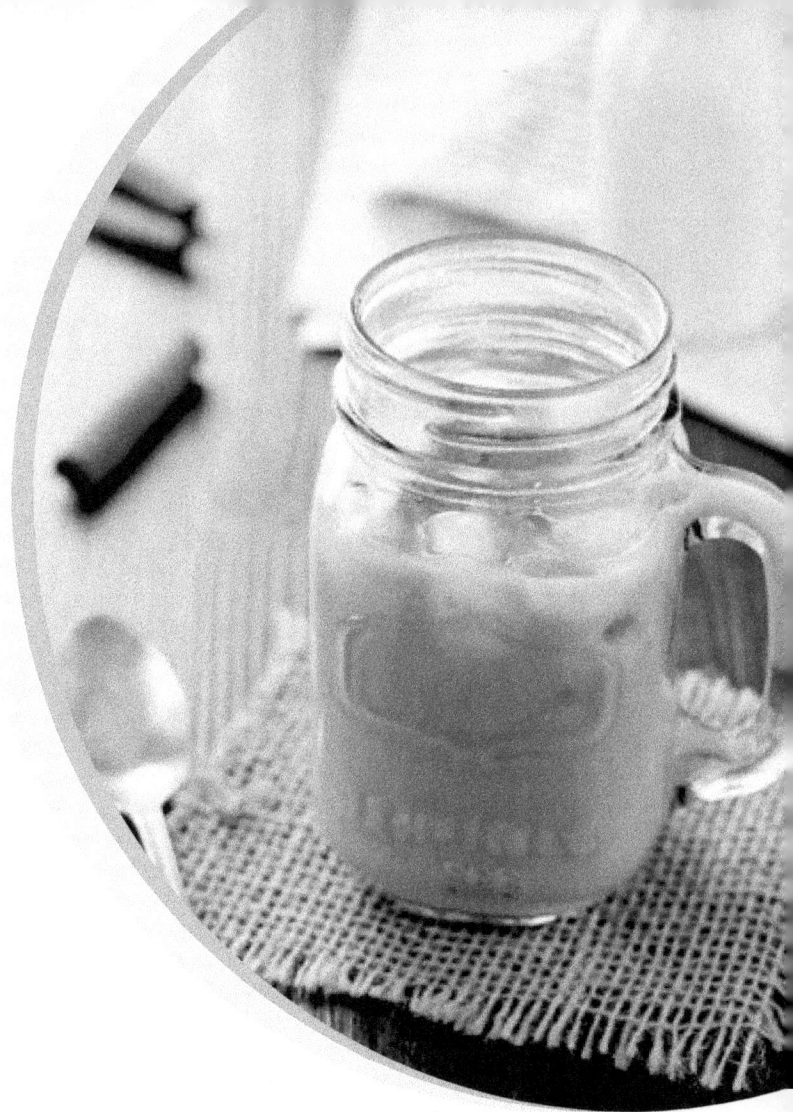

113 CINNAMON SMOOTHIE

Preparation Time: 5 minutes

Cooking Time: 5 minutes

Servings: 2

INGREDIENTS:

- 1 large banana
- 150g plain or Greek yogurt
- 300ml milk
- 2 tbsp smooth peanut butter
- 1/4 tsp Schwartz
  Ground Cinnamon

DIRECTIONS:

1. Add all the ingredients to a blender and blitz until smooth.
2. Serve immediately.

NUTRITION:

Calories: 88
Fat: 4.3g
Carbs: 3g
Protein: 8g
Sodium: 187mg
Potassium: 241mg
Phosphorus: 20mg

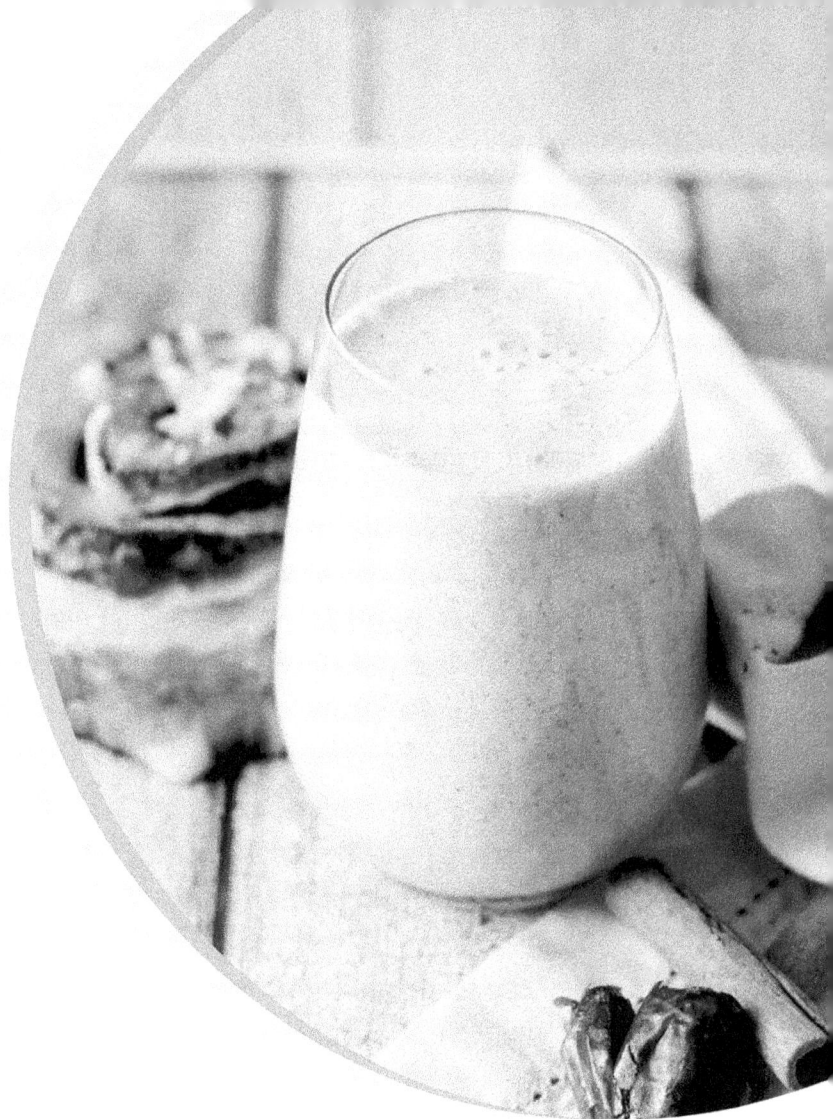

114 CITRUS SMOOTHIE

Preparation Time: 5 minutes

Cooking Time: 2 minutes

Servings: 2

INGREDIENTS:

- 1 large orange, peeled, halved
- ¼ lemon, peeled, seeded
- ½ cup (85 g) pineapple, peeled, cubed
- ¼ cup (60 g) frozen mango
- 1 cup (130 g) ice cubes

DIRECTIONS:

1. Prepare all ingredients into the container and secure lid.
2. Turn machine on and slowly increase speed to high.
3. Blend for 1 minute or until the desired consistency is reached.

NUTRITION:

Calories: 280
Fat: 0g
Carbs: 67g
Protein: 4g
Sodium: 30mg
Potassium: 570mg
Phosphorus: 0mg

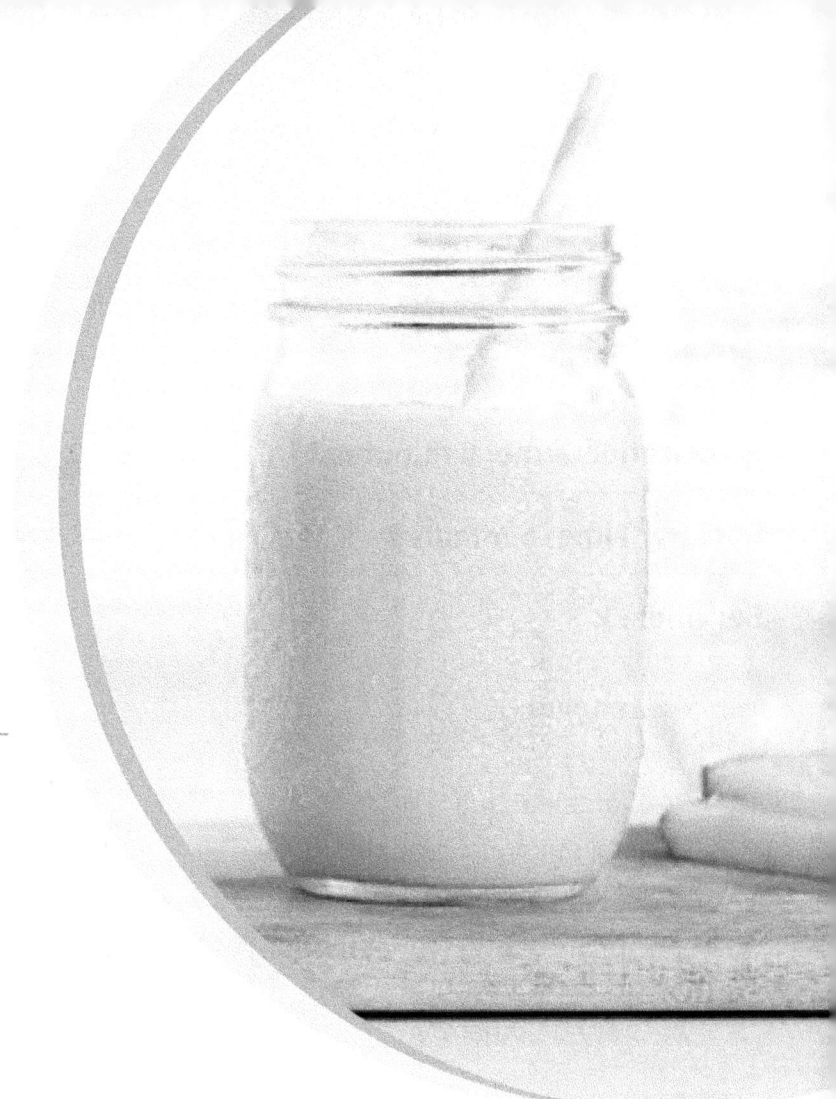

115 PINEAPPLE PROTEIN SMOOTHIE

Preparation Time: 5 minutes

Cooking Time:

Servings: 1

INGREDIENTS:

1. 1/2 cup cottage cheese
2. 1/2 frozen banana
3. 1/2 cup frozen pineapple chunks
4. 1/2 tsp brown sugar (optional)
5. 1/4 tsp vanilla extract
6. 1 Tbsp ground flaxseed (optional)
7. 1 cup milk of choice (unsweetened almond milk)

DIRECTIONS:

1. Place all of the ingredients into a blender, and then blend until smooth.
2. Serve immediately.

NUTRITION:

Calories: 220
Carbohydrates: 29g
Protein: 24g
Fat: 0.5g
Sodium: 195mg
Potassium: 325mg
Phosphorus: 0mg

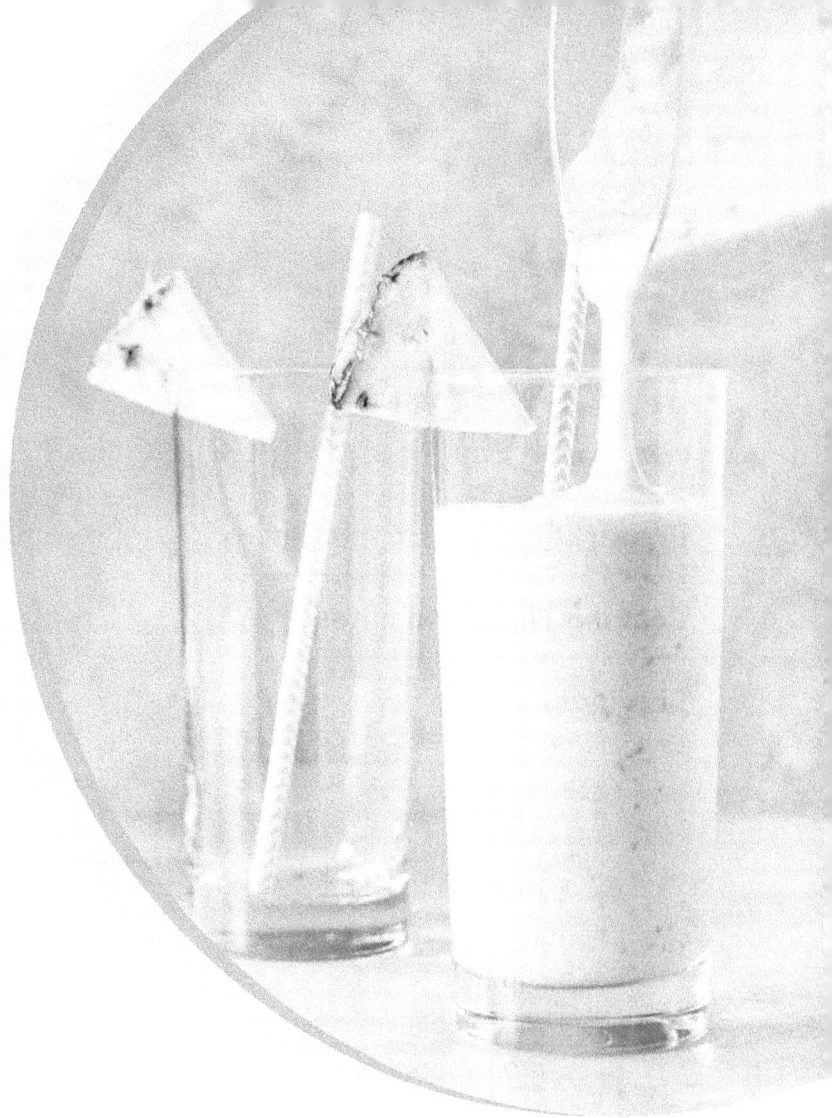

116 HAZELNUT CINNAMON COFFEE

Preparation Time: 5 minutes

Cooking Time: 2 minutes

Servings: 1

INGREDIENTS:

- 1 1/2 cups fresh brewed Toasted Hazelnut Blend
- 1 cup half & half
- 1/4 cup chocolate syrup
- 2 tablespoons hazelnut syrup
- 1/8 teaspoon ground cinnamon

DIRECTIONS:

1. Add hot coffee to a 1-quart saucepan.
2. Steadily add all remaining ingredients, then stir.
3. Cook at medium temperature.
4. Put a sprinkle of cinnamon on top and enjoy.

NUTRITION:

Calories: 161
Fat: 7g
Carbs: 23g
Protein: 2g
Sodium: 34.6mg
Potassium: 219mg
Phosphorus: 100mg

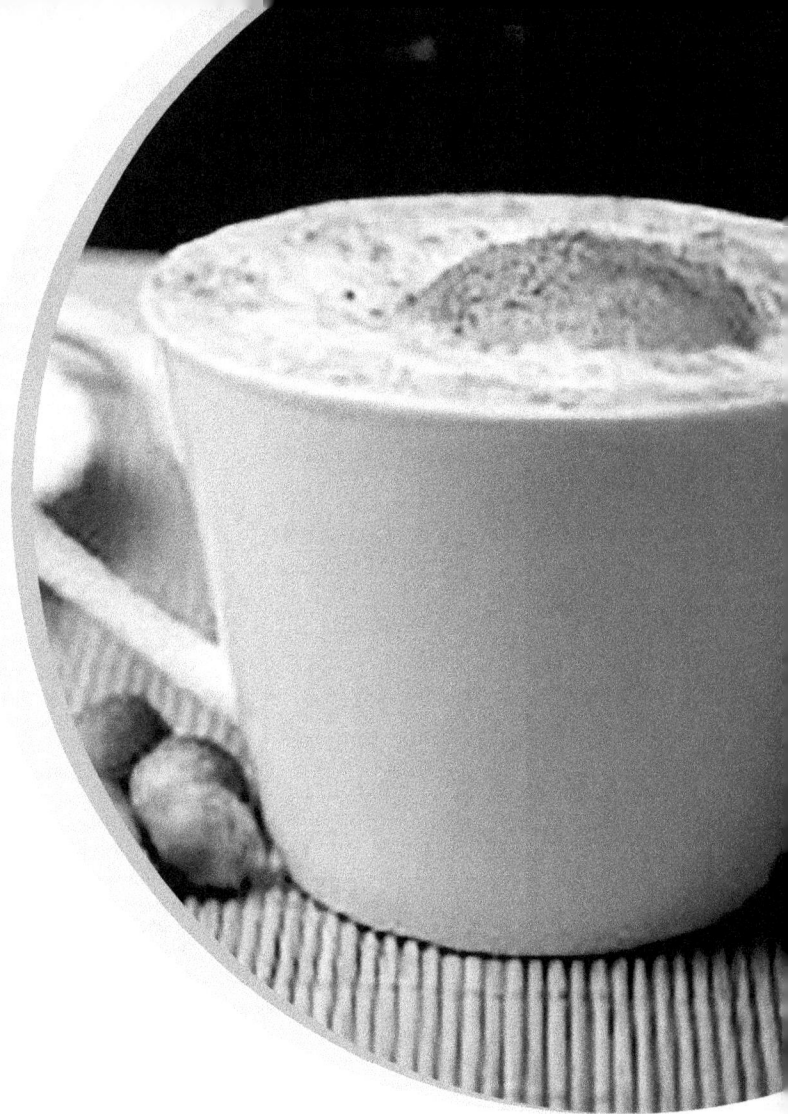

117 PINA COLADA PROTEIN SMOOTHIE

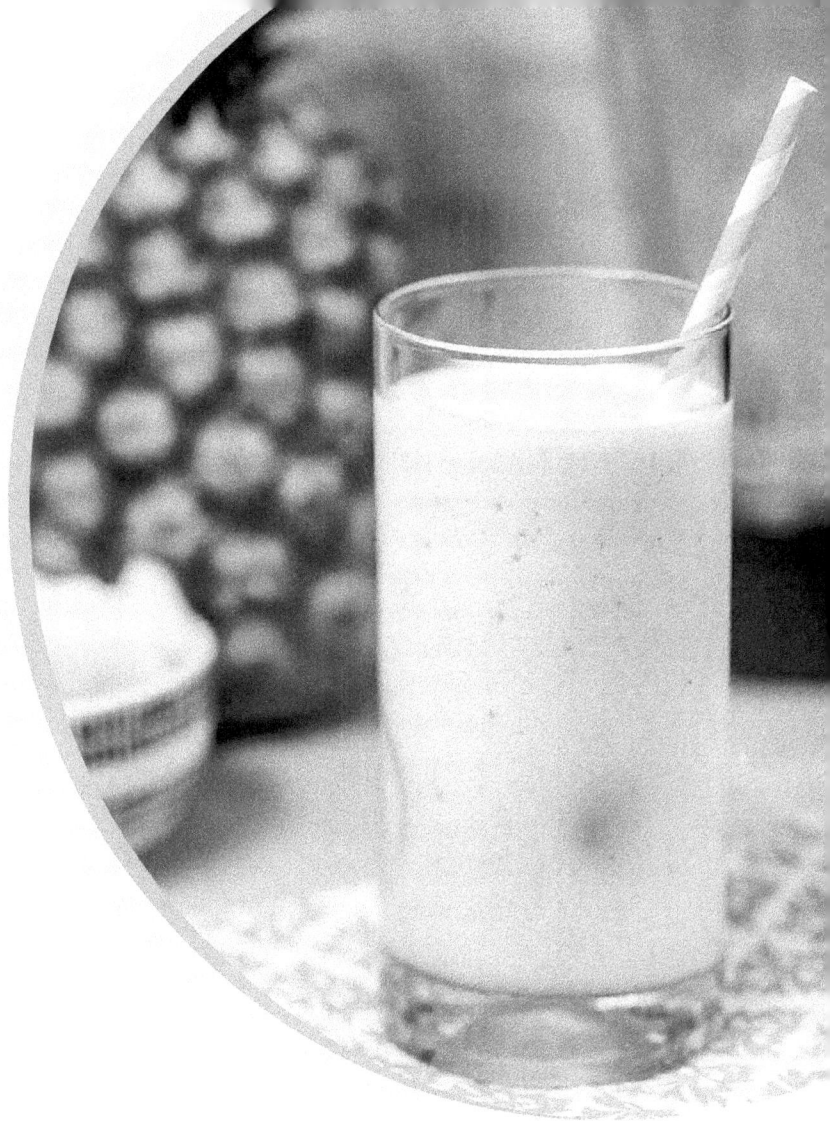

Preparation Time: 5 minutes

Cooking Time: 2 minutes

Servings: 1

INGREDIENTS:

- 1/2 cup unsweetened vanilla almond milk
- 1/2 cup unsweetened coconut milk
- 3/4 cup frozen pineapple chunks
- 1 scoop vanilla protein powder
- 1 tsp raw honey
- 1 tsp vanilla

DIRECTIONS:

1. Place almond milk, coconut milk, pineapple, vanilla protein powder, honey, and vanilla in a blender.
2. Blend until smooth. Serve immediately.

NUTRITION:

Calories: 241

Fat: 7g

Carbs: 20g

Protein: 26g

Sodium: 420mg

Potassium: 205mg

Phosphorus: 10mg

118 HOLIDAY CIDER

Preparation Time: 10 minutes

Cooking Time: 2 hours

Servings: 8

INGREDIENTS:

- 1 orange
- 2 teaspoons whole clove
- 1 apple
- 1 teaspoon whole allspice
- 4 cinnamon sticks
- 1 gal apple cider (4 L)
- ½ cup brown sugar (110 g)
- 1 teaspoon nutmeg
- whiskey, or rum, optional

DIRECTIONS:

1. Season orange with cloves. (If you have an infuser, tea bag or cheese cloth, you can use that to keep the spices under control).
2. Pierce apple with allspice.
3. Put the orange, apple, cinnamon sticks, apple cider, brown sugar and nutmeg into
4. your slow cooker.
5. Turn on high for 2 hours, then keep warm on low until you're ready to drink.
6. Drink as is or with a shot (or two) of whiskey, rum, etc. Enjoy.

NUTRITION:

Calories: 98

Fat: 0.3g

Carbs: 27g

Protein: 1g

Sodium: 2.6mg

Potassium: 84.6mg

Phosphorus: 16mg

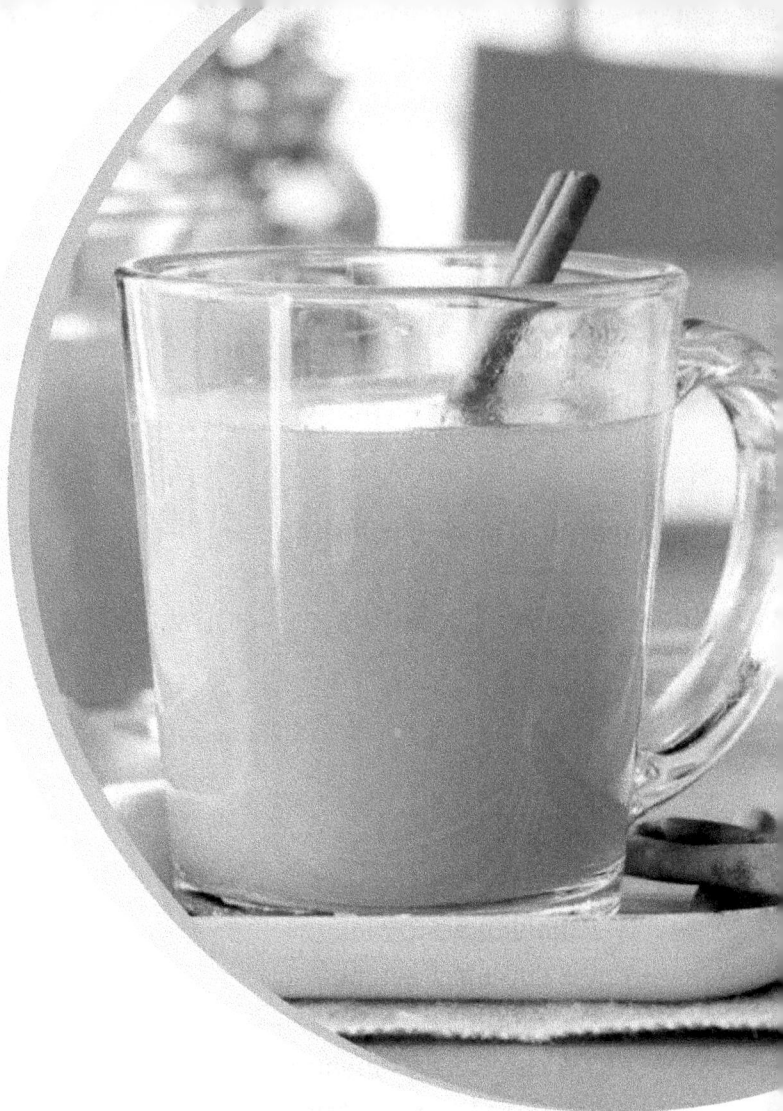

119 CARROT PEACH WATER

Preparation Time: 5 minutes

Cooking Time: 10 minutes

Servings: 10

INGREDIENTS:

- 2 peaches, peeled, pitted, and chopped
- 1 large carrot, peeled and grated
- 1-inch piece peeled fresh ginger, lightly crushed
- 3 fresh thyme sprigs
- 10 c. water

DIRECTIONS:

1. Place the peaches, carrot, ginger, and thyme in a large pitcher.
2. Pour in the water and stir the mixture.
3. Place the pitcher in the refrigerator and leave to infuse, overnight if possible.
4. Serve cold.

NUTRITION:

Calories: 140
Fat: 0g
Carbs: 36g
Protein: 0g
Sodium: 30mg
Potassium: 0mg
Phosphorus: 0mg

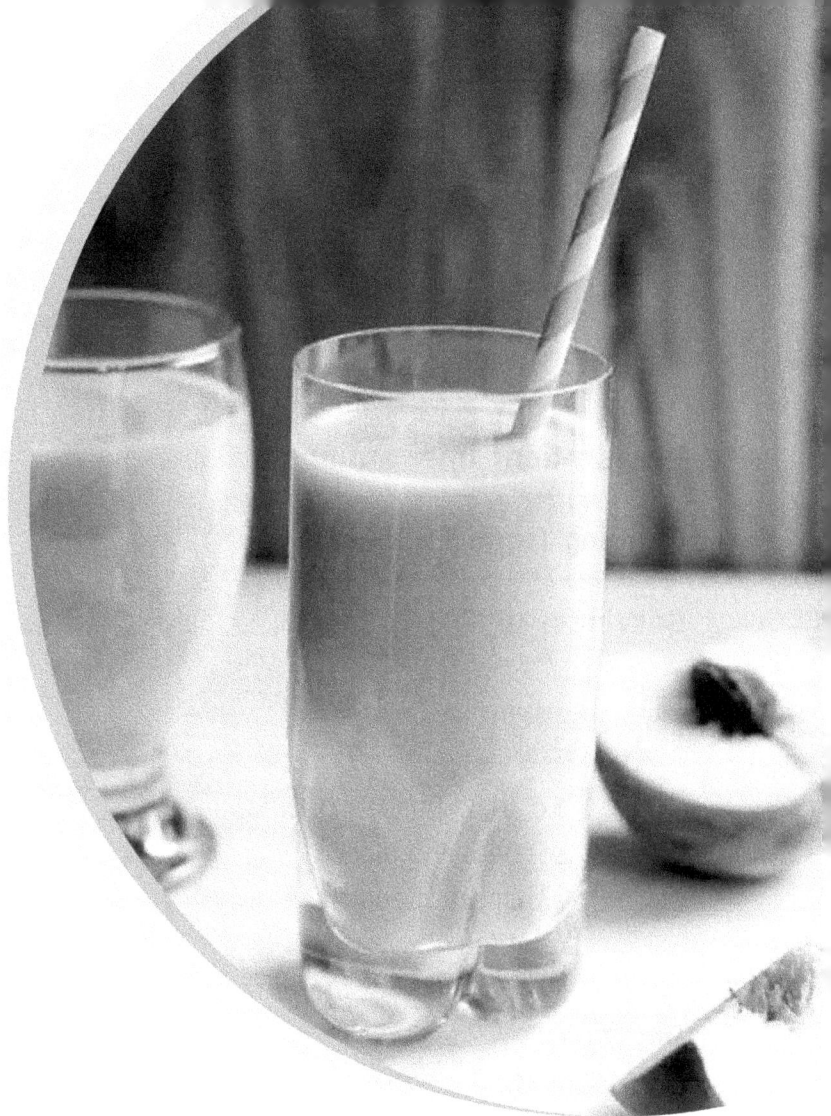

120 PAPAYA MINT WATER

Preparation Time: 5 minutes

Cooking Time: 5 minutes

Servings: 10

INGREDIENTS:

- 1 c. fresh papaya, peeled, seeded, and diced
- 2 tbsp. chopped fresh mint leaves
- 10 c. distilled or filtered water

Directions:

1. Place the papaya and mint in a large pitcher. Pour in the water.
2. Stir and place the pitcher in the refrigerator to infuse, overnight if possible.
3. Serve cold.

NUTRITION:

Calories: 5
Fat: 1g
Carbs: 1g
Protein: 2g
Sodium: 15mg
Potassium: 0mg
Phosphorus: 0mg

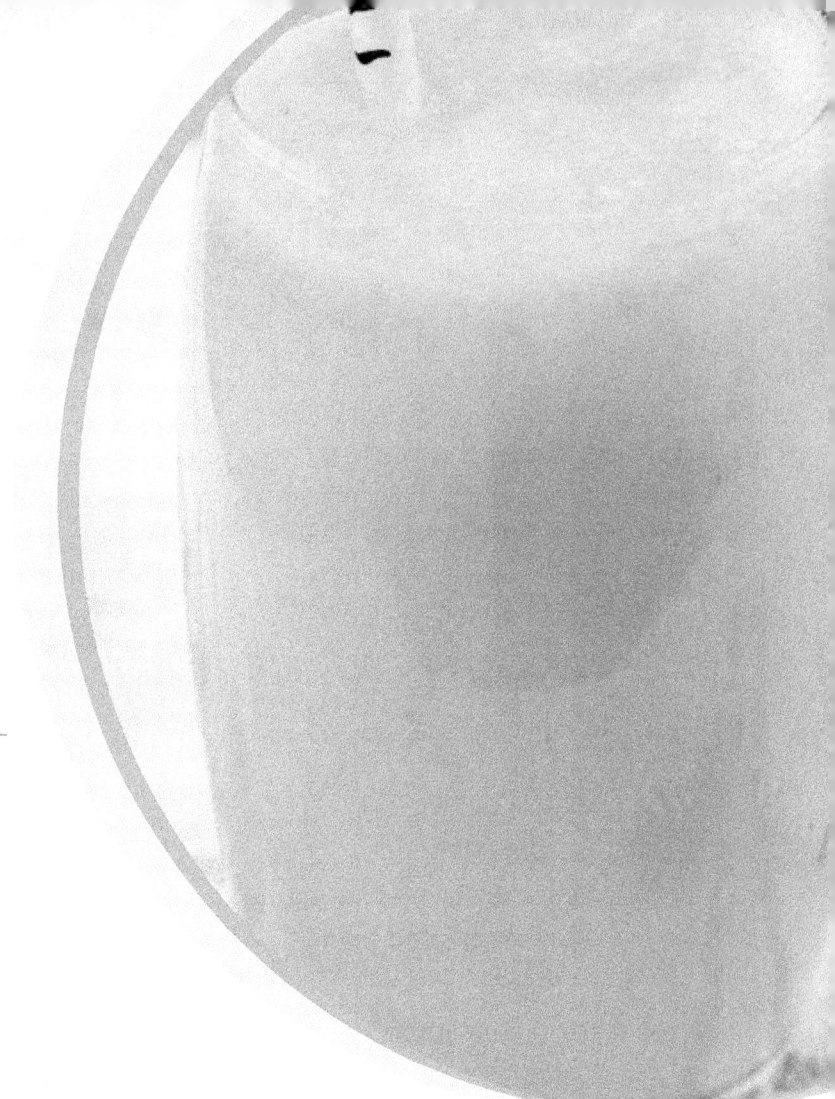

121 RASPBERRY CUCUMBER SMOOTHIE

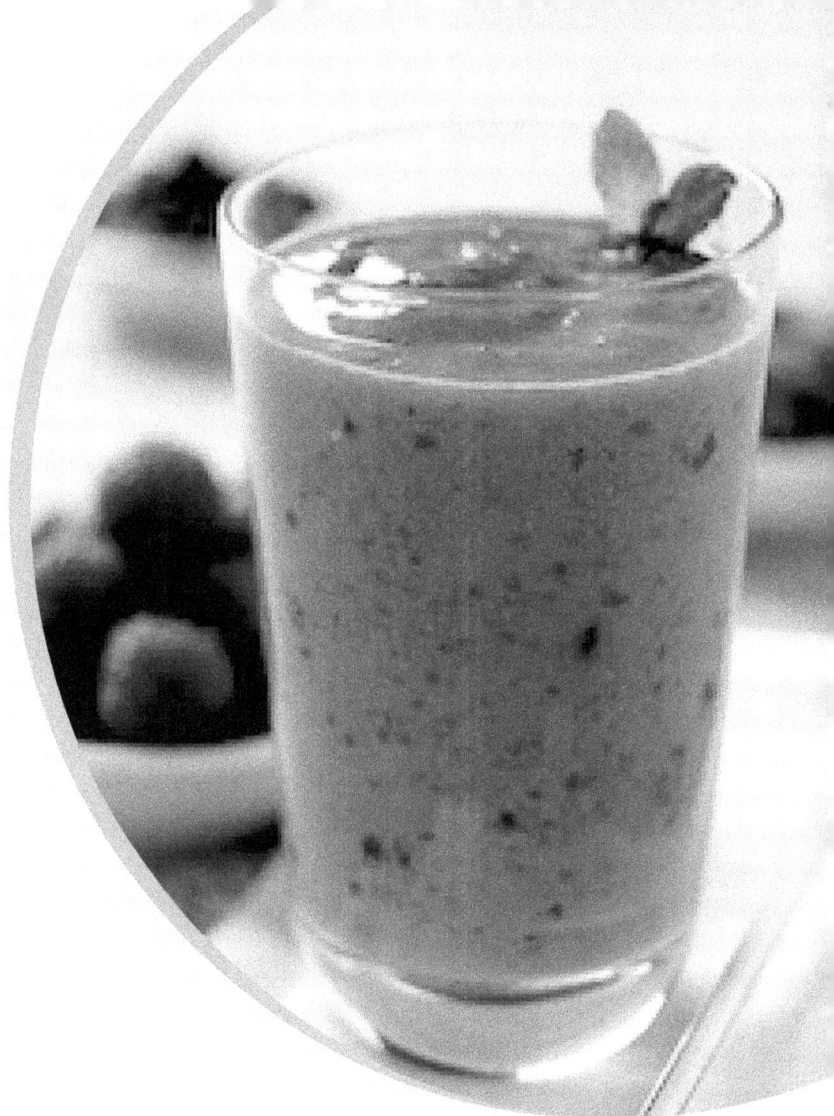

Preparation Time: 5 minutes

Cooking Time: 5 minutes

Servings: 2

INGREDIENTS:

- 1 c. fresh or frozen raspberries
- ½ c. diced English cucumber
- 1 c. Homemade Rice Milk (or use unsweetened store-bought) or almond milk
- 2 tsp. chia seeds
- 1 tsp. honey
- 3 ice cubes

DIRECTIONS:

1. Place the raspberries, cucumber, rice milk, chia seeds, and honey in a blender. Then, blend until smooth.
2. Add the ice cubes. Then, blend until thick and smooth.
3. Pour into two tall glasses. Serve immediately.

NUTRITION:

Calories: 125
Fat: 1.1g
Carbs: 23.5g
Protein: 6g
Sodium: 44mg
Potassium: 199mg
Phosphorus: 54mg

122 SUNNY PINEAPPLE SMOOTHIE

Preparation Time: 5 minutes

Cooking Time: 5 minutes

Servings: 2

INGREDIENTS:

- 1/2 c. frozen pineapple chunks
- 2/3 c. almond milk
- 1/2 tsp. ginger powder
- 1 tbsp. agave syrup

DIRECTIONS:

1. Prepare a blender and mix everything until nice and smooth (around 30 seconds).
2. Transfer into a tall glass or Mason jar.
3. Serve and enjoy.

NUTRITION:

Calories: 144
Fat: 0.36g
Carbs: 37g
Protein: 1.6g
Sodium: 354mg
Potassium: 1000mg
Phosphorus: 40mg

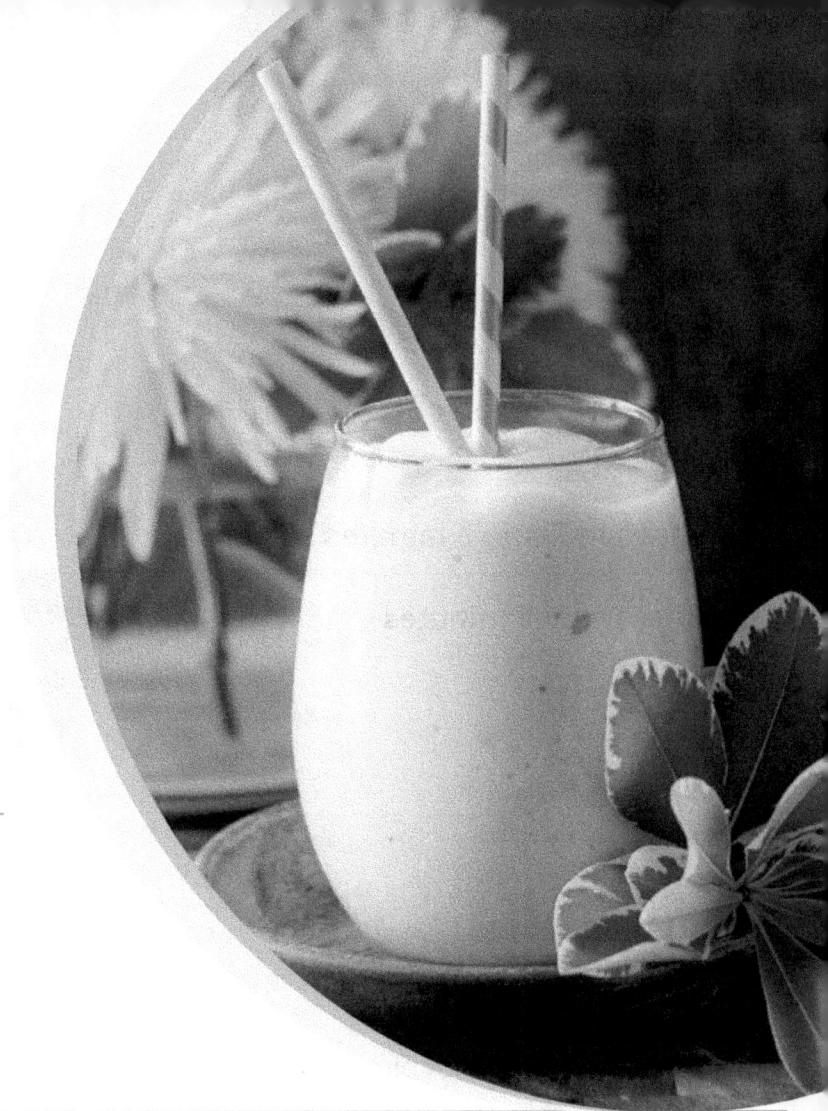

123 MANGO CHEESECAKE SMOOTHIE

Preparation Time: 5 minutes

Cooking Time: 5 minutes

Servings: 2

INGREDIENTS:

- 1 c. Homemade Rice Milk
- ½ ripe fresh mango, peeled and chopped
- 2 tbsp. cream cheese, at room temperature
- 1 tsp. honey
- ½ vanilla bean split and seeds scraped out
- Pinch ground nutmeg
- 3 ice cubes

DIRECTIONS:

1. Place the rice milk, mango, cream cheese, honey, vanilla bean seeds, and nutmeg in a blender, and blend until smooth and thick.
2. Add the ice cubes and blend.
3. Serve in two glasses immediately.

NUTRITION:

Calories: 177
Fat: 4g
Carbs: 10g
Protein: 24g
Sodium: 346mg
Potassium: 66mg
Phosphorus: 62mg

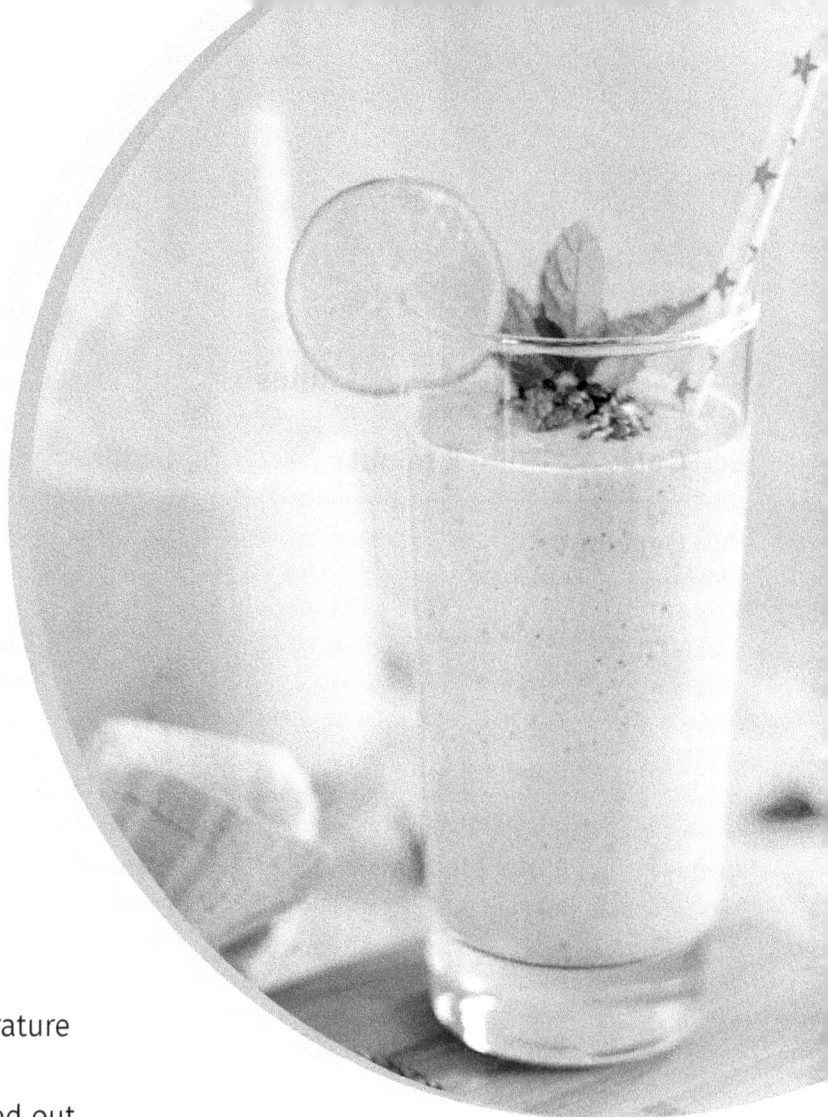

124 HOT COCOA

Preparation Time: 5 minutes

Cooking Time: 5 minutes

Servings: 1

INGREDIENTS:

- 1 tbsp. cocoa powder, unsweetened
- 2 tsp. Splenda granulated sugar
- 3 tbsp. whipped dessert topping
- 1 c. water, at room temperature
- 2 tbsp. water, cold

DIRECTIONS:

1. Place a saucepan over medium heat and let it heat until hot.
2. Take a cup, place cocoa powder and sugar in it, pour in cold water, and mix well.
3. Then slowly stir in hot water until cocoa mixture dissolves and top with whipped topping.
4. Serve straight away.

NUTRITION:

Calories: 120
Fat: 3g
Carbs: 23g
Protein: 1g
Sodium: 110mg
Potassium: 199mg
Phosphorus: 88mg

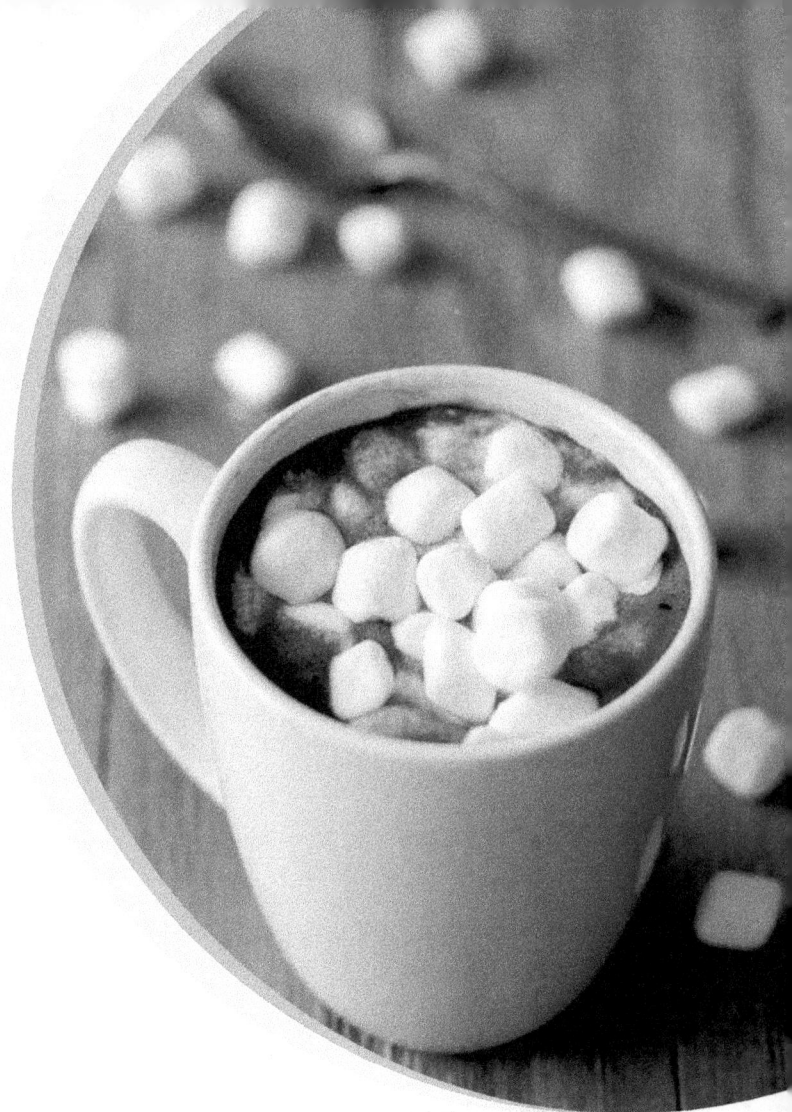

125 RICE MILK

Preparation Time: 2 minutes

Cooking Time: 2 minutes

Servings: 2

INGREDIENTS:

- 1 c. rice milk, unenriched, chilled
- 1 scoop vanilla whey protein

DIRECTIONS:

1. Pour milk in a blender, add whey protein, and then pulse until well blended.
2. Distribute the milk into two glasses and serve.

NUTRITION:

Calories: 120
Fat: 2g
Carbs: 24g
Protein: 0g
Sodium: 86mg
Potassium: 27mg
Phosphorus: 56mg

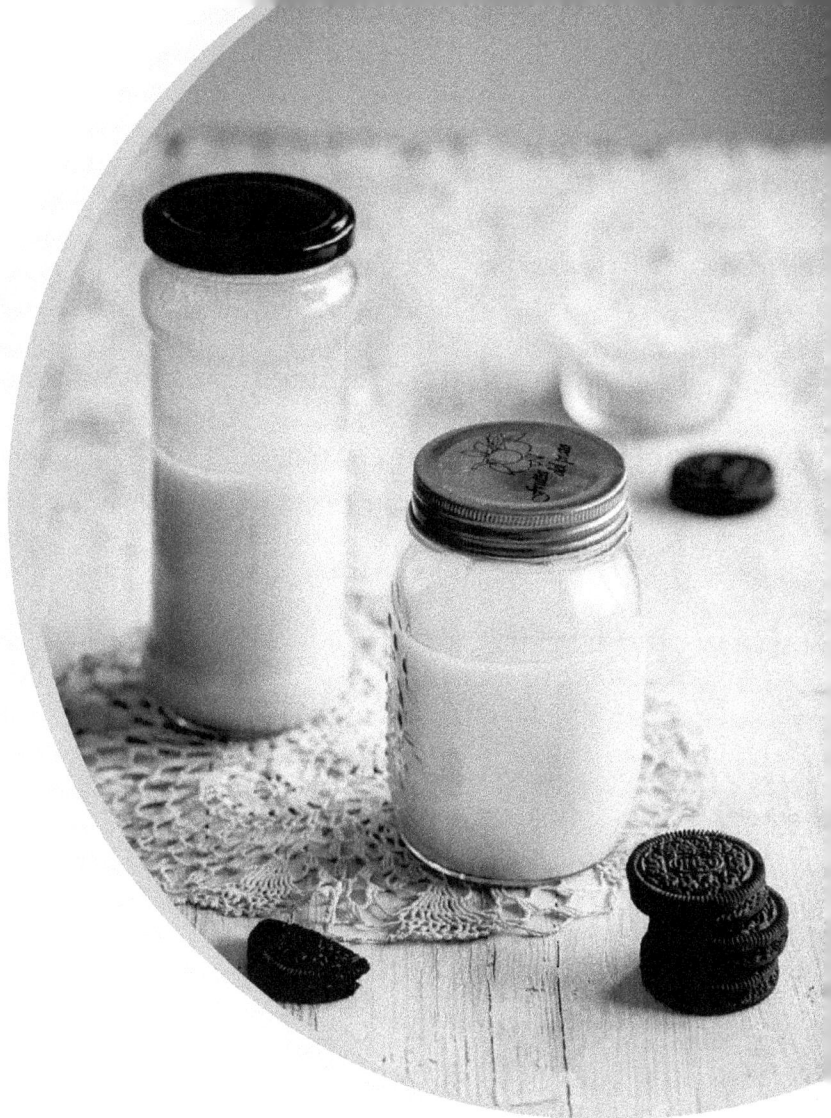

126 ALMOND MILK

Preparation Time: 3 minutes

Cooking Time: 2 minutes

Servings: 3

INGREDIENTS:

- 1 c. almonds, soaked in warm water for 10 minutes
- 1 tsp. vanilla extract, unsweetened
- 3 c. filtered water

DIRECTIONS:

1. Drain the soaked almonds, place them into the blender, pour in water, and blend for 2 minutes until almonds are chopped.
2. Strain the milk by passing it through cheesecloth into a bowl, discard almond meal, and then stir vanilla into the milk.
3. Cover the milk, refrigerate until chilled, and when ready to serve, stir it well, pour the milk evenly into the glasses and then serve.

NUTRITION:

Calories: 30
Fat: 2.5g
Carbs: 1g
Protein: 1g
Sodium: 170mg
Potassium: 140mgmg
Phosphorus: 30mg

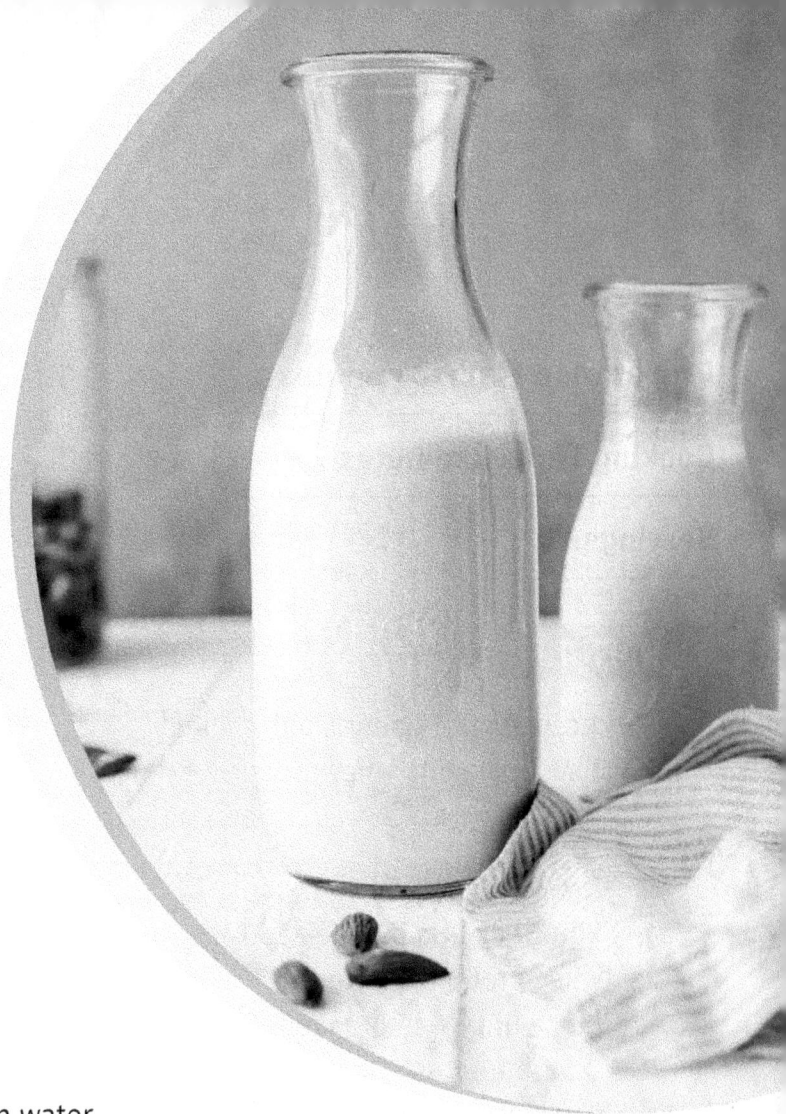

127 CUCUMBER AND LEMON-FLAVORED WATER

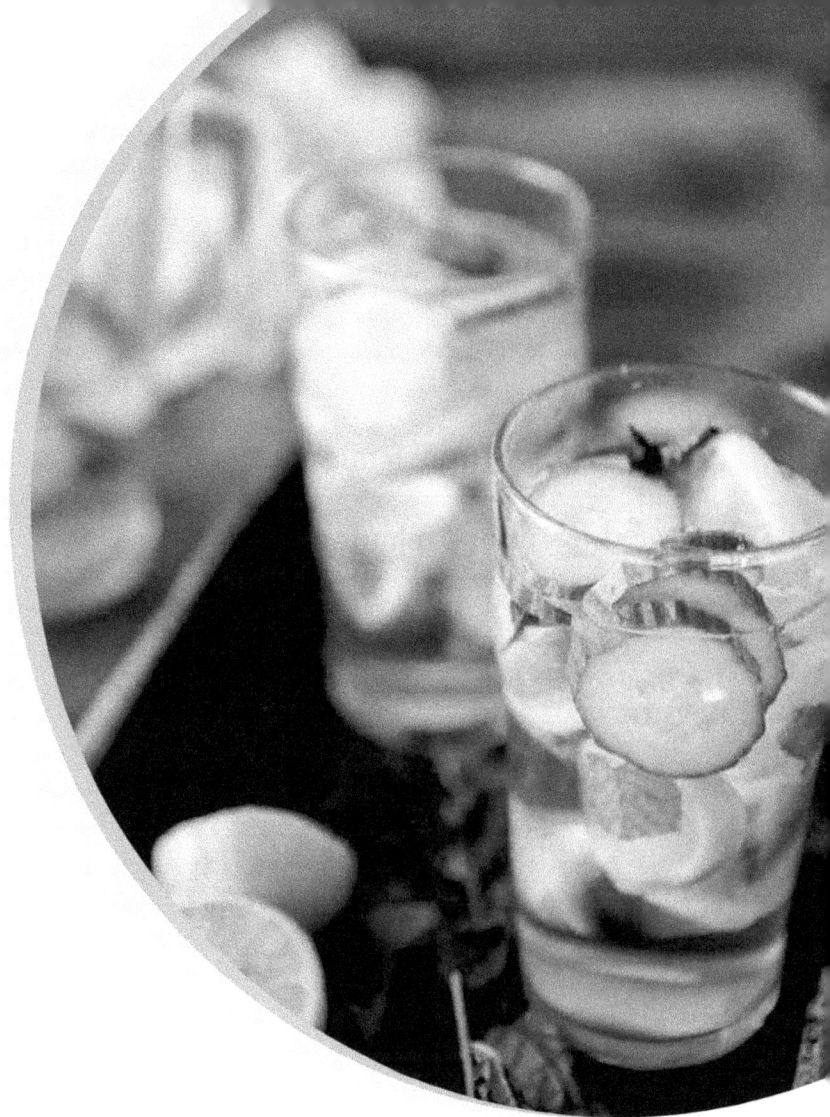

Preparation Time: 5 minutes

Cooking Time: 3 hours

Servings: 10

INGREDIENTS:

- · 1 lemon, deseeded, sliced
- · ¼ c. fresh mint leaves, chopped
- · 1 medium cucumber, sliced
- · ¼ c. fresh basil leaves, chopped
- · 10 c. water

DIRECTIONS:

1. Place the papaya and mint in a large pitcher. Pour in the water.
2. Stir and place the pitcher in the refrigerator to infuse, overnight if possible.
3. Serve cold.

NUTRITION:

Calories: 10
Fat: 0g
Carbs: 2.25g
Protein: 0.12g
Sodium: 2.5mg
Potassium: 8.9mg
Phosphorus: 10mg

BLUEBERRY SMOOTHIE

Preparation Time: 5 minutes

Cooking Time: 2 minutes

Servings: 4

INGREDIENTS:

- 1 c. frozen blueberries
- 6 tbsp. protein powder
- 8 packets Splenda
- 14 oz. apple juice, unsweetened
- 8 cubes of ice

DIRECTIONS:

1. Take a blender and place all the ingredients (in order) in it. Process for 1 minute until smooth.
2. Distribute the smoothie between four glasses and then serve.

NUTRITION:

Calories: 162
Fat: 0.5g
Carbs: 30g
Protein: 8g
Sodium: 123.4mg
Potassium: 223mg
Phosphorus: 109mg

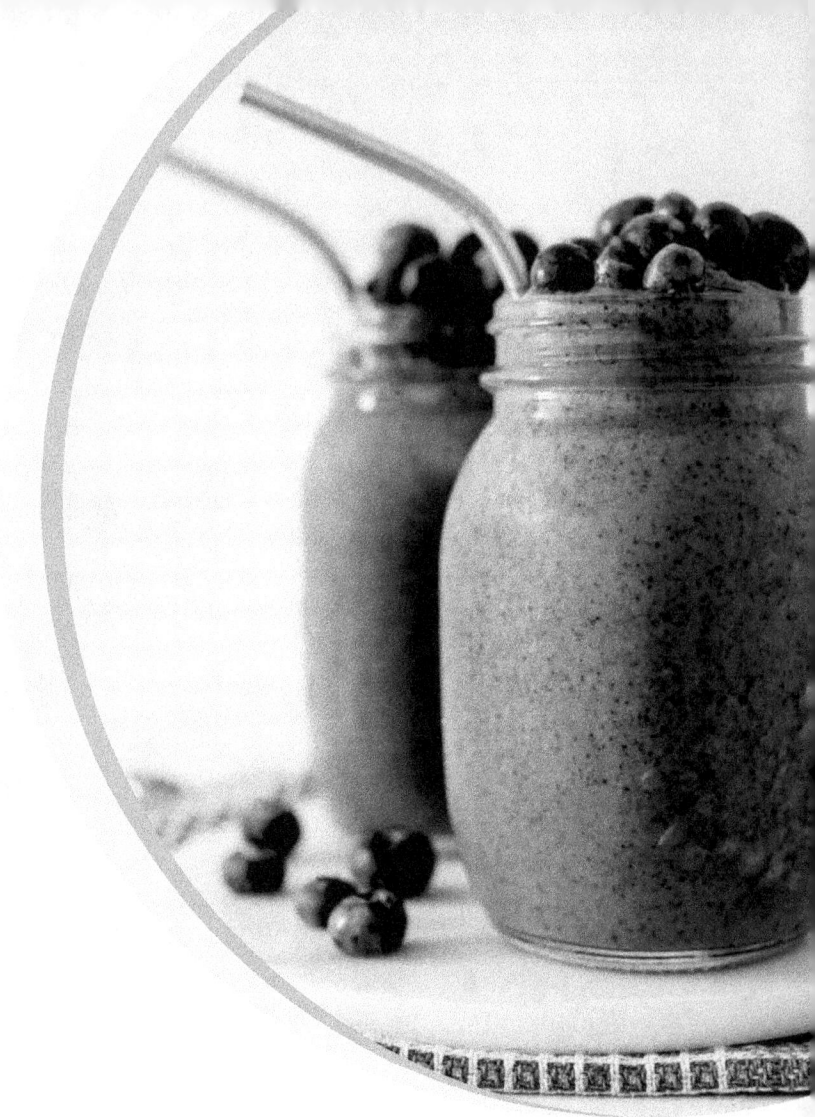

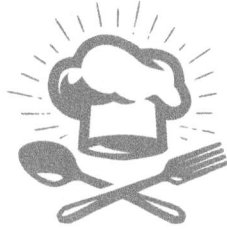

CHAPTER 18

FISH AND SEAFOOD

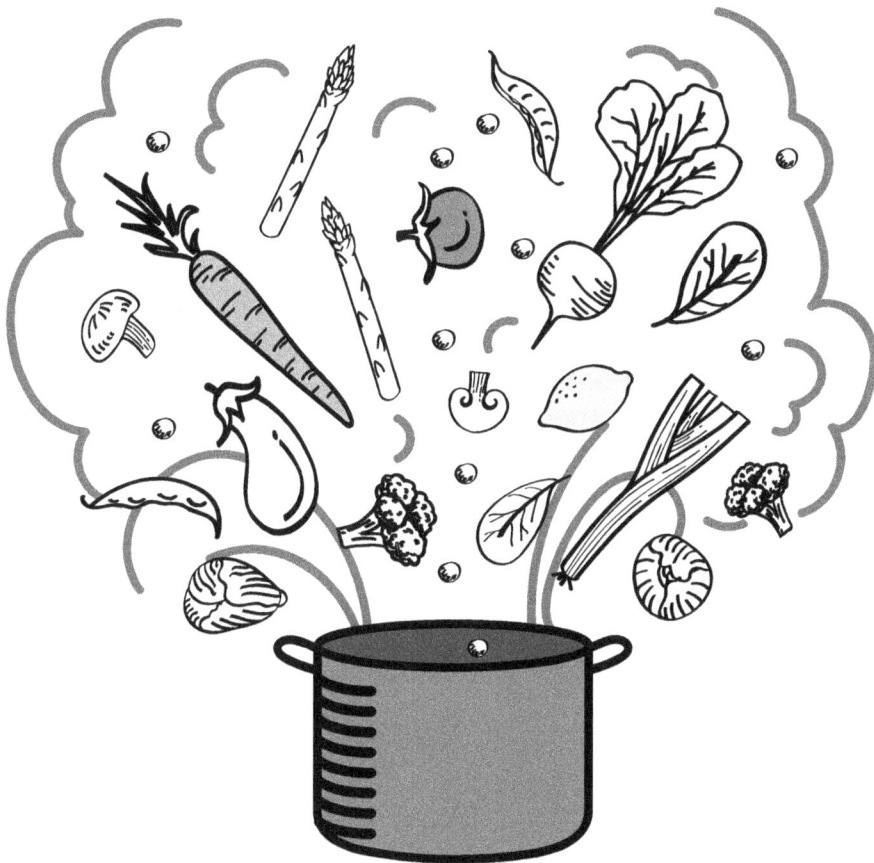

129 SHRIMP SCAMPI LINGUINE

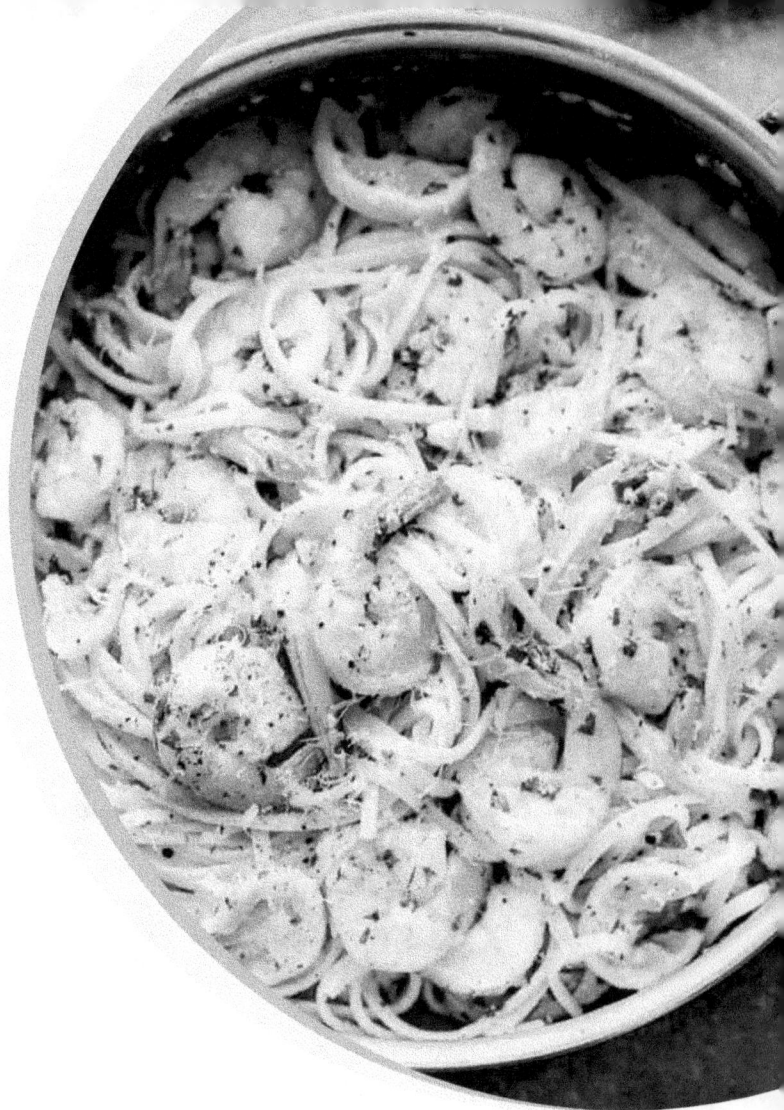

Preparation Time: 15 minutes

Cooking Time: 15 minutes

Serving: 4

INGREDIENTS:

- 4 ounces Uncooked linguine
- 1 tsp. Olive oil
- 2 tsp Minced garlic
- 4 ounces peeled and chopped Shrimp
- ½ cup Dry white wine
- Juice of 1 lemon
- 1 tbsp Chopped fresh basil
- ½ cup Heavy whipping cream
- Ground black pepper

DIRECTIONS:

1. Prepare the linguine according to package instructions.
2. Heat the olive oil in a skillet.
3. Sauté the garlic and shrimp for 6 minutes or until the shrimp is opaque and just cooked through.
4. Add the lemon juice, wine, and basil. Cook for 5 minutes.
5. Stir in the cream and simmer for 2 minutes more.
6. Add the linguine to the skillet and toss to coat.
7. Divide the pasta onto 4 plates to serve.

NUTRITION:

Calories: 219

Fat: 7g

Carb: 21g

Protein: 12g

Sodium: 42mg

Potassium: 155mg

Phosphorus: 119mg

130 GRILLED SHRIMP WITH CUCUMBER LIME SALSA

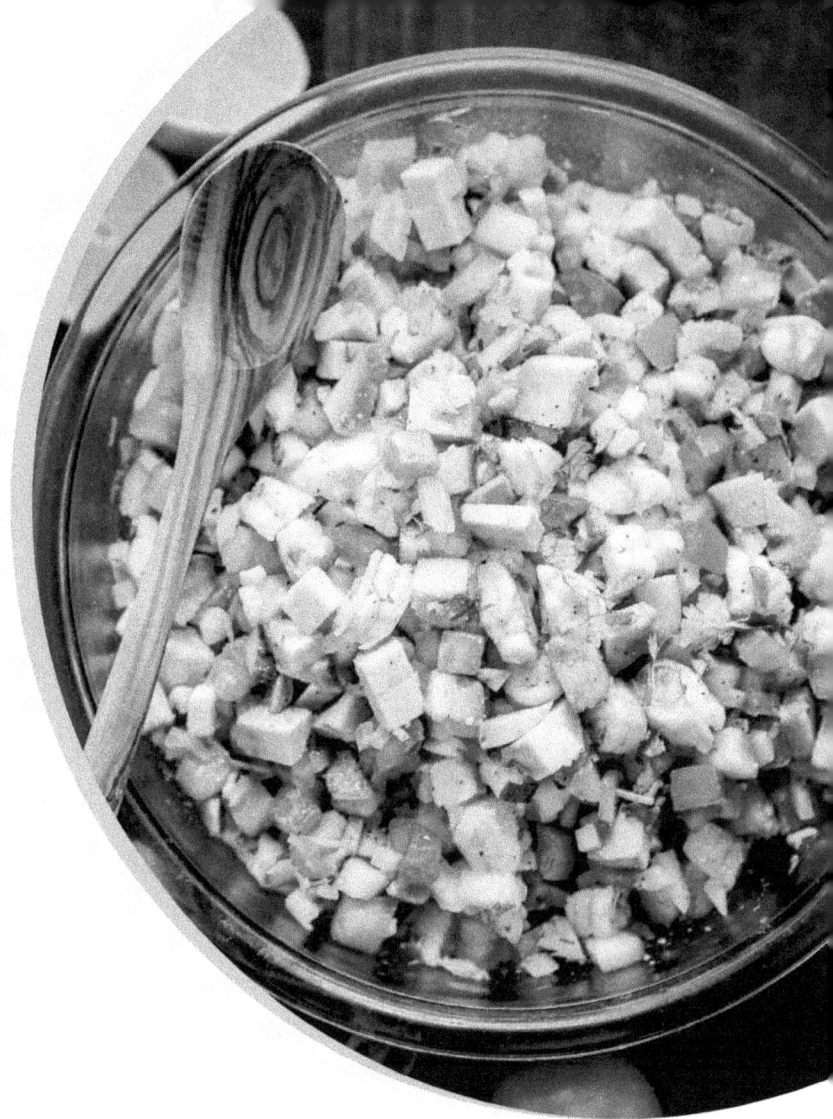

Preparation Time: 15 minutes

Cooking Time: 10 minutes

Serving: 4

INGREDIENTS:

- 2 tbsp. Olive oil
- 6 ounces, peeled and deveined, tails left on Large shrimp
- 1 tsp Minced garlic
- ½ cup Chopped English cucumber
- ½ cup Chopped mango
- Zest of 1 lime
- Juice of 1 lime
- Ground black pepper
- Lime wedges for garnish

DIRECTIONS:

1. Soak 4 wooden skewers in water for 30 minutes.
2. Preheat the barbecue to medium heat.
3. In a bowl, toss together the olive oil, shrimp, and garlic.
4. Thread the shrimp onto the skewers, about 4 shrimp per skewer.
5. In a bowl, stir together the mango, cucumber, lime zest, and lime juice and season the salsa lightly with pepper. Set aside.
6. Grill the shrimp for 10 minutes, turning once or until the shrimp is opaque and cooked through.
7. Season the shrimp lightly with pepper.
8. Serve the shrimp on the cucumber salsa with lime wedges on the side.

NUTRITION:

Calories: 120   Carb: 4g   Sodium: 60mg   Phosphorus: 91mg
Fat: 8g   Protein: 9g   Potassium: 129mg

131 CRAB CAKES WITH LIME SALSA

Preparation Time: 20 minutes

Cooking Time: 20 minutes

Serving: 4

INGREDIENTS:

For the Salsa
- ½, diced English cucumber
- 1, chopped Lime
- ½ cup Boiled and chopped red bell pepper
- 1 tsp Chopped fresh cilantro
- Ground black pepper

For the crab cakes
- 8 ounces Queen crab meat
- ¼ cup Breadcrumbs
- 1 Small egg
- ¼ cup Boiled and chopped red bell pepper
- 1, both green and white parts, minced Scallion
- 1 tbsp Chopped fresh parsley
- Splash hot sauce
- Olive oil spray, for the pan

DIRECTIONS:

1. Combine the lime, cucumber, red pepper, and cilantro in a small bowl to make the salsa. Season with pepper and set aside.
2. To make the crab cakes, mix the breadcrumbs, crab, red pepper, egg, scallion, parsley, and hot sauce until it holds together in a bowl. Add more if necessary.

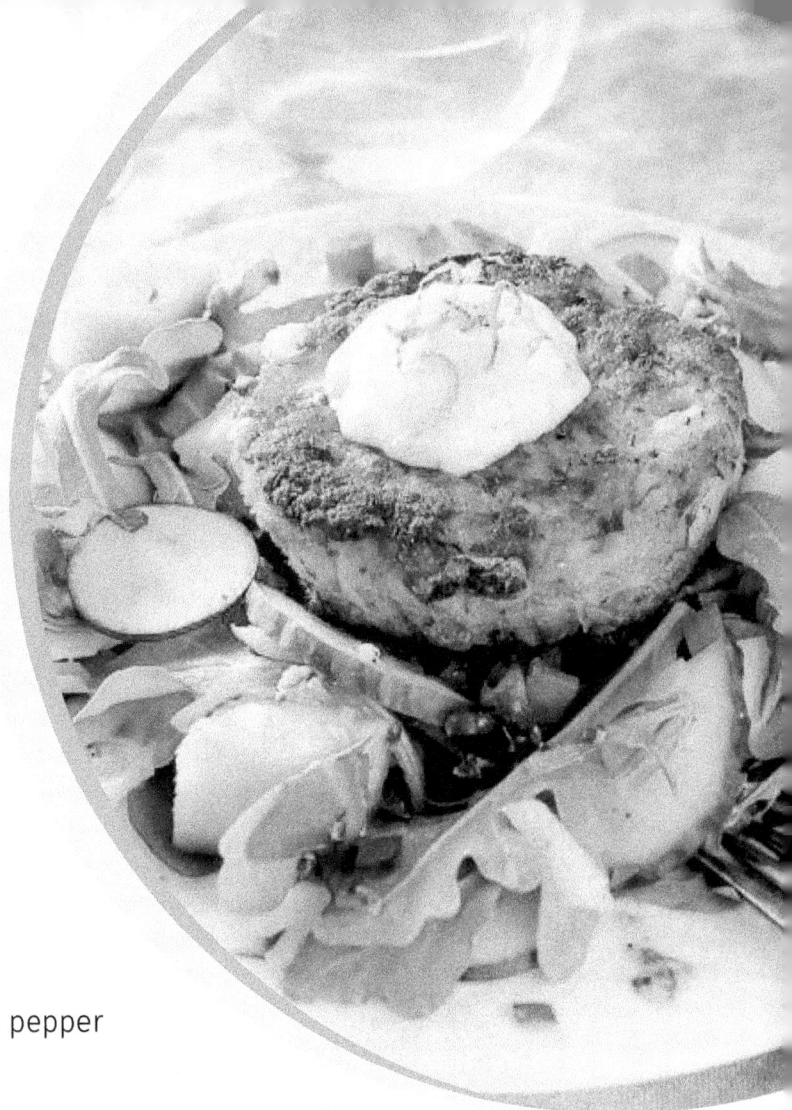

3. Form the crab mixture into 4 patties.
4. Refrigerate for 1 hour to firm them.
5. Place the skillet on medium heat and spray with olive oil.
6. Cook the crab cakes in batches, turning, for about 5 minutes per side or until golden brown.
7. Serve the crab cakes with salsa.

NUTRITION:

Calories: 115
Fat: 2g
Carb: 7g
Protein: 16g
Sodium: 421mg
Potassium: 200mg
Phosphorus: 110mg

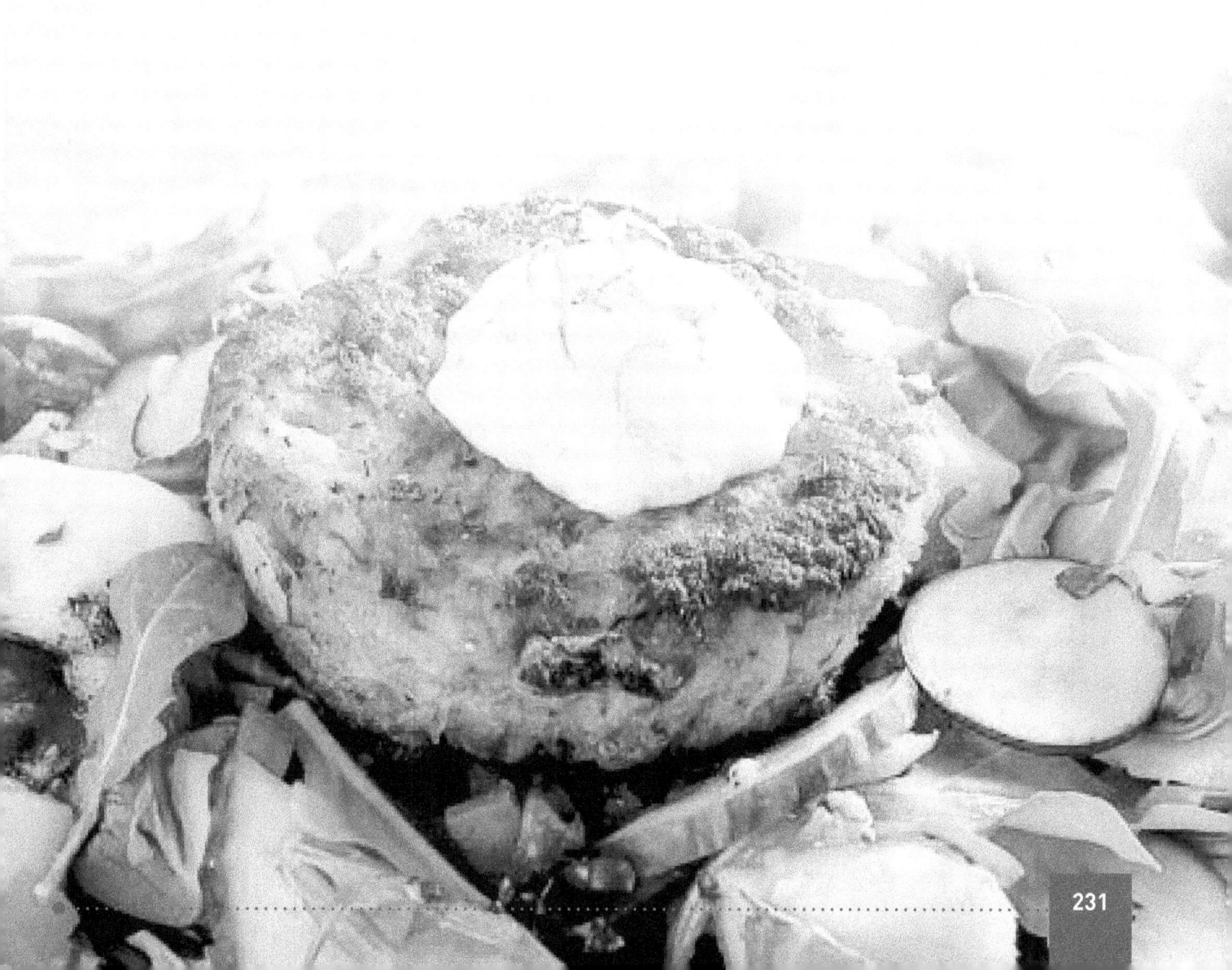

132 SWEET GLAZED SALMON

Preparation Time: 10 minutes

Cooking Time: 10 minutes

Serving: 4

INGREDIENTS:

- · 2 tbsp Honey
- · 1 tsp Lemon zest
- · ½ tsp Ground black pepper
- · 4 (3-ounce) each
  Salmon fillets
- · 1 tbsp Olive oil
- · ½, white and green parts, chopped Scallion

DIRECTIONS:

1. In a bowl, stir together the lemon zest, honey, and pepper.
2. Wash the salmon and pat dry with paper towels.
3. Rub the honey mixture all over each fillet.
4. In a large skillet, heat the olive oil.
5. Add the salmon fillets and cook the salmon for 10 minutes, turning once, or until it is lightly browned and just cooked through.
6. Serve topped with chopped scallion.

NUTRITION:

Calories: 240

Fat: 15g

Carb: 9g

Protein: 17g

Sodium: 51mg

Potassium: 317mg

Phosphorus: 205mg

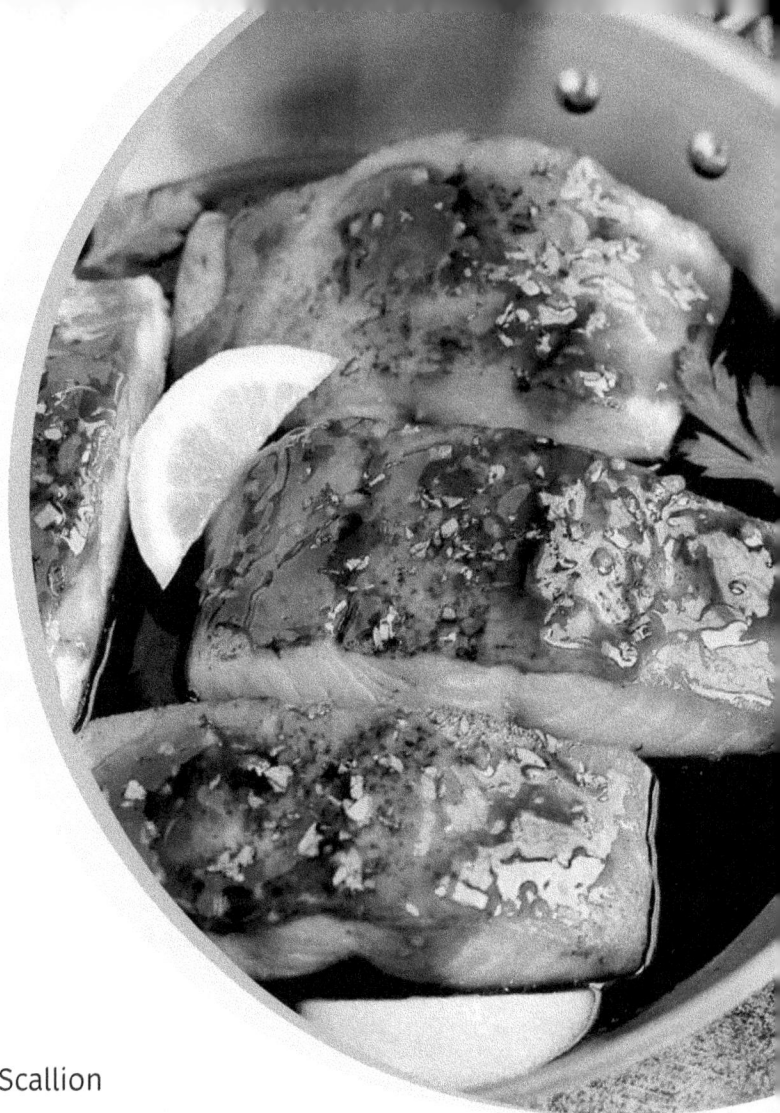

133 HERB-CRUSTED BAKED HADDOCK

Preparation Time: 10 minutes

Cooking Time: 20 minutes

Serving: 4

INGREDIENTS:

- ½ cup Breadcrumbs
- 3 tbsp Chopped fresh parsley
- 1 tbsp Lemon zest
- 1 tsp Chopped fresh thyme
- ¼ tsp Ground black pepper
- 1 tbsp Melted unsalted butter
-

  12-ounces, deboned and skinned Haddock fillets

DIRECTIONS:

1. Preheat the oven to 350F.
2. In a bowl, stir together the parsley, breadcrumbs, lemon zest, thyme, and pepper until well combined.
3. Add the melted butter and toss until the mixture resembles coarse crumbs.
4. Place the haddock on a baking sheet and spoon the bread crumb mixture on top, pressing down firmly.
5. Bake the haddock in the oven for 20 minutes or until the fish is just cooked through and flakes off in chunks when pressed.

NUTRITION:

Calories: 143
Fat: 4g
Carb: 10g
Protein: 16g

Sodium: 281mg
Potassium: 285mg
Phosphorus: 216mg

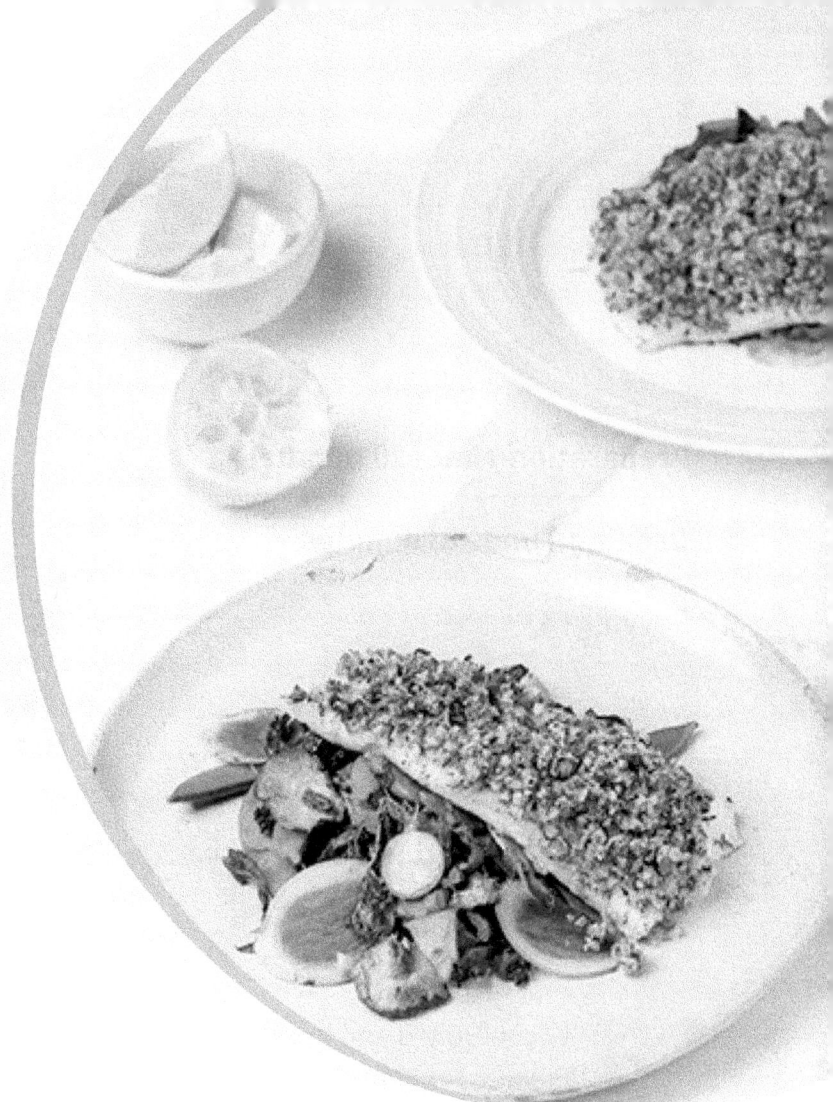

BAKED COD WITH SALSA

Preparation Time: 20 minutes

Cooking Time: 10 minutes

Serving: 4

INGREDIENTS:

For the salsa
- ½, chopped English cucumber
- 2 tbsp.   Chopped fresh dill
- Juice of 1 lime
- Zest of 1 lime
- ¼ cup Boiled and minced red bell pepper
- ½ tsp.   Granulated sugar

For the fish
- 12 ounces, deboned and cut into 4 servings Cod fillets
- Juice of 1 lemon
- ½ tsp Ground black pepper
- 1 tsp Olive oil

DIRECTIONS:

1. To make the cucumber salsa: in a bowl, mix the salsa ingredients and set aside.
2. To make the fish: preheat the oven to 350F.
3. Put the fish on a pie plate and add the lemon juice over the fillets.
4. Sprinkle with pepper and drizzle the olive oil evenly over the fillets.
5. Bake the fish for 6 minutes or until it flakes easily with a fork.
6. Transfer the fish to 4 plates and serve topped with cucumber salsa.

NUTRITION:

Calories: 110
Fat: 2g
Carb: 3g

Protein: 20g
Sodium: 67mg

Potassium: 275mg
Phosphorus: 120mg

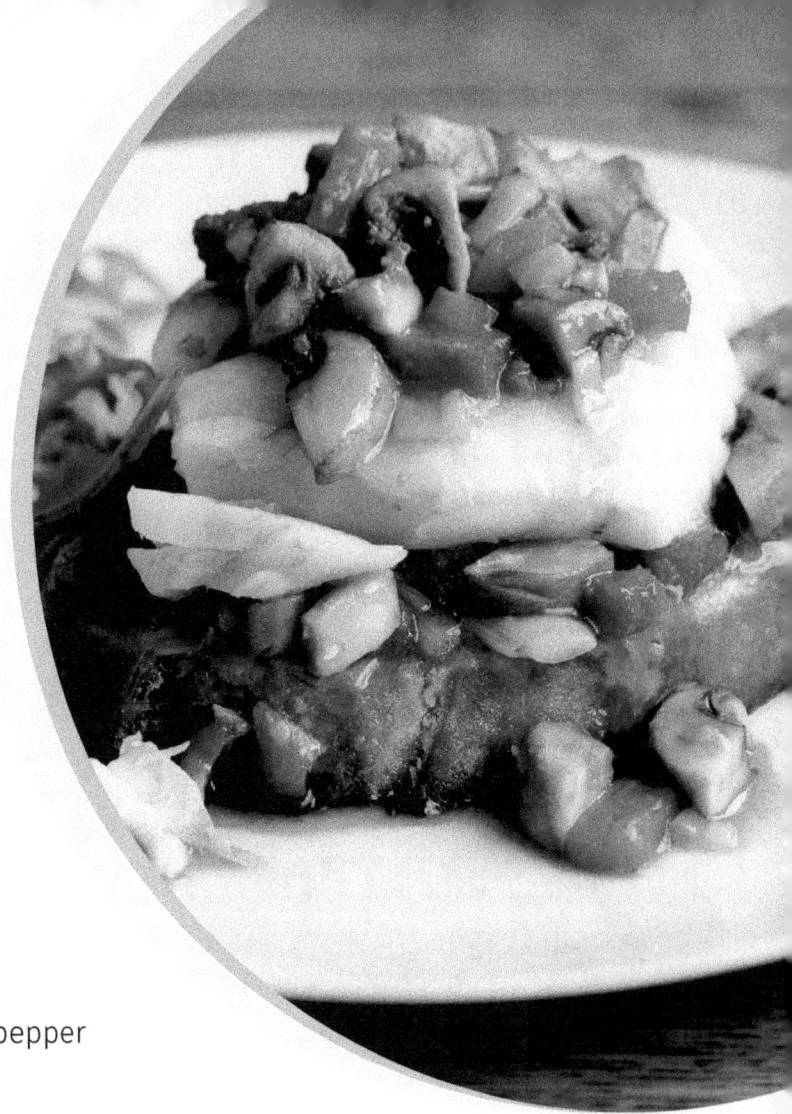

135 CILANTRO-LIME FLOUNDER

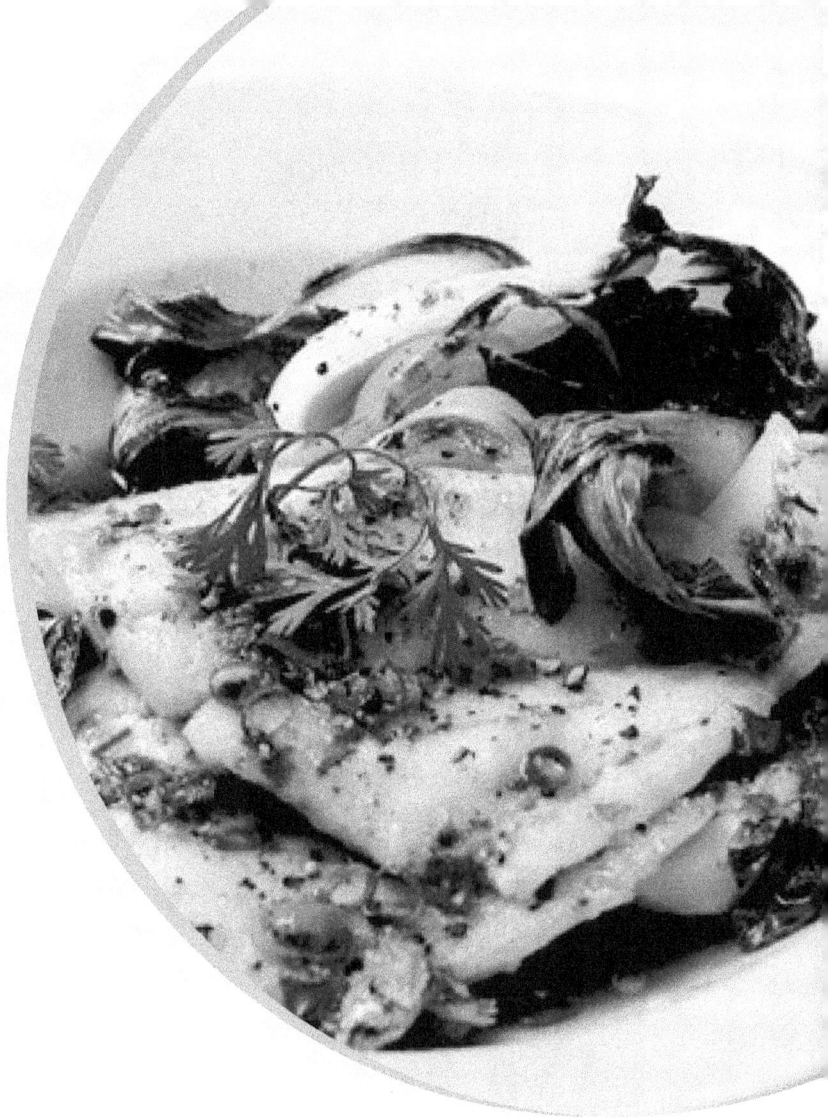

Preparation Time: 20 minutes

Cooking Time: 5 minutes

Serving: 4

INGREDIENTS:

- ¼ cup Homemade mayonnaise
- Juice of 1 lime
- Zest of 1 lime
- ½ cup Chopped fresh cilantro
- 4 (3-ounce) Flounder fillets
- Ground black pepper

DIRECTIONS:

1. Preheat the oven to 400F.
2. In a bowl, stir together the cilantro, lime juice, lime zest, and mayonnaise.
3. Place 4 pieces of foil, about 8 by 8 inches square, on a clean work surface.
4. Place a flounder fillet in the center of each square.
5. Top the fillets evenly with the mayonnaise mixture.
6. Season the flounder with pepper.
7. Fold the foil's sides over the fish, create a snug packet and place the foil packets on a baking sheet.
8. Bake the fish 5 minutes.
9. Unfold the packets and serve.

NUTRITION:

Calories: 92

Fat: 4g

Carb: 2g

Protein: 12g

Sodium: 267mg

Potassium: 137mg

Phosphorus: 208mg

136 COOKED TILAPIA WITH MANGO SALSA

Preparation Time: 2 hours

Cooking Time: 10 minutes

Serving: 2

INGREDIENTS:

- 2 (3 oz. each) Fresh tilapia fillets
- ½, diced Red onion
- ½, diced Red bell pepper
- 2 tbsp Fresh cilantro
- ¼ cup Olive oil
- 1 tsp Black pepper
- 1 Lime
- 4 Crackers/slices of melba toast

DIRECTIONS:

1. Preheat the broiler on medium heat.
2. Cut tilapia into small bite-size pieces.
3. Place tilapia under the broiler for 7 to 10 minutes or until cooked through.
4. Remove and allow to cool in a bowl. Then squeeze the juice from the lime over the top and mix well.
5. Mix the onion, bell pepper, cilantro, mango, pepper, and oil with the cooked tilapia and marinate for 2 hours in the refrigerator.
6. Divide into two bowls and serve with crackers.

NUTRITION:

Calories: 389

Fat: 29g

Carb: 18g

Protein: 17g

Sodium: 134mg

Potassium: 217mg

Phosphorus: 183mg

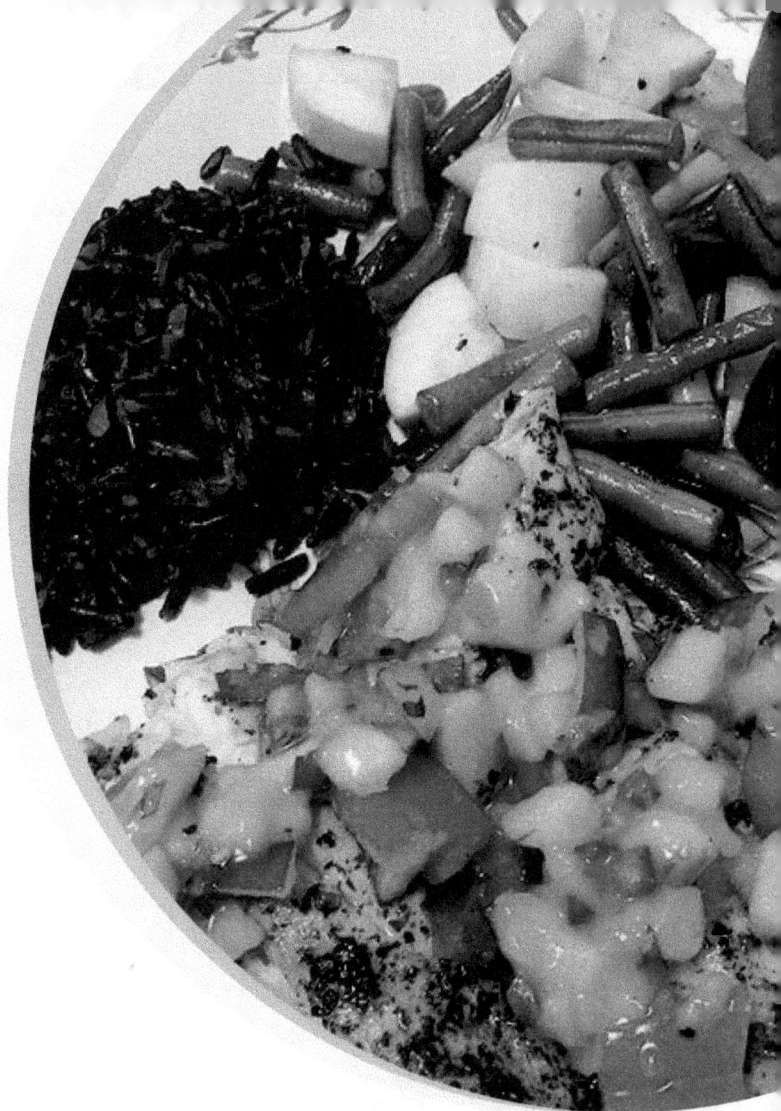

137 CILANTRO AND CHILI INFUSED SWORDFISH

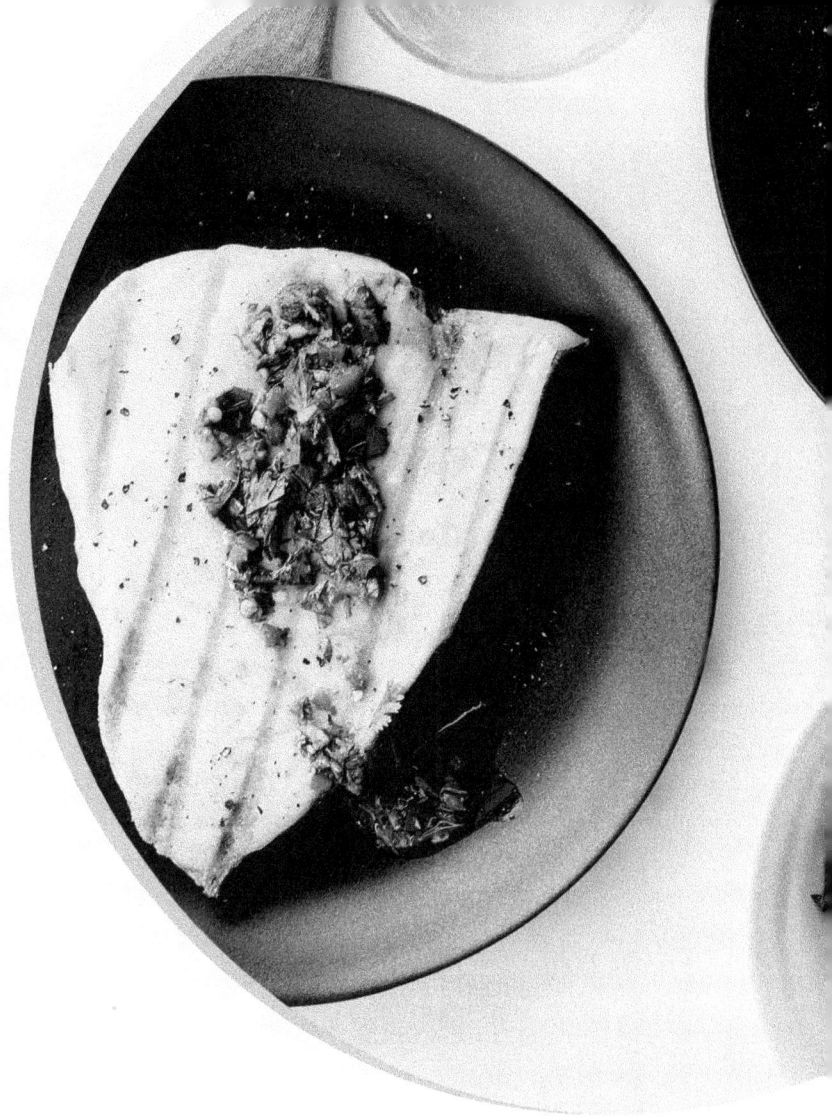

Preparation Time: 30 minutes

Cooking Time: 15 minutes

Serving: 2

INGREDIENTS:

- 2 (30 oz.) Swordfish fillets
- 4 tsp Fresh cilantro
- 1, finely diced Onion
- 1 tsp Brown sugar
- 1 diced Red chili
- 1 Lemon
- 1 tbsp Extra virgin olive oil
- 1 clove, minced Garlic

DIRECTIONS:

1. Soak vegetables in warm water.
2. Meanwhile, add fish to an ovenproof baking dish.
3. Whisk onion, cilantro, chili, sugar, lemon juice, oil, and garlic in another bowl.
4. Pour the marinade over the swordfish and turn the fish over to coat both sides.
5. Cover and marinate in the refrigerator for 30 minutes or more.
6. Preheat the broiler to medium heat.
7. Place oven dish under the broiler for 6 to 7 minutes on each side or until fish flakes easily with a fork. Serve hot.

NUTRITION:

Calories: 340
Fat: 16g
Carb: 25g

Protein: 23g
Sodium: 258mg

Potassium: 243mg
Phosphorus: 284mg

138 CITRUS TUNA CEVICHE

Preparation Time: 5 minutes

Cooking Time: 0 minutes

Serving: 2

INGREDIENTS:

- 1 (5 oz.) drained and rinsed Low-sodium water-packed tuna
- 1 tbsp Cilantro
- ½, diced Red onion
- 1 tsp Black pepper
- 1 Lemon
- 1 tsp Red wine vinegar
- 1, chopped Red bell pepper

DIRECTIONS:

1. Add tuna together with the rest of the ingredients into a serving bowl, mix well and cover plastic wrap.
2. Marinate as long as possible.
3. Serve with a salad or sandwich.

NUTRITION:

Calories: 127
Fat: 1g
Carbs: 10g
Protein: 21g
Sodium: 278mg
Potassium: 149mg
Phosphorus: 116mg

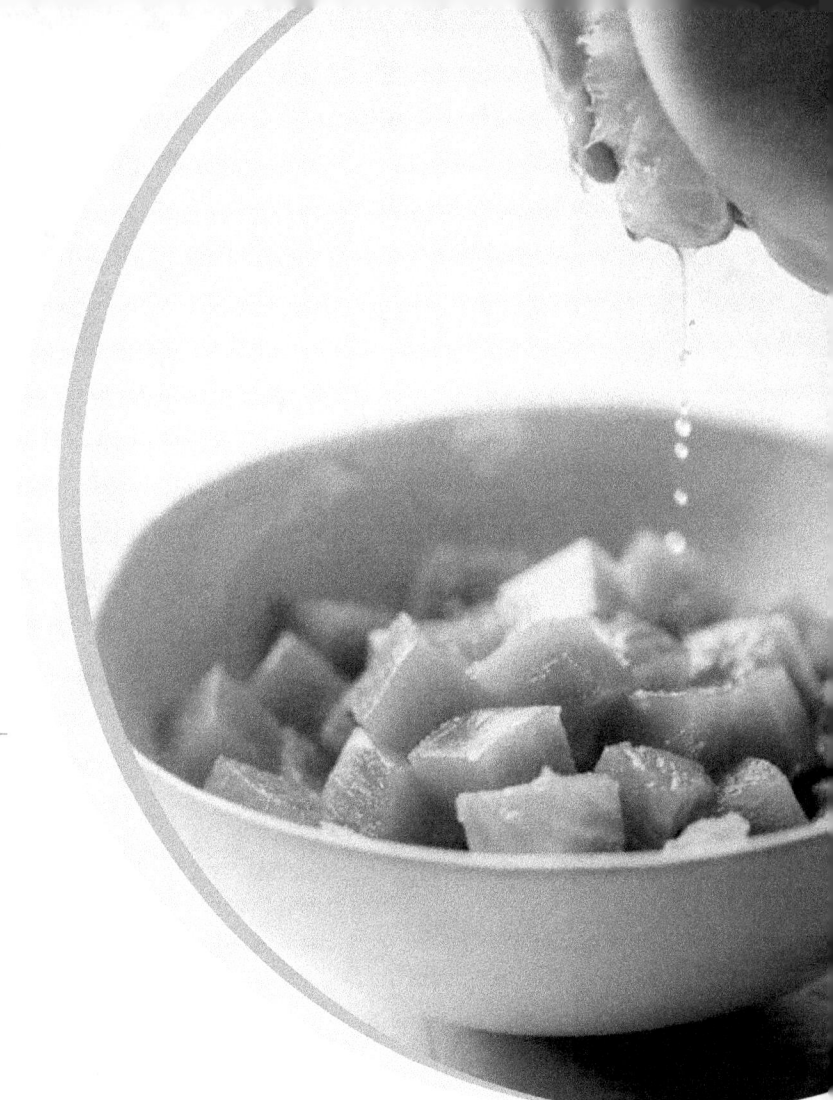

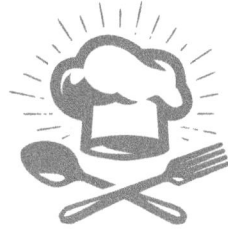

CHAPTER 19

SAUCE RECIPES

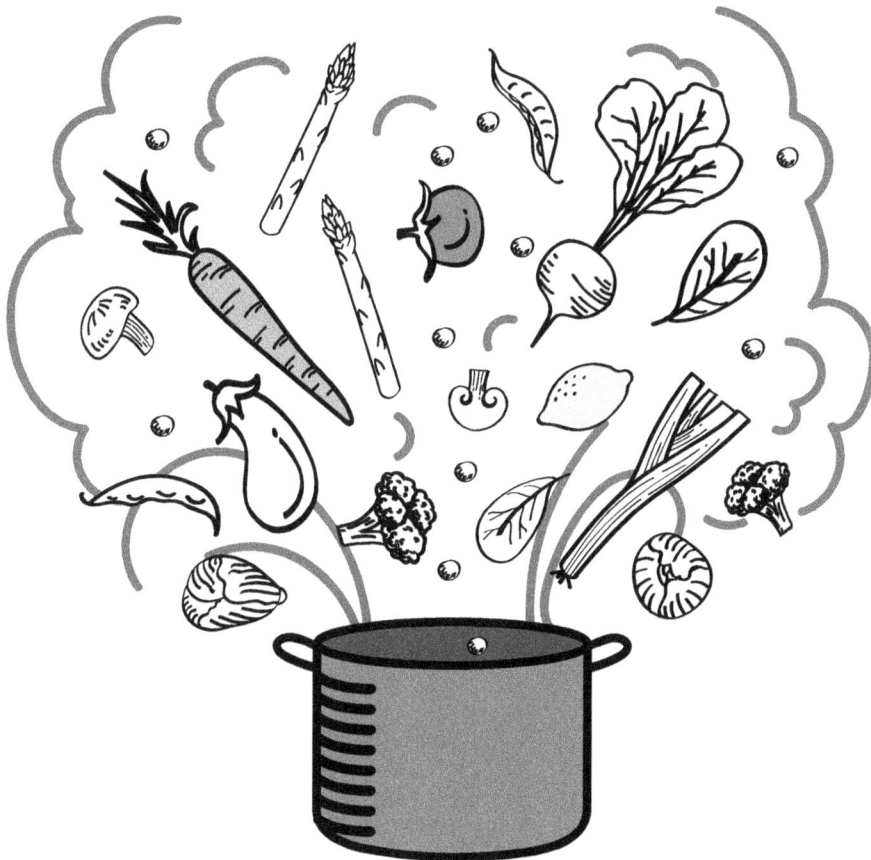

139 LEMON CAPER SAUCE

Preparation Time: 5 minutes

Cooking time: 7 minutes

Servings: 6

INGREDIENTS:

- 2 tablespoons butter, unsalted
- 1 1/2 teaspoon all-purpose flour
- 1/2 cup reduced-sodium chicken broth
- 1/4 cup white wine
- 2 tablespoons lemon juice
- 1 teaspoon capers
- 1/4 teaspoon white pepper

DIRECTIONS:

1. Set a suitable skillet over low heat and add the butter to melt.
2. Gradually stir in the flour and mix well for 1 minute.
3. Pour in the broth and continue mixing for another 1 minute.
4. Stir in the pepper, lemon juice, wine, capers, and lemon juice.
5. Mix well and cook by stirring for 5 minutes until it thickens.
6. Allow the sauce to cool down. Serve.

NUTRITION:

Calories 48
Fat 4g
Carbohydrate 0.9g
Protein 0.6g

Sodium 107mg
Phosphorous 63mg
Potassium 36mg

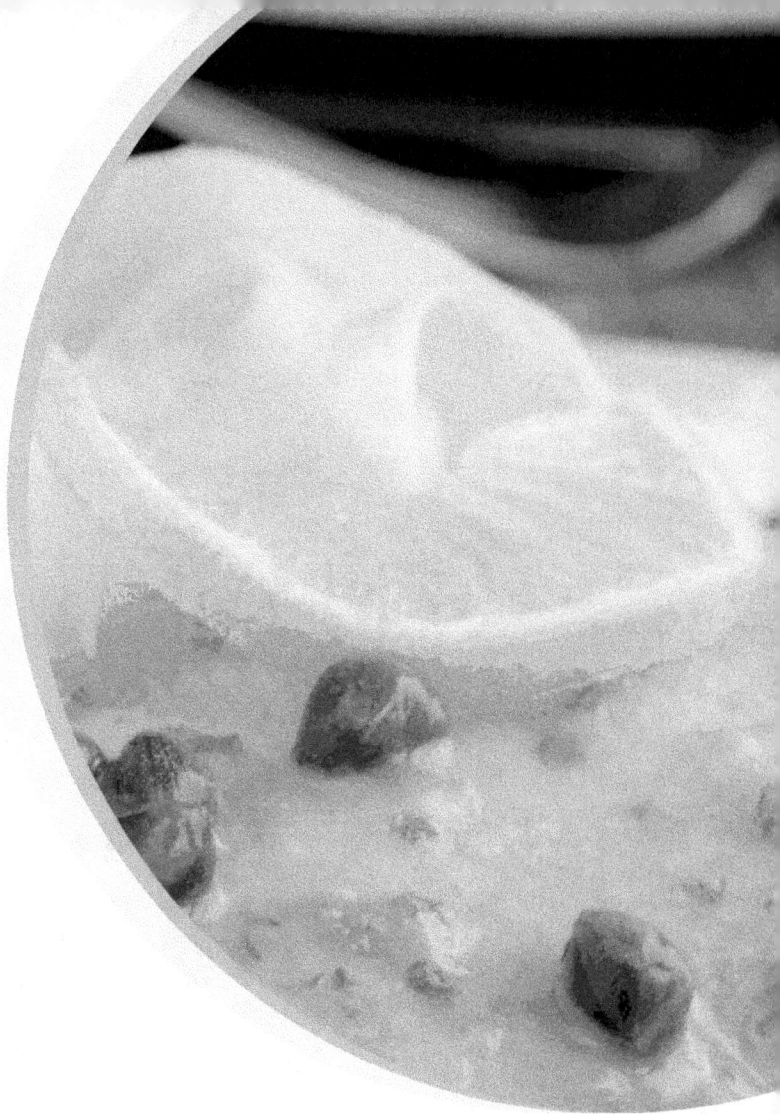

140 ALFREDO SAUCE

Preparation Time: 5 minutes

Cooking time: 5 minutes

Servings: 4

INGREDIENTS:

- 4 oz. cream cheese
- 1/2 cup grated Parmesan cheese
- 3/4 cup low-fat milk
- 1/4 cup butter
- 1/4 teaspoon white pepper
- 1/8 teaspoon garlic powder

DIRECTIONS:

1. Set a 2-quart saucepan over moderate heat and add the Parmesan cheese, cream cheese, butter, milk, garlic powder, and white pepper.
2. Stir and cook this mixture for 5 minutes until the cheese is melted. Serve.

NUTRITION:

Calories 311
Fat 27.8g
Carbohydrate 4.2g
Protein 12.8g
Sodium 446mg
Potassium 108mg
Phosphorous 43mg

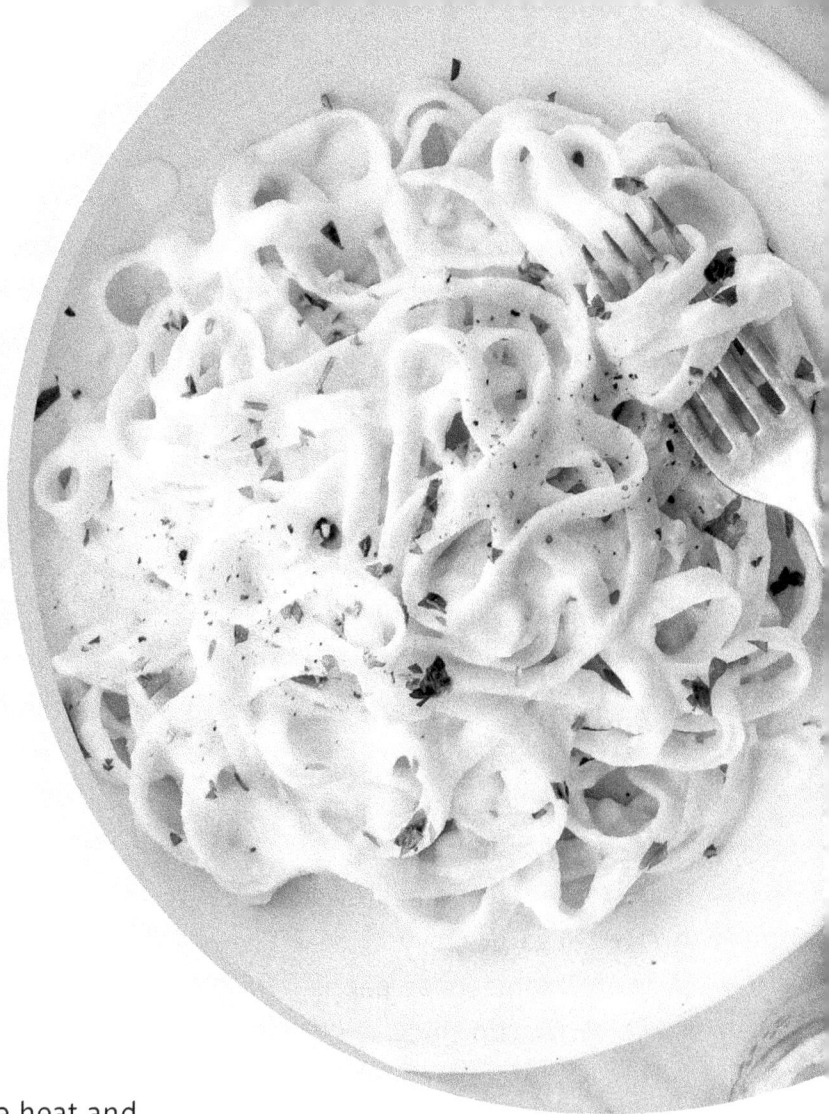

141 BARBEQUE SAUCE

Preparation Time: 10 minutes

Cooking time: 20 minutes

Servings: 8

INGREDIENTS:

- 1/3 cup corn oil
- 1/2 cup tomato juice
- 1 tablespoon brown Swerve
- 1 garlic clove
- 1 tablespoon paprika
- 1/4 cup vinegar
- 1 teaspoon pepper
- 1/3 cup water
- 1/4 teaspoon onion powder

DIRECTIONS:

1. Toss all the ingredients into a suitable saucepan.
2. Cook this sauce for 20 minutes with occasional stirring. Serve.

NUTRITION:

Calories 93
Fat 9.2g
Carbohydrate 0.5g
Protein 0.3g
Sodium 42mg
Potassium 68mg
Phosphorous 31mg

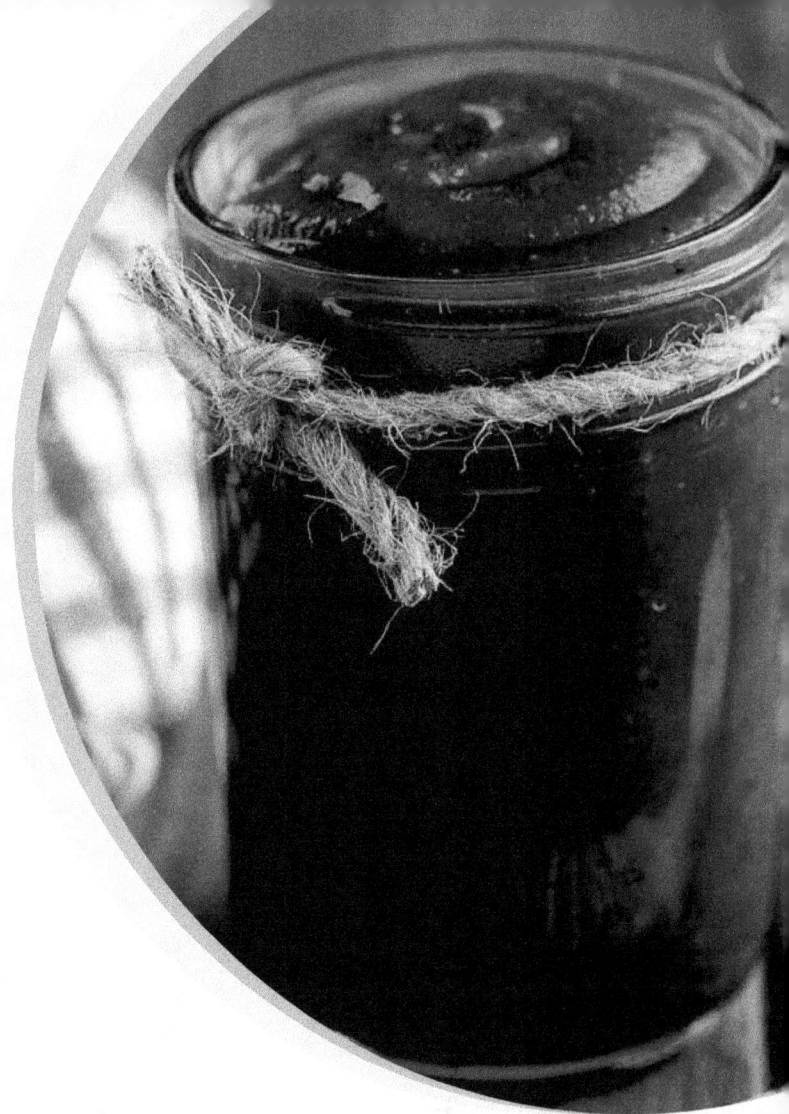

142 APPLE BUTTER

Preparation Time: 5 minutes

Cooking time: 2 hours

Servings: 20

INGREDIENTS:

- 4 1/2 cups apple sauce
- 2 cups granulated Swerve
- 1/4 cup vinegar
- 1/2 teaspoon ground cloves
- 1/2 teaspoon cinnamon

DIRECTIONS:

1. Whisk the apple sauce, Swerve, vinegar, ground cloves, and cinnamon in a small roasting pan.
2. Bake the mixture for 2 hours at 350 degrees F in a preheated oven until it thickens.
3. Mix well and transfer to a mason jar.

NUTRITION:

Calories 97
Fat 0g
Carbohydrate 9.6g
Protein 0.1g
Sodium 1mg
Potassium 40mg
Phosphorous 110mg

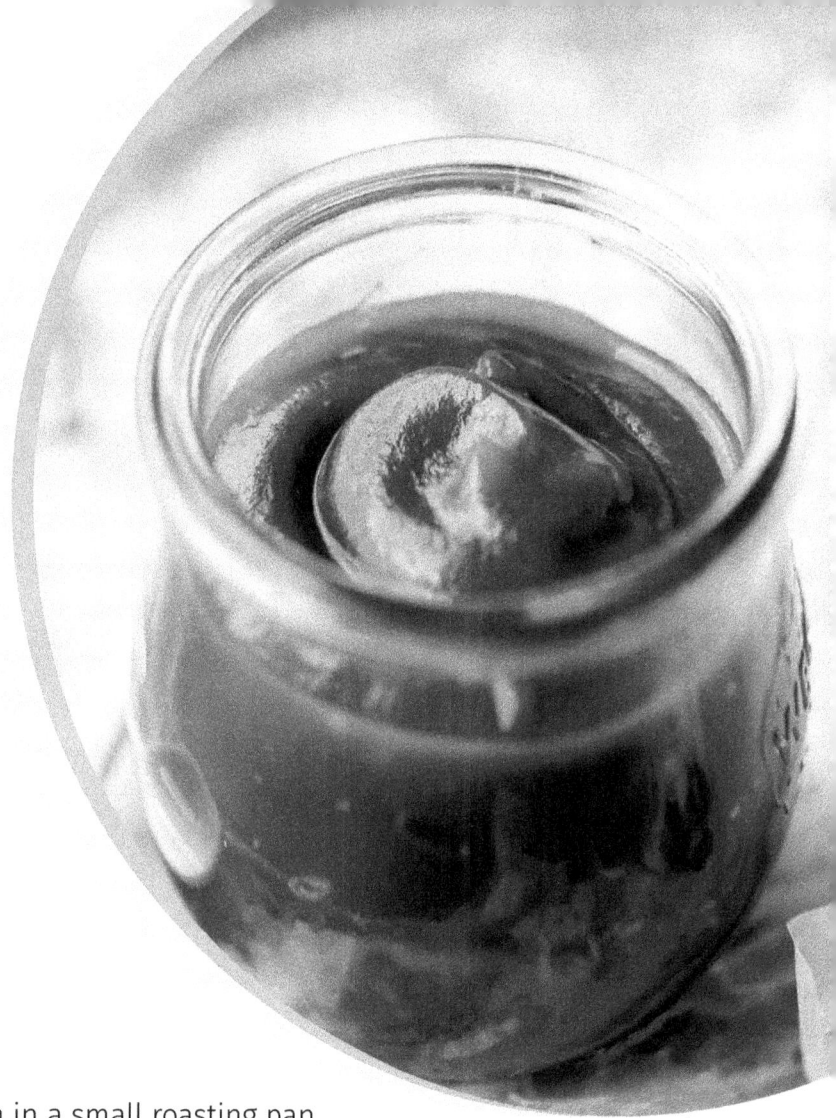

143 BLACKBERRY SAUCE

Preparation Time: 5 minutes

Cooking time: 10 minutes

Servings: 10

INGREDIENTS:

- 5 cups blackberries
- 1/2 tablespoon stevia
- 1 tablespoon arrowroot powder
- 1 tablespoon lemon juice
- 1 cup water

DIRECTIONS:

1. Crush the berries in a saucepan and add the stevia and a cup of water.
2. Bring the berries to a boil, then lower the heat to a simmer.
3. Whisk the arrowroot powder with 2 tablespoons of water in a bowl and add it to the berries.
4. Stir and cook the berries for 1 minute until the sauce thickens.
5. Remove the cooked berry sauce from heat and stir in lemon juice. Serve.

NUTRITION:

Calories 60
Fat 0.4g
Carbohydrate 14.8g
Protein 1g
Sodium 1mg
Potassium 119mg
Phosphorous 72mg

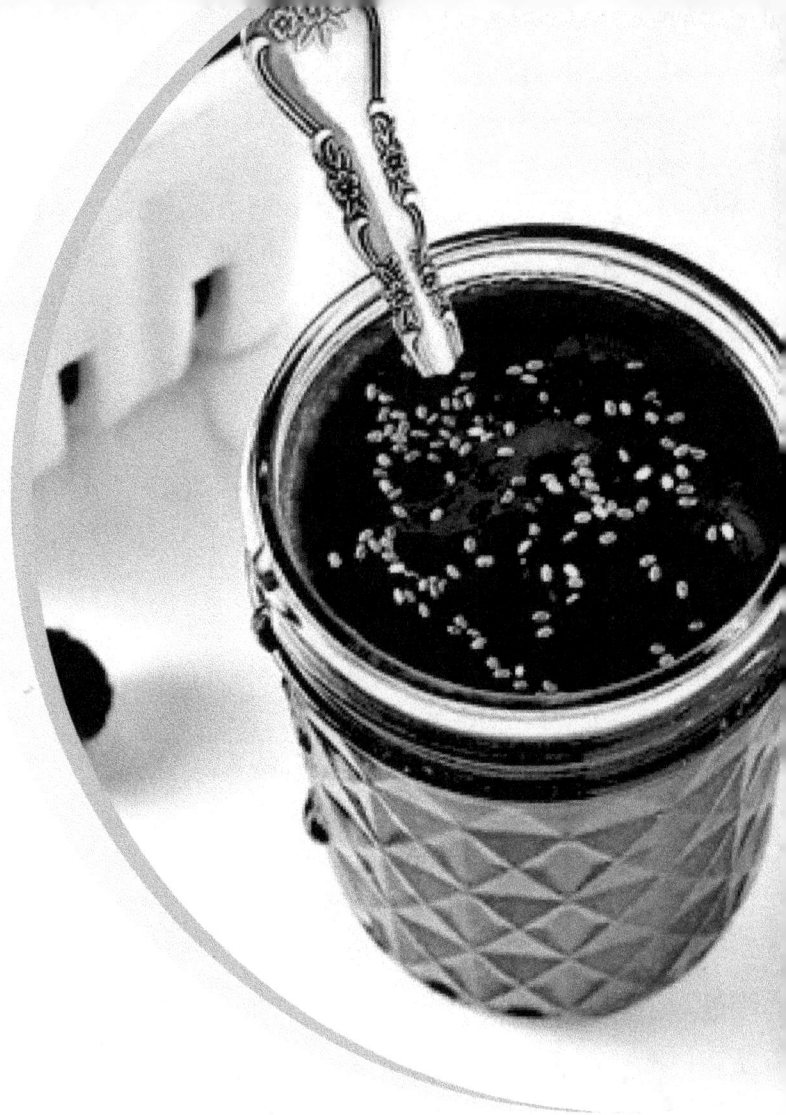

144 BLUEBERRY SALSA

Preparation Time: 5 minutes

Cooking time: 0 minutes

Servings: 4

INGREDIENTS:

- 1 cup blueberries
- 1 cup raspberries
- 1/4 cup red onion
- 2 tablespoons lime juice
- 1 tablespoon basil

DIRECTIONS:

1. Add the berries, lime juice, onion, and basil to a food processor.
2. Pulse until all ingredients are finely chopped into a salsa.
3. Serve.

NUTRITION:

Calories 45
Fat 0.4g
Carbohydrate 11.5g
Protein 0.8g
Sodium 1mg
Potassium 112mg
Phosphorous 53mg

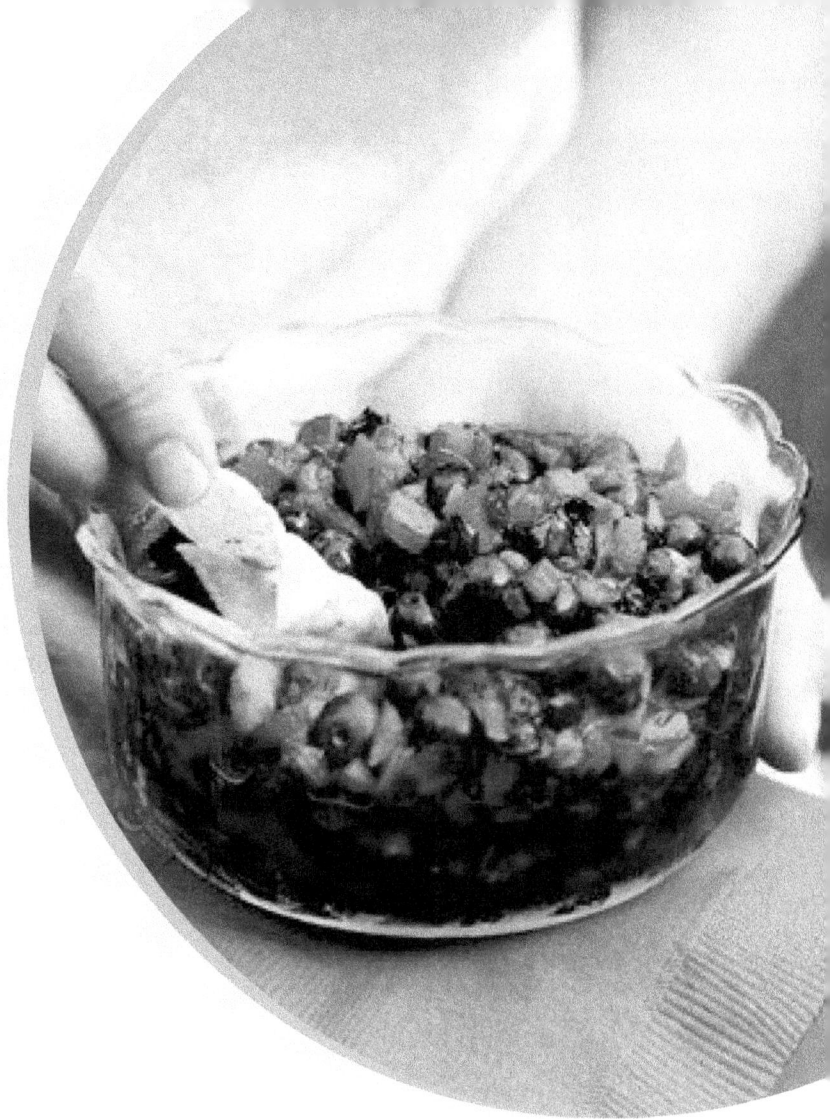

145 CRANBERRY SALSA

Preparation Time: 5 minutes

Cooking time: 0 minutes

Servings: 4

INGREDIENTS:

- 16 oz. canned whole cranberries, chopped
- 8 oz. canned pineapple, crushed
- 10 oz. frozen strawberries, chopped
- 1/2 cup apple sauce

DIRECTIONS:

1. Toss the pineapple with the strawberries, cranberries, and apple sauce in a salad bowl.
2. Refrigerate the salsa for 2 hours or until ready to use.
3. Serve.

NUTRITION:

Calories 127
Fat 0.1g
Carbohydrate 29.3g
Protein 0.9g
Sodium 2.3mg
Potassium 278mg
Phosphorous 61mg

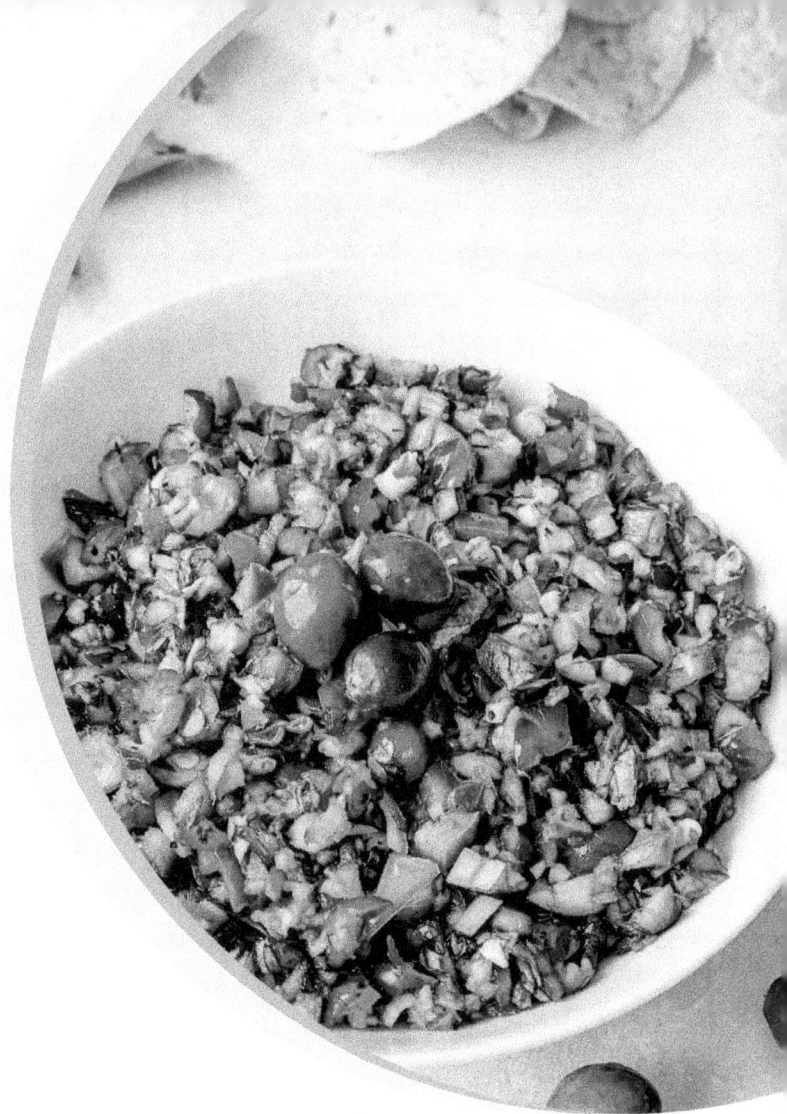

146 STRAWBERRY SALSA

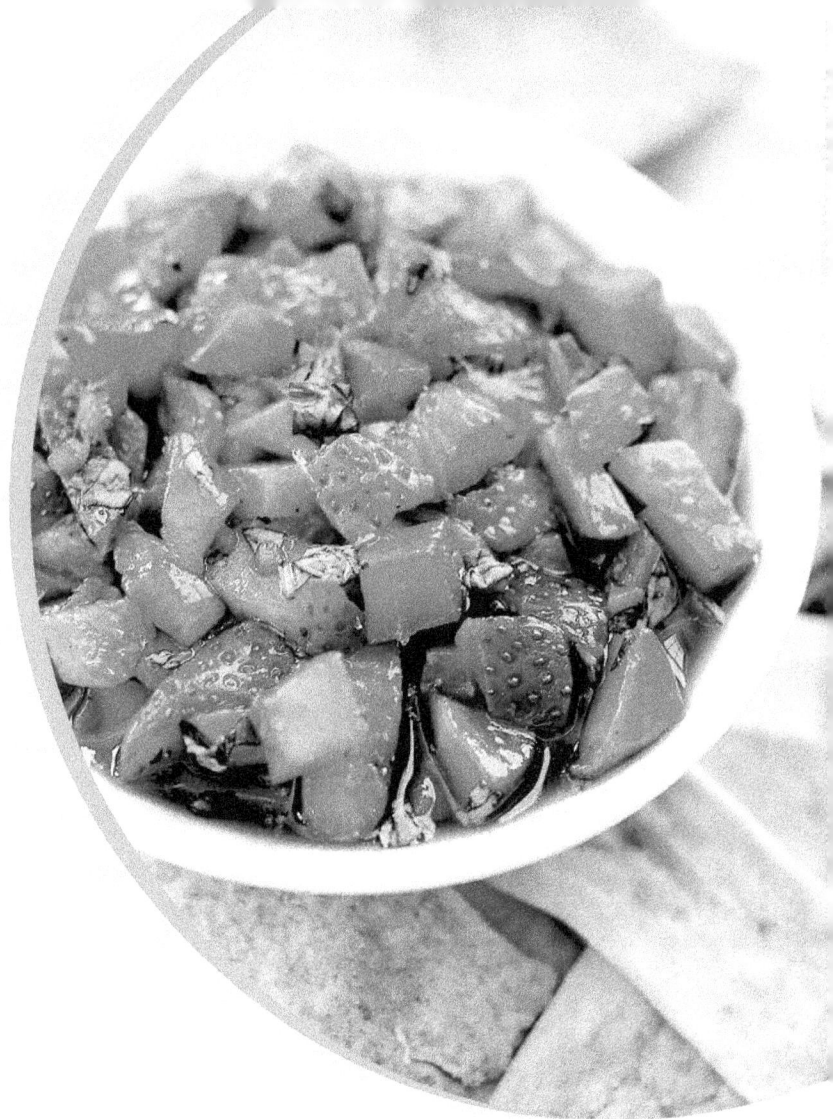

Preparation Time: 5 minutes

Cooking time: 0 minutes

Servings: 4

INGREDIENTS:

- 1 1/2 cups strawberries
- 1/2 cup cucumber
- 1/2 cup red onion
- 2 tablespoons jalapeño pepper, halved and seeded
- 1 tablespoon mint
- 1 teaspoon lime rind
- 2 tablespoons lime juice
- 1 tablespoon orange juice
- 1 tablespoon honey

DIRECTIONS:

1. Add the red onion, cucumber, strawberries, mint, and jalapeño to a food processor.
2. Pulse until all the ingredients are chopped into a salsa.
3. Add the lime juice, orange juice, honey, and mix well. Serve.

NUTRITION:

Calories 49
Fat 0.2g
Carbohydrate 13.2g
Protein 0.8g
Sodium 3mg
Potassium 161mg
Phosphorous 113mg

147 GARLIC SAUCE

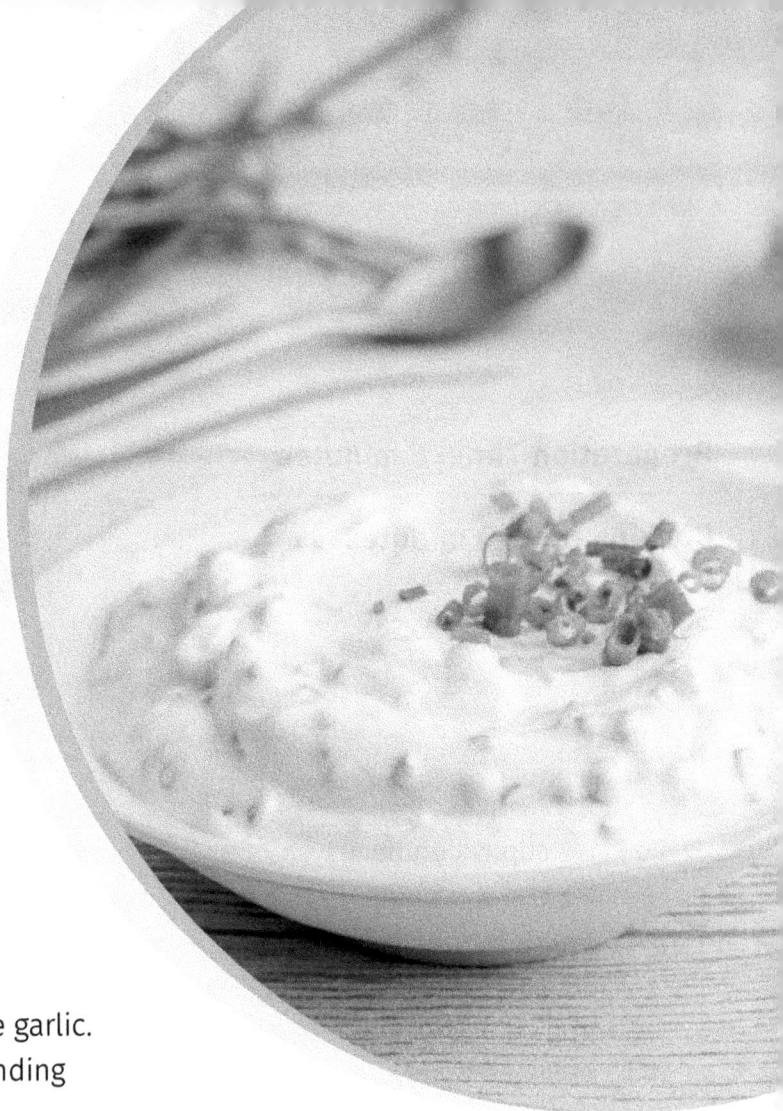

Preparation Time: 3 minutes

Cooking time: 0 minutes

Servings: 6

INGREDIENTS:

- 1 garlic head, cloves peeled
- 2 tablespoons lemon juice
- 1 cup olive oil

DIRECTIONS:

1. Add the garlic and lemon juice to a blender and blend to puree the garlic.
2. Slowly stir in the olive oil while blending the garlic mixture.
3. Serve.

NUTRITION:

Calories 290
Fat 33.6g
Carbohydrate 0.7g
Protein 0.2g
Sodium 1mg
Potassium 14mg
Phosphorous 20mg

148 CRANBERRY SAUCE

Preparation Time: 3 minutes

Cooking time: 10 minutes

Servings: 6

INGREDIENTS:

- 1 cup granulated Swerve
- 12 oz. whole cranberries
- 1 cup water

DIRECTIONS:

1. Set a 2-quart saucepan over medium-high heat and add the Swerve and 1 cup water.
2. Bring the Swerve up to a boil, add the cranberries and reduce the heat to a simmer.
3. Cook, stirring gently for 10 minutes, then pass the mixture through a fine sieve over a mixing bowl.
4. Spread the berries in the sieve using the back of a spoon.
5. Mix well the strained sauce. Serve.

NUTRITION:

Calories 25

Fat 0g

Carbohydrate 7g

Protein 0g

Sodium 1mg

Potassium 44mg

Phosphorous 7mg

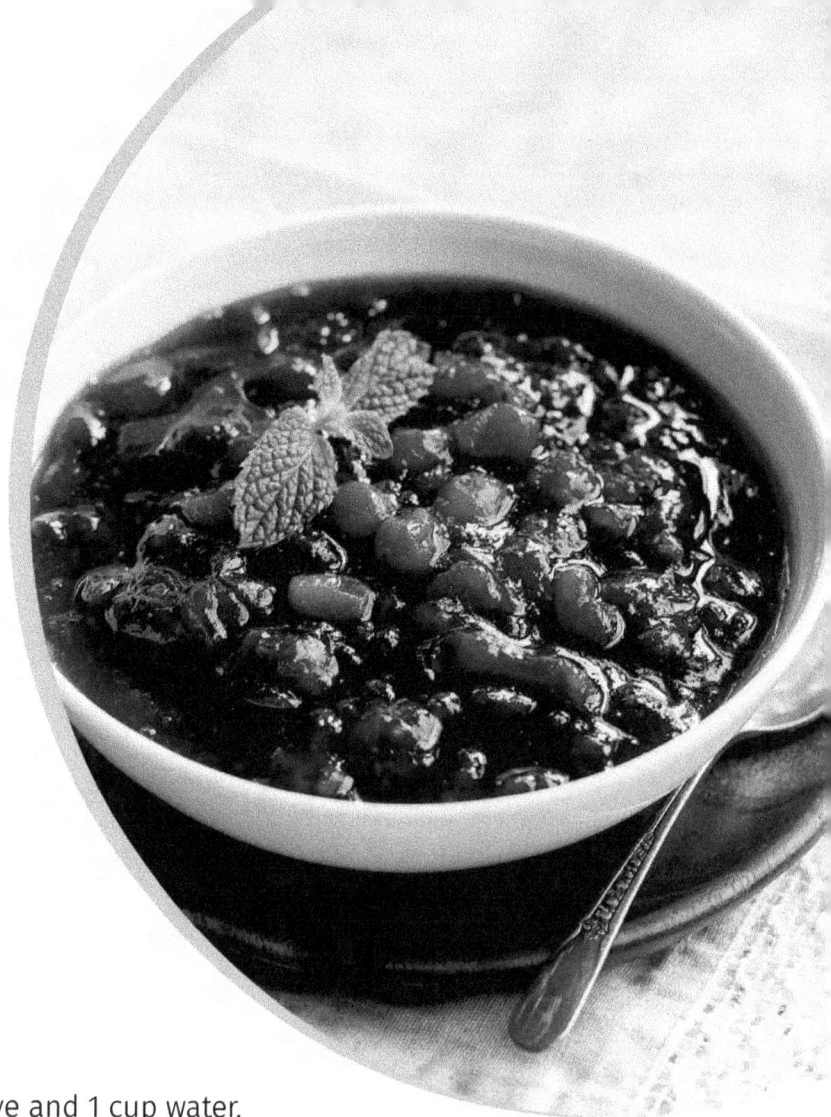

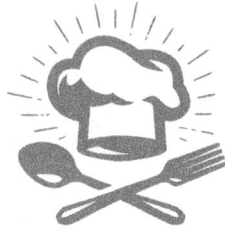

CHAPTER 20

LOW POTASSIUM RECIPES

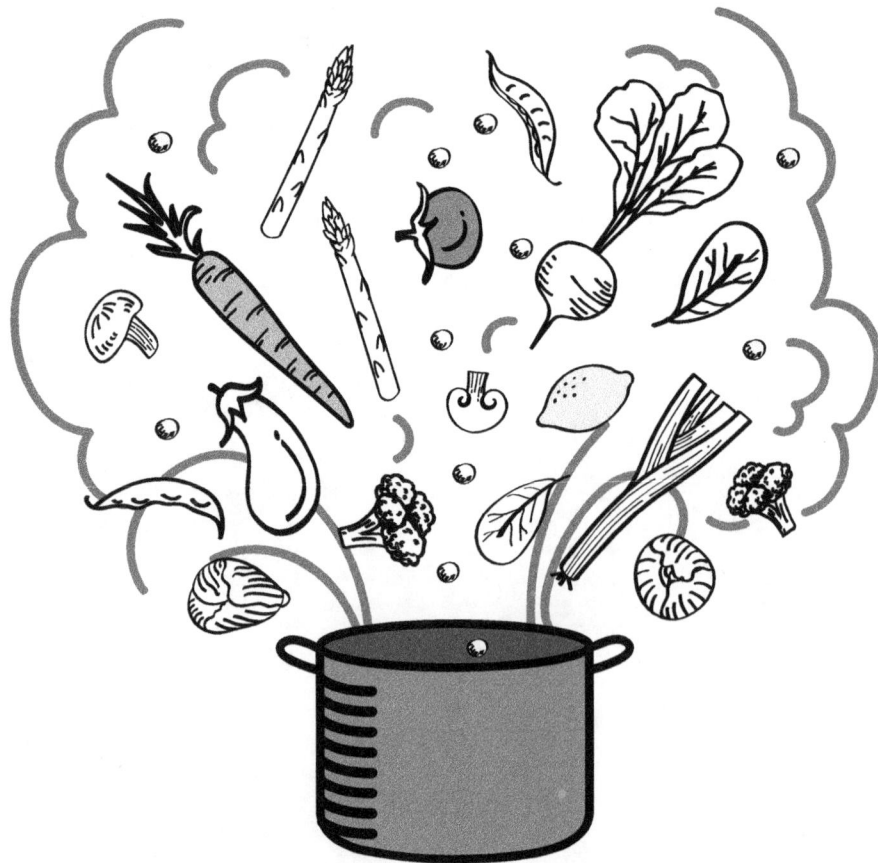

149 STRAWBERRY JELLY STUFFED FRENCH TOAST

Preparation Time: 15 minutes

Cooking Time: 1 hour

Servings: 6

INGREDIENTS:

- 8 ounces Cream cheese
- 1-pound Loaf of day-old French bread
- 8 tbsp. Strawberry jelly
- 6 large Eggs
- 1 cup 1% low-fat milk
- 1 tsp. Vanilla extract

DIRECTIONS:

1. Slice the French bread loaf into 16 slices.
2. Bring cream cheese to room temperature, spread 1 tablespoon on each slice of bread.
3. Top it with 1 tablespoon strawberry jelly. Spread evenly. Add another bread slice to make a sandwich.
4. Repeat on the remaining sandwiches.
5. Place all the sandwiches in the baking dish.
6. In a mixing bowl beat egg. Add milk and vanilla extract and whisk the mixture well.
7. Pour the egg mixture over bread sandwiches.
8. Cover and refrigerate overnight or at least 8 to 12 hours.
9. Preheat your oven to 359 F.
10. Bake for one hour or 55 minutes.
11. Once done, remove the foil, and put the dish back to give a nice golden color to the sandwiches.
12. Let it cool. Garnish with strawberry slices and dust with powdered sugar.

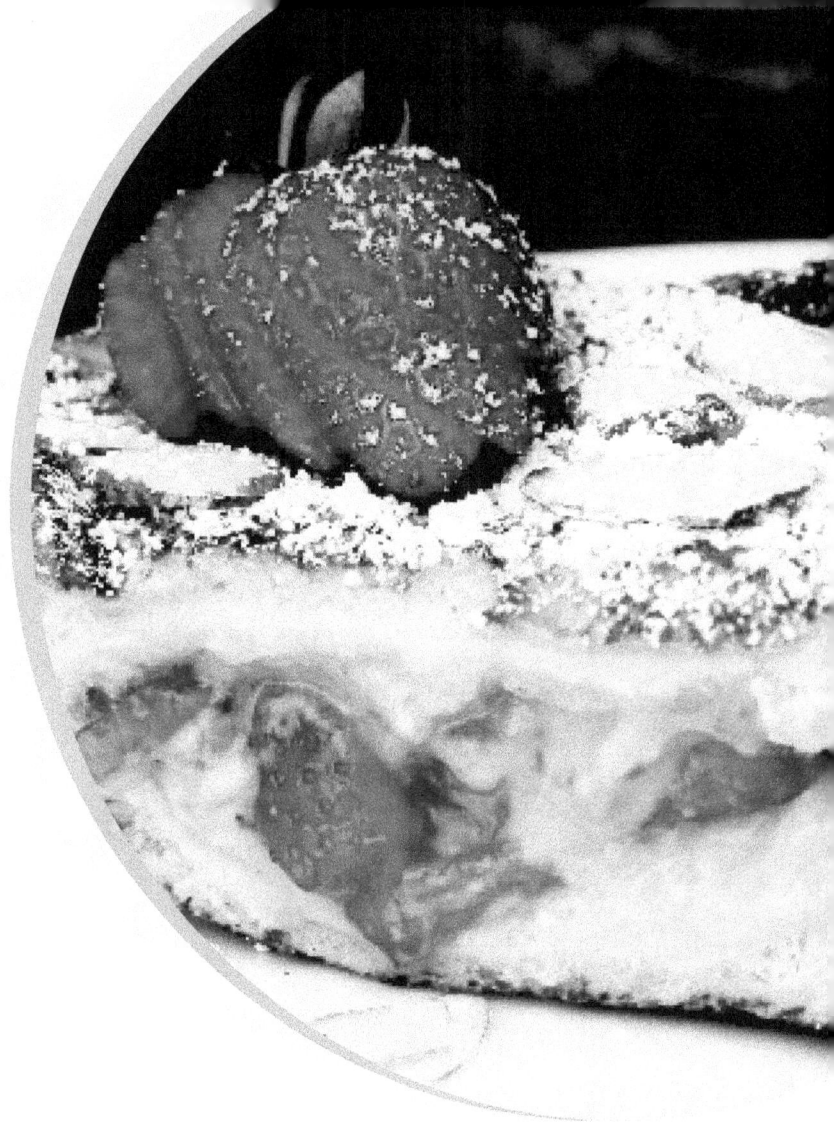

Calories: 250
Fat: 2g
Carbs: 46g
Protein: 12g
Sodium: 540mg
Potassium: 200mg
Phosphorus: 78mg

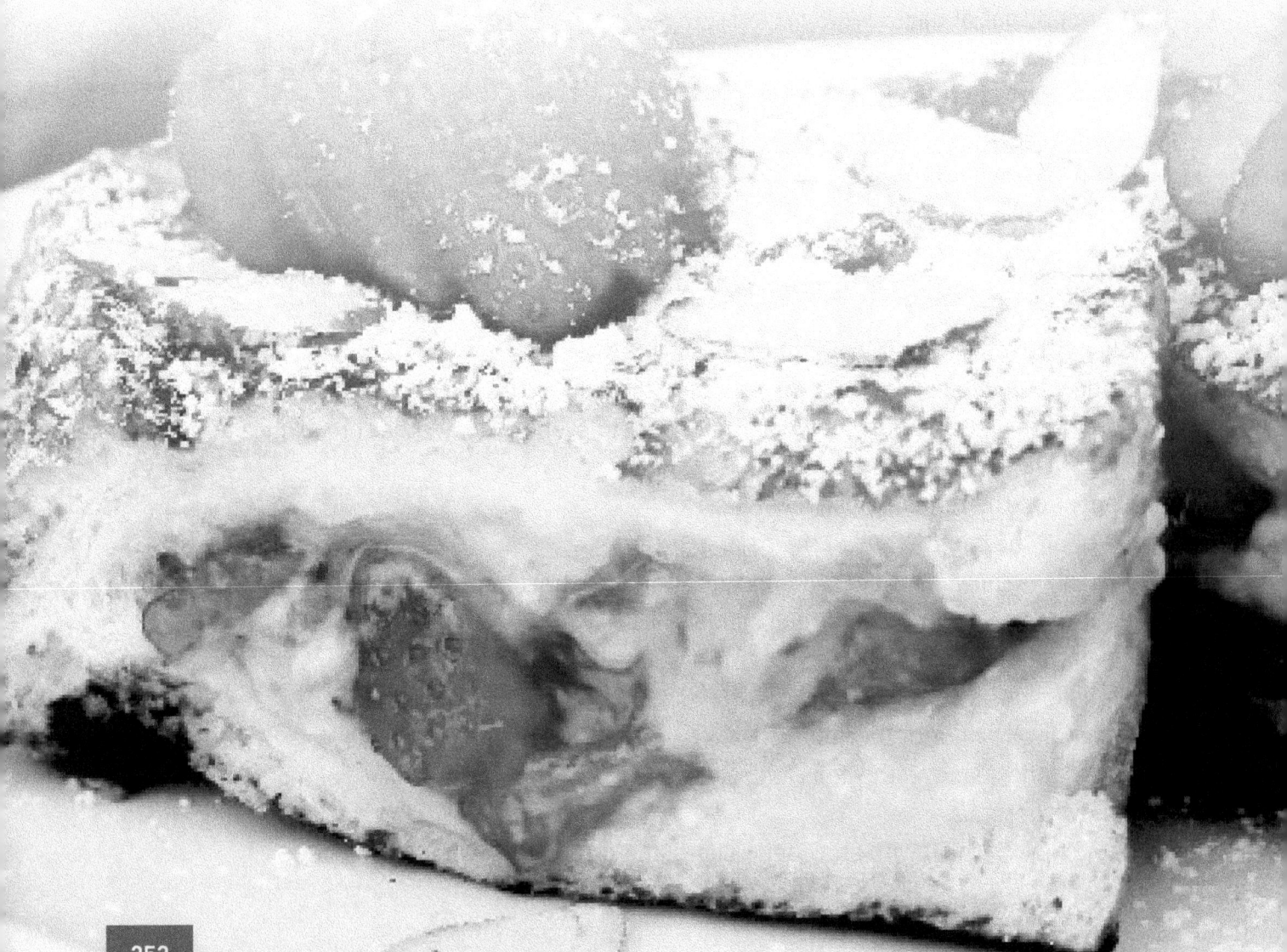

150 MINCED BEEF SAMOSA

Preparation Time: 20 minutes

Cooking Time: 25 minutes

Servings: 8

INGREDIENTS:

- 1-pound Minced beef
- ¼ cup Onion
- 1 tsp. Ginger root
- 1 clove Garlic
- 2 tbsp. Cilantro
- ½ cup   Green peas (fresh)
- 3 tbsp. Canola oil
- 1 tbsp. Coriander powder
- ½ tsp. Turmeric powder
- ¼ tsp.   Pepper
- 1 tsp. Lemon juice
- 1 tsp. Allspice powder
- 24 pastries Samosa pastries
- 2 tbsp. Flour
- 1 ½ tbsp. Water

DIRECTIONS:

1. Chop ginger, garlic, and cilantro finely.
2. Chop the onion finely and set aside.
3. Take a large saucepan and heat 3 tablespoon oil.
4. Add garlic, ginger, and onion and sauté for 2 to 3 minutes.
5. Add coriander powder, turmeric powder, and cayenne pepper stir for one minute.
6. Add ground beef and allspice powder and until beef is cooked.
7. Include green peas and cook the mixture to dry
8. Top with lemon juice and cilantro and evenly stir.

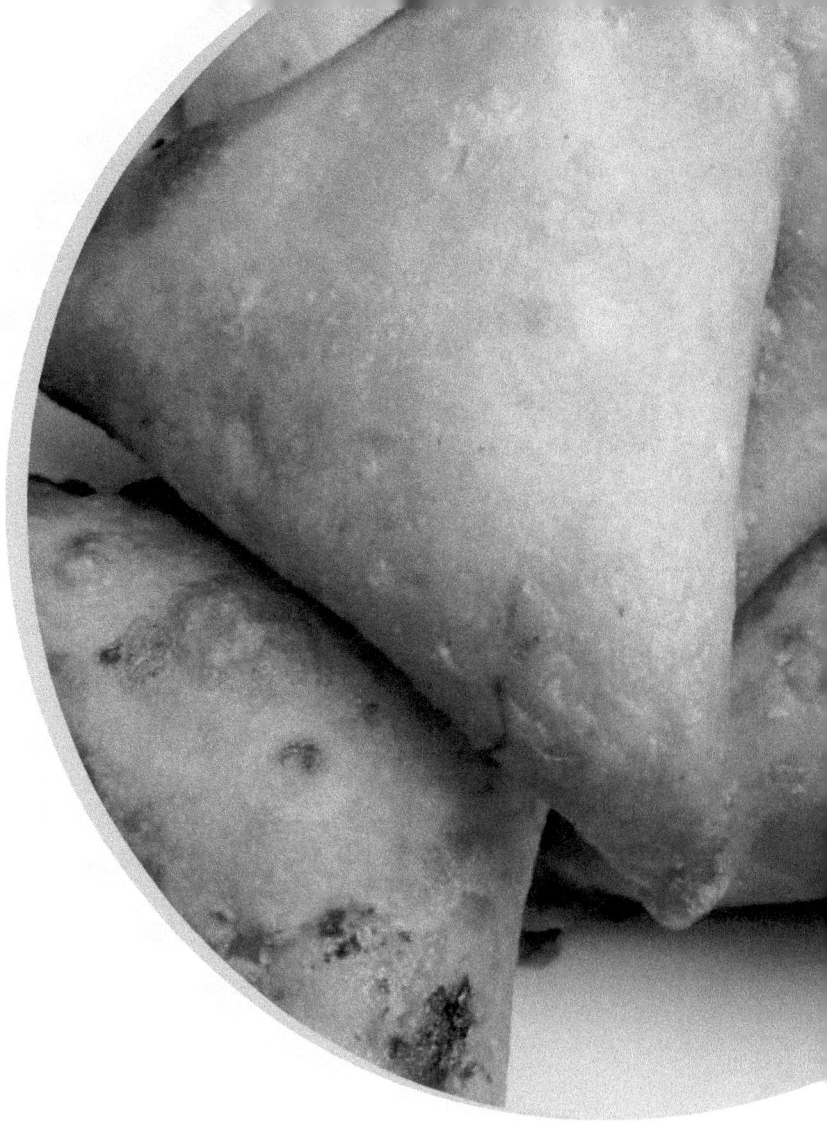

9. In a small bowl, make a thin paste with 1 tablespoon of flour and enough water.
10. Spread remaining flour on a board and roll out the pastry on it.
11. In the center of the pastry, put 2 tablespoons of the beef mixture and fold diagonally to make a triangular shape.
12. Close edges with water and flour paste.
13. Repeat the procedure with all pastries.
14. Deep fry until light golden brown.

NUTRITION:

Calories: 210
Fat: 11g
Carbs: 20g
Protein: 7g
Sodium: 346mg
Potassium: 196mg
Phosphorus: 0mg

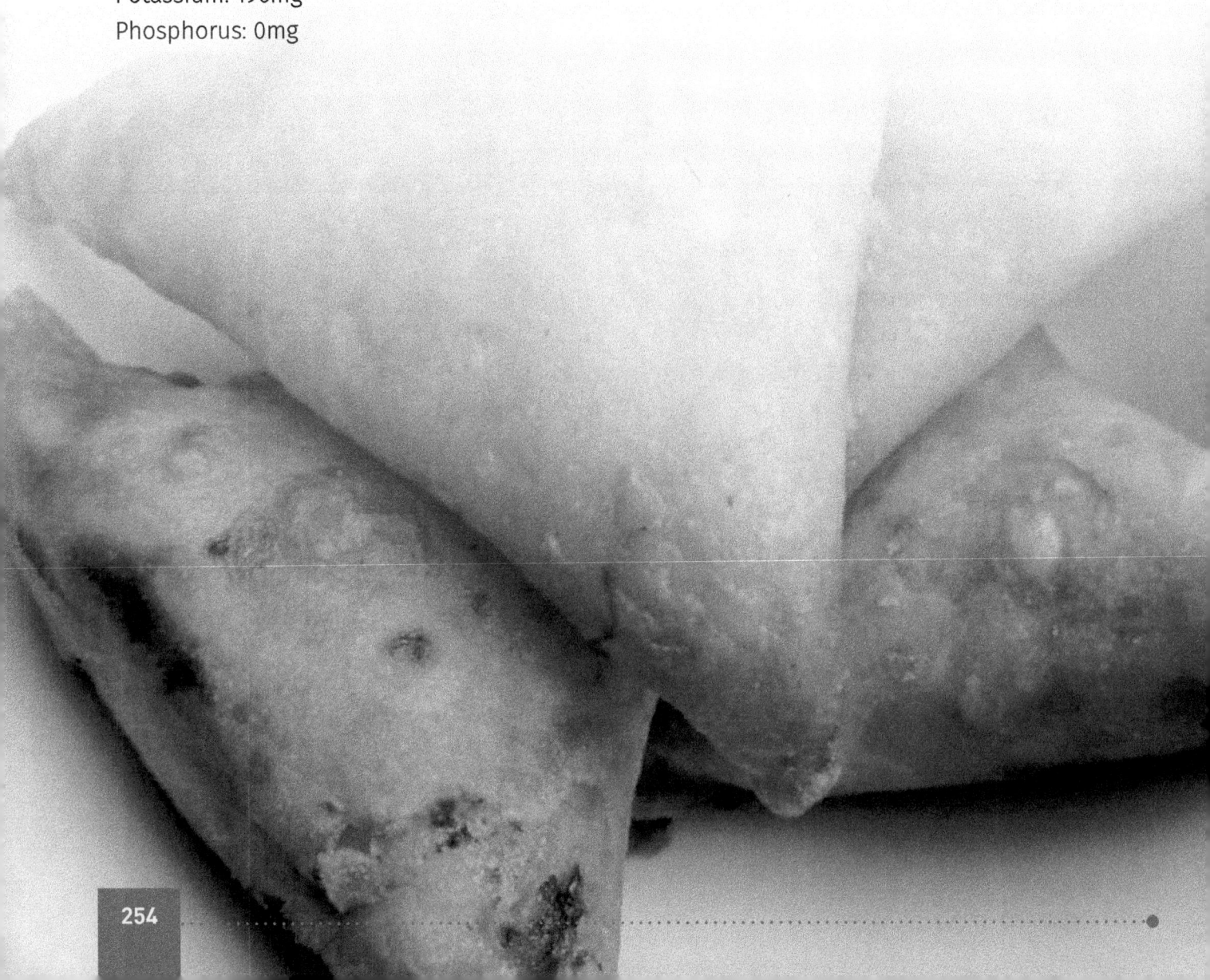

151 APPLE PIE

Preparation Time: 20 minutes

Cooking Time: 1 hour

Servings: 6

INGREDIENTS:

- · 6 medium Apples
- · ½ cup Granulated sugar
- · 1 tsp. Cinnamon powder
- · 6 tbsp. Butter
- · 2 to 2/3 cups All-purpose flour
- · 1 shortening
- · 6 tbsp. Water

DIRECTIONS:

1. Heat up oven to 400 F.
2. Peel all apples, core them, and cut into slightly thin slices.
3. In a large bowl, put apple slices, add cinnamon powder, and sugar it.
4. Mix all the ingredients carefully so that all apple slices are covered with cinnamon powder and sugar.
5. Take another large bowl, put flour in it. With the help of a pastry blender, carefully mix shortening with flour.
6. Add chilled water to the mixture slowly at a time.
7. Knead the dough until it forms a ball.
8. Roll one portion of the kneaded dough.
9. Place this rolled dough in an inch pie pan.
10. Stir cinnamon and apple mixture and pour it into the pie pan.
11. Refrigerate the pie pan for at least 15 minutes.
12. Bake until pie crust turns to golden brown (45-60 minutes).

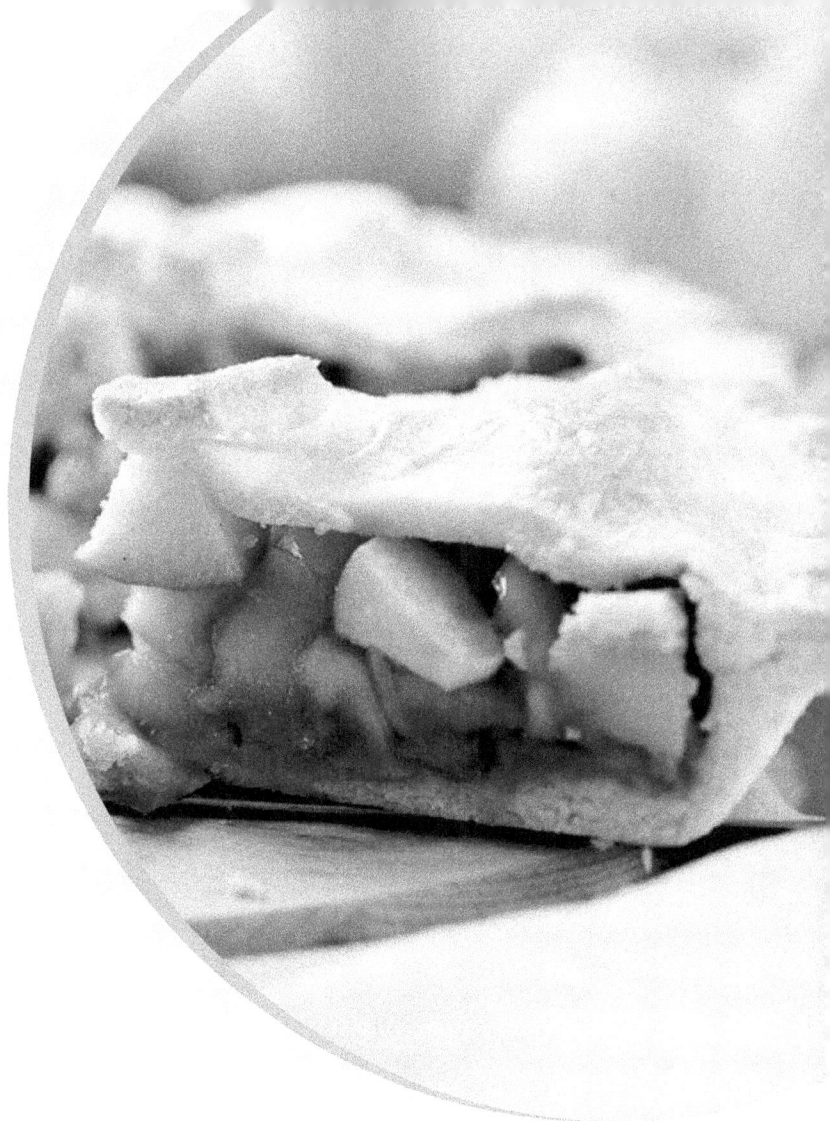

Calories: 140
Fat: 4g
Carbs: 24g
Protein: 2g
Sodium: 105mg
Potassium: 112mg
Phosphorus: 11mg

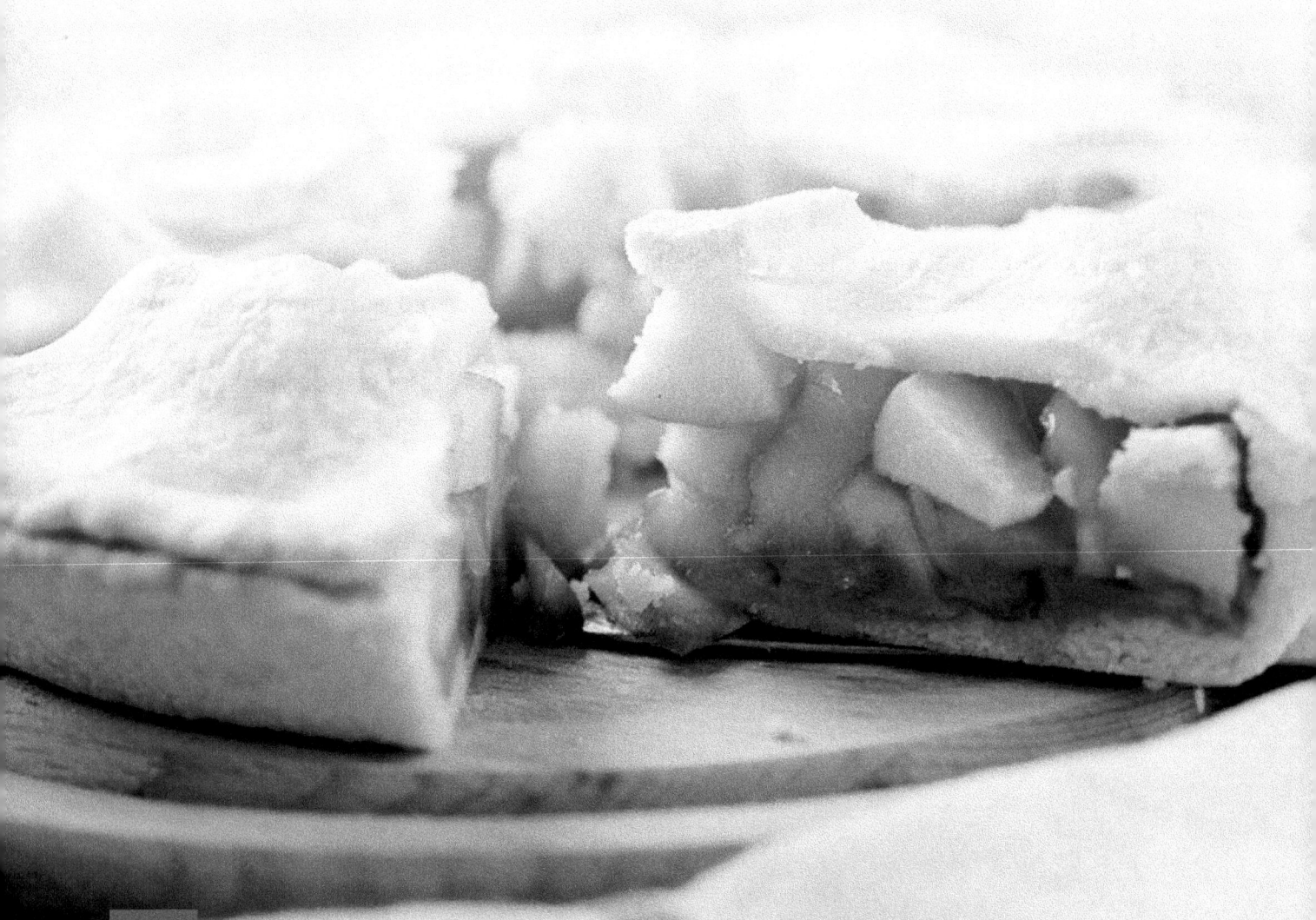

152 EGGPLANT AND BELL PEPPER CASSEROLE

Preparation Time: 15 minutes

Cooking Time: 40 minutes

Servings: 2

INGREDIENTS:

- 2 medium Eggplant
- 1 Tbsp. Olive oil
- ¼ cup   Butter
- ½ cup Onion
- ¼ cup Green bell pepper
- 5 cloves Garlic
- ½ tsp. Cayenne paper
- ½ tsp. Black pepper
- ½ tsp. Ground thyme
- 1 large Egg
- ½ cup Plain breadcrumbs

DIRECTIONS:

1. Preheat oven to 350 F.
2. Cut eggplants into cubes.
3. Chop garlic, pepper, and onion finely.
4. Beat egg in a separate bowl.
5. Sauté onion, garlic, and green pepper in heated oil.
6. Add in black pepper and cayenne pepper and sauté for a while.
7. Add eggplant and thyme and cook until eggplant softens.
8. Add the remaining breadcrumbs to the eggplant. Cook for 15 minutes.
9. Add the beaten egg to the mixture.

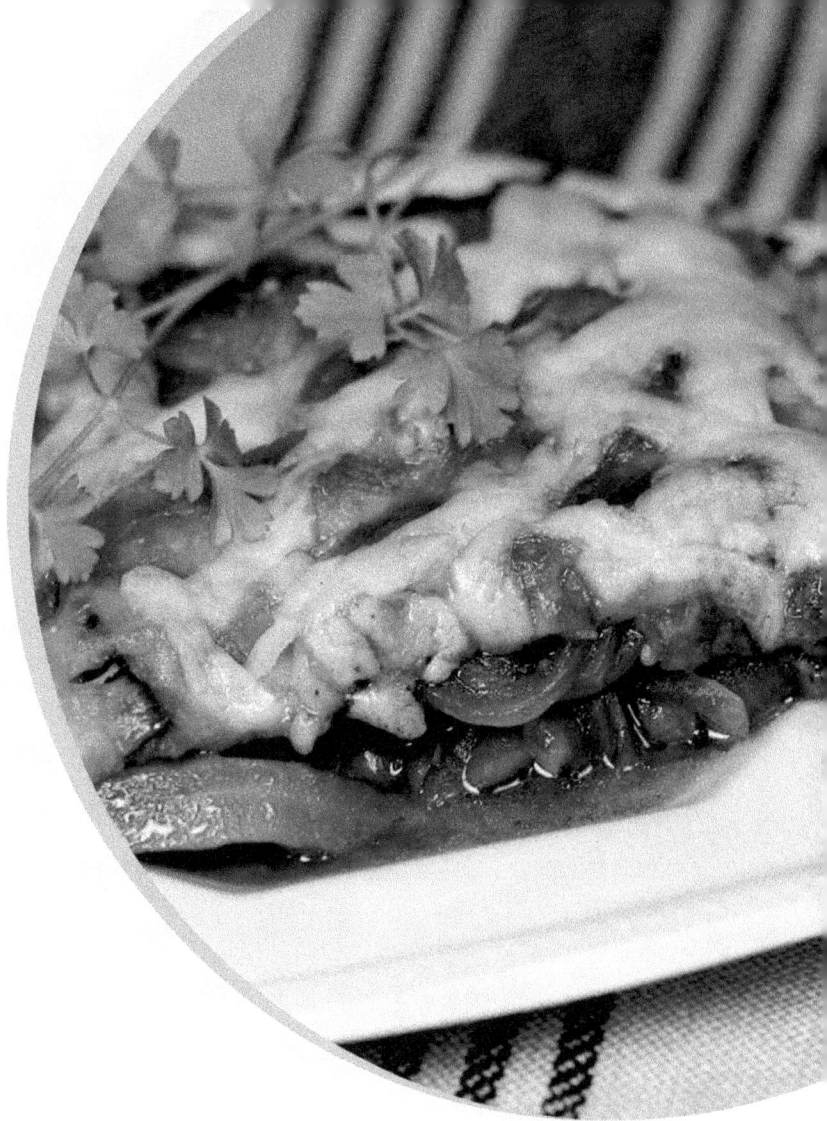

10. Place in a casserole dish.
11. Bake for 25 minutes. Serve.

NUTRITION:

Calories: 140
Fat: 3g
Carbs: 27g
Protein: 4g
Sodium: 400mg
Potassium:718 mg
Phosphorus: 83mg

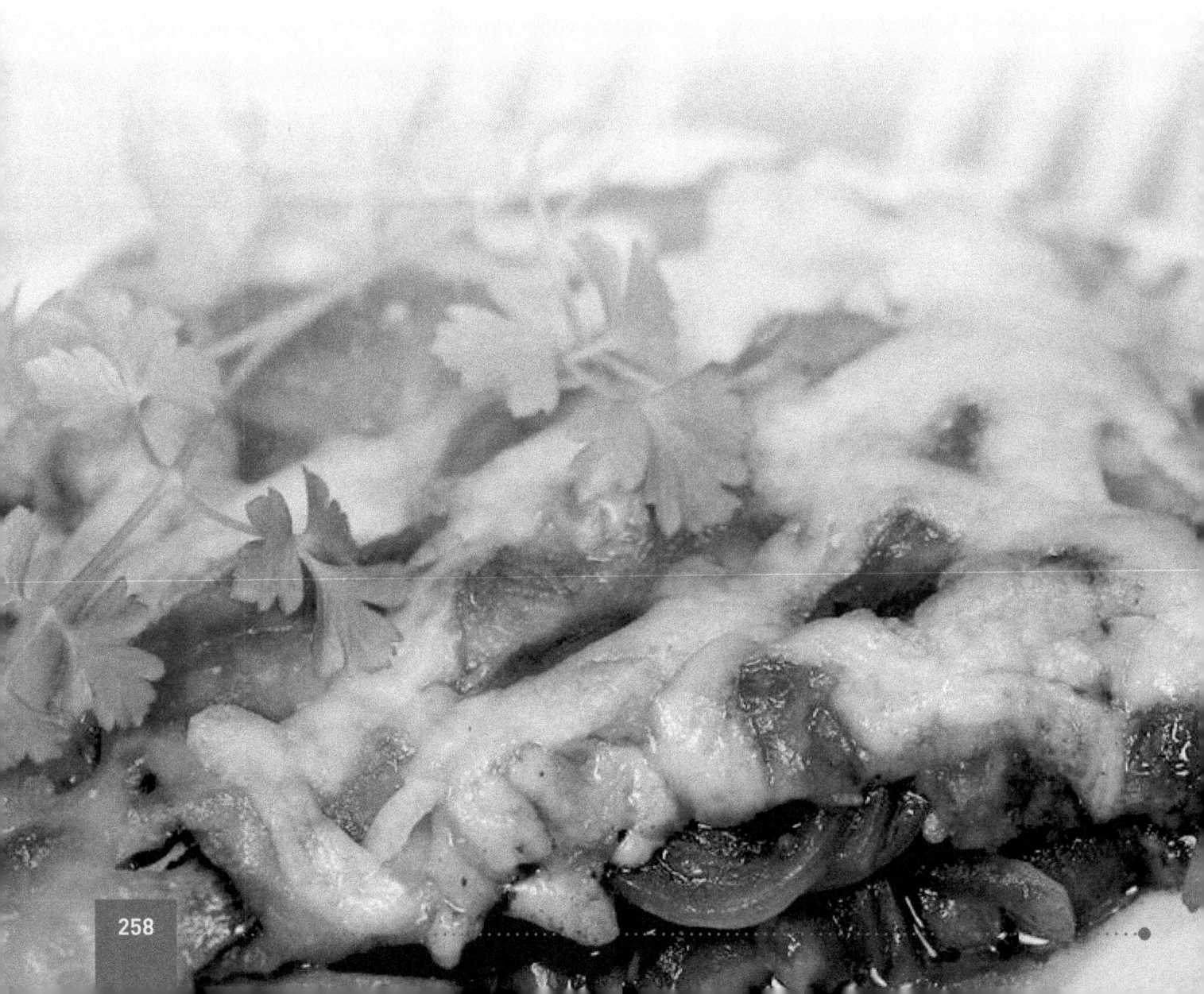

153 GLAZED CHICKEN WINGS

Preparation Time: 15 minutes

Cooking Time: 1 hour

Servings: 6

INGREDIENTS:

- 7 pounds Chicken wings
- 4 medium Green onion chopped
- 2 tbsp. soya sauce
- ¼ cup Honey
- 2 Tbsp. Granulated sugar
- ¼ cup Brown sugar
- 2 tsp. All spice powders
- 2 tsp. Dried thyme
- 1 tsp. Ginger chopped
- 1 tsp. Minced garlic
- ¼ cup Apple cider vinegar
- ¼ cup Lime juice
- ¼ cup Cranberry juice

DIRECTIONS:

1. In a large mixing bowl, add all ingredients and mix well to make a marinade.
2. Reserve ¾ cup of marinade for glaze.
3. Pour the marinade over wings.
4. Keep in refrigerator for 6 to 8 hours.
5. Preheat oven to 375 F.
6. On a baking sheet place all chicken wings.
7. Bake for 20 minutes.
8. To prepare glaze take a small saucepan and add reserved ¾ cup marinade in it.
9. Bring it to boil. Cook on medium low flame until it thickens slightly to a glaze.

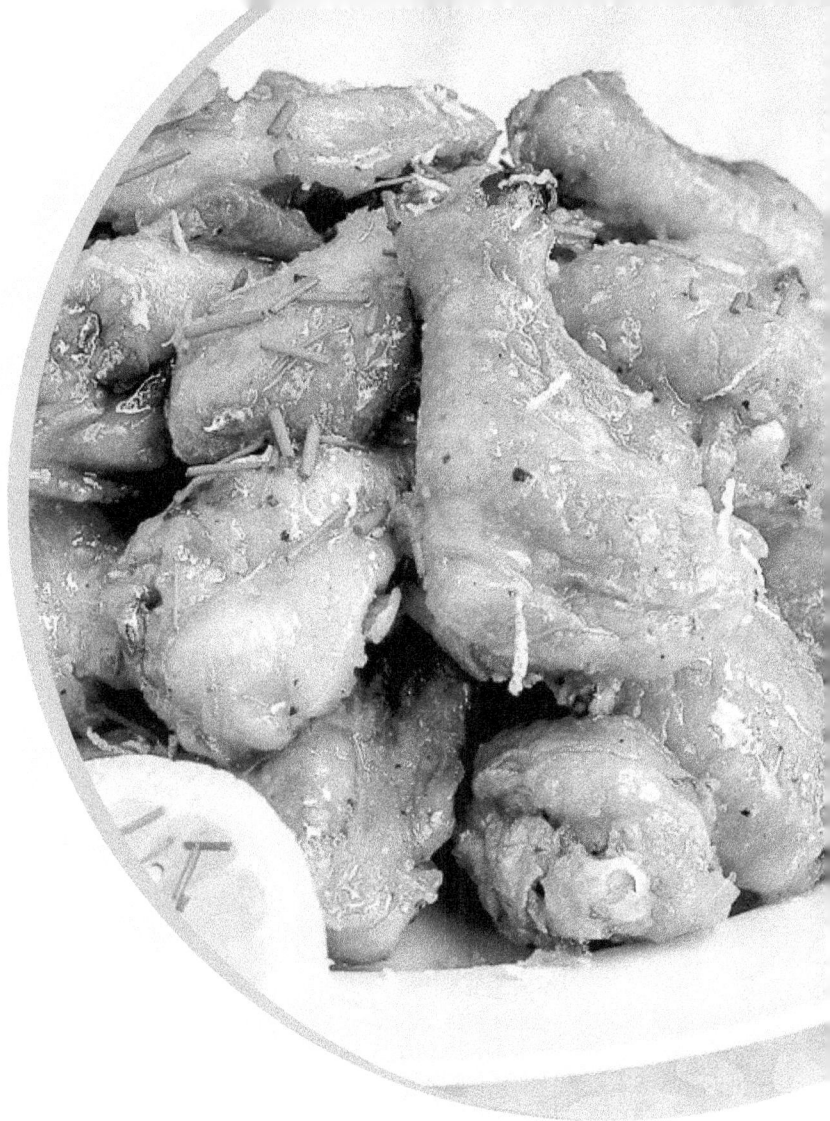

10. Remove chicken wings from oven after 20 minutes and brush all the wings with the glaze.
11. Raise your oven temperature to 400 F.
12. Place chicken wings in oven and cook about another 20 minutes or until done.
13. Garnish with chopped green onion and serve.

NUTRITION:

Calories: 170
Fat: 9g
Carbs: 12g
Protein: 11g
Sodium: 400mg
Potassium: 110mg
Phosphorus: 58mg

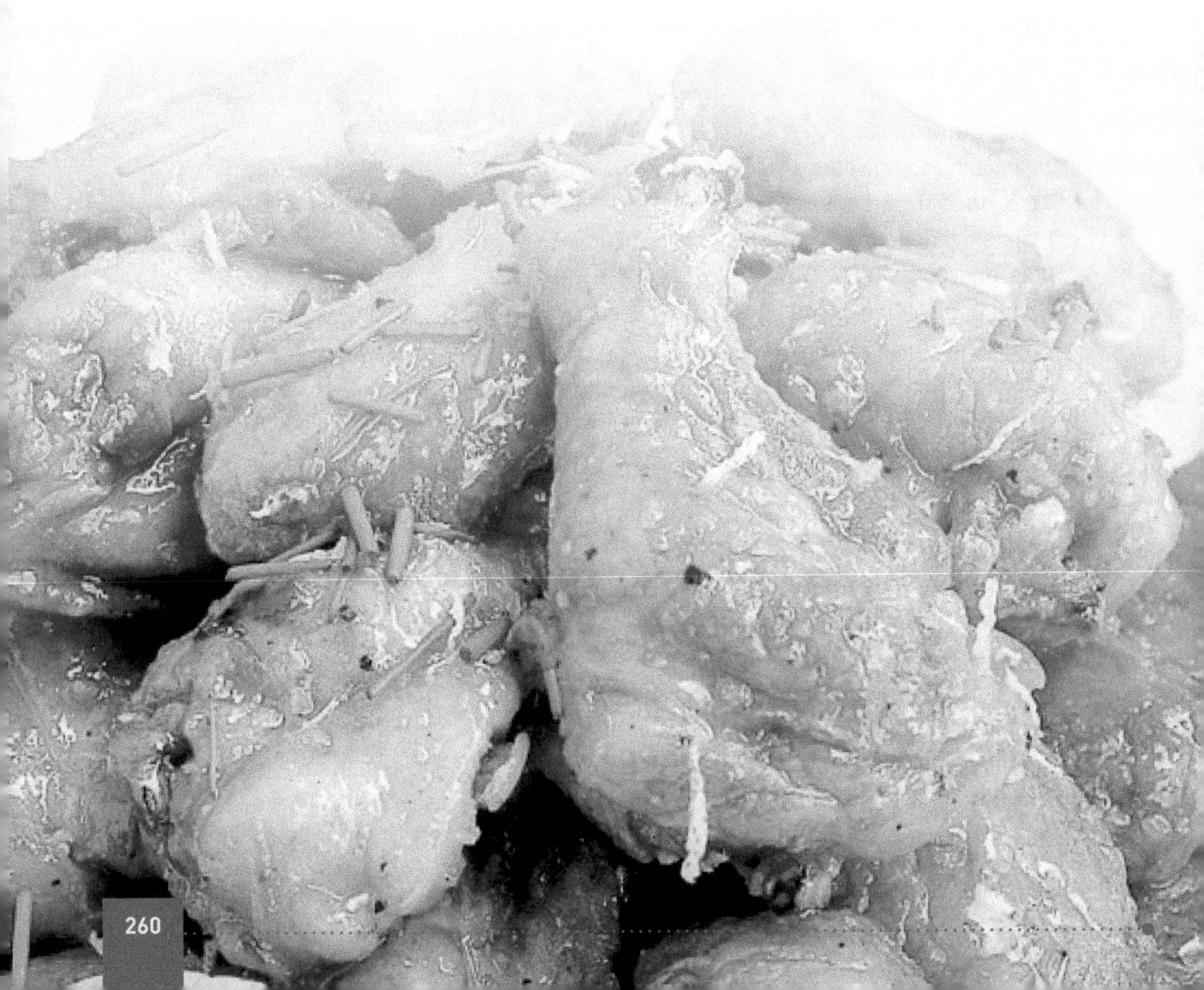

154 CUCUMBER AND DILL COLD SOUP

Preparation Time: 15 minutes

Cooking Time: 1 hour

Servings: 3

INGREDIENTS:

- 2 medium Cucumbers
- 1/3 cup Sweet white onion
- 1 medium Green onion
- ¼ cup Fresh mint leaves
- 2 Tbsp. Fresh dill
- 2 Tbsp. Lemon juice
- 2/3 cup Water
- ½ cup Half and half cream
- 1/3 cup Sour cream
- ½ tsp. Pepper

DIRECTIONS:

1. Peel and remove the seeds from cucumber and cut them into small cubes.
2. Chop mint leaves, sweet onion, and dill.
3. Place ingredients in blender.
4. Blend well until smooth.
5. Cover and keep it in refrigerator for 4 hours or until chilled.
6. Garnish this yummy cool soup with dill sprigs and serve.

NUTRITION:

Calories: 70
Fat: 3g
Carbs: 10g
Protein: 4g

Sodium: 88mg
Potassium: 388mg
Phosphorus: 100mg

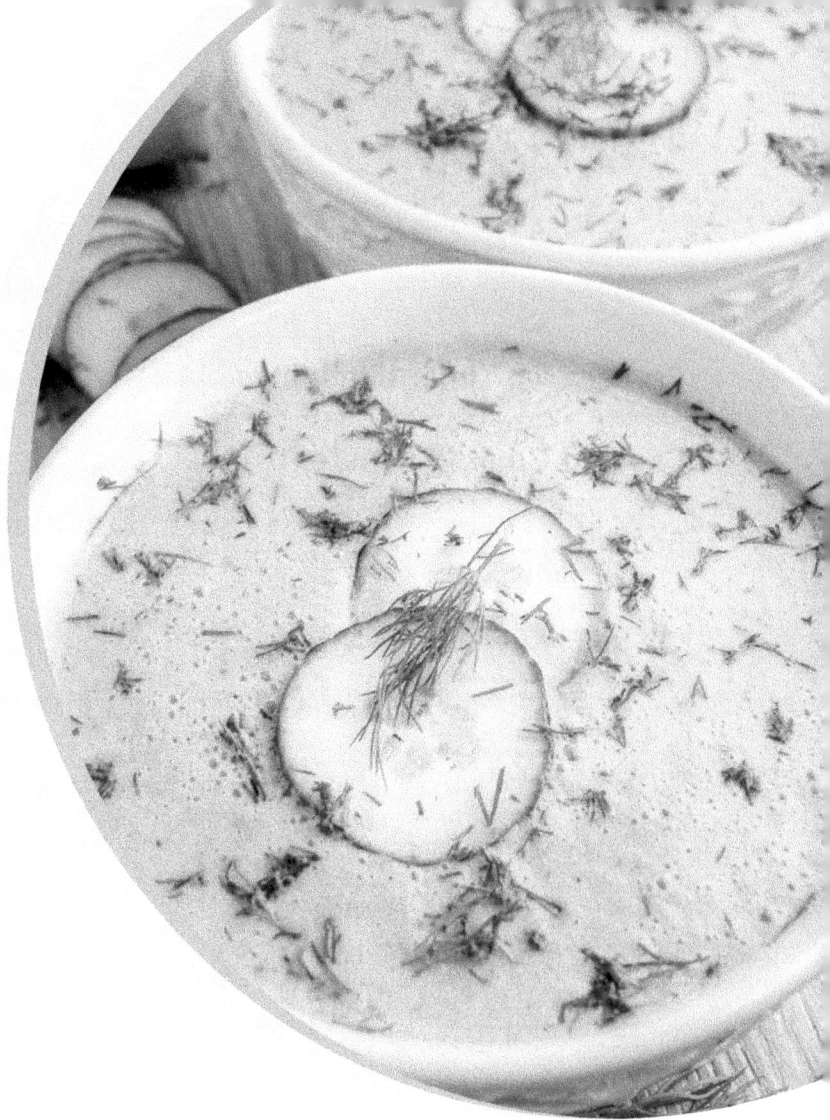

155 THAI FISH SOUP

Preparation Time: 15 minutes

Cooking Time: 10 minutes

Servings: 3

INGREDIENTS:

- 5 cups Water
- 2 fillets frozen
- 1 cup Green onion chopped
- 2 cloves Chopped garlic
- 1 Tbsp. Minced ginger
- 1 cup Carrots diced
- 1 cup Celery diced
- Basil to taste
- 1 Tbsp. Cilantro
- ½ tsp. or to taste Black pepper powder
- 1 Tbsp. Lime juice
- 1 cup Bean sprouts
- 1 cup Long grain rice cooked
- 1 small de-seeded and finely chopped Red chili
- 1 Tbsp. Oil

DIRECTIONS:

1. Boil water in a pan.
2. In a pan add 1 Tbsp. oil sauté garlic, ginger, green onion, and celery over medium high heat.
3. Add boiling water, carrots, and fish.
4. Simmer until fish is cooked.
5. Add basil, cilantro, black pepper, and chopped red chili. Simmer for 5 minutes.
6. Add bean sprouts and cooked rice and cook for 4 to 6 minutes.
7. Garnish with chopped cilantro and squeeze lime juice.

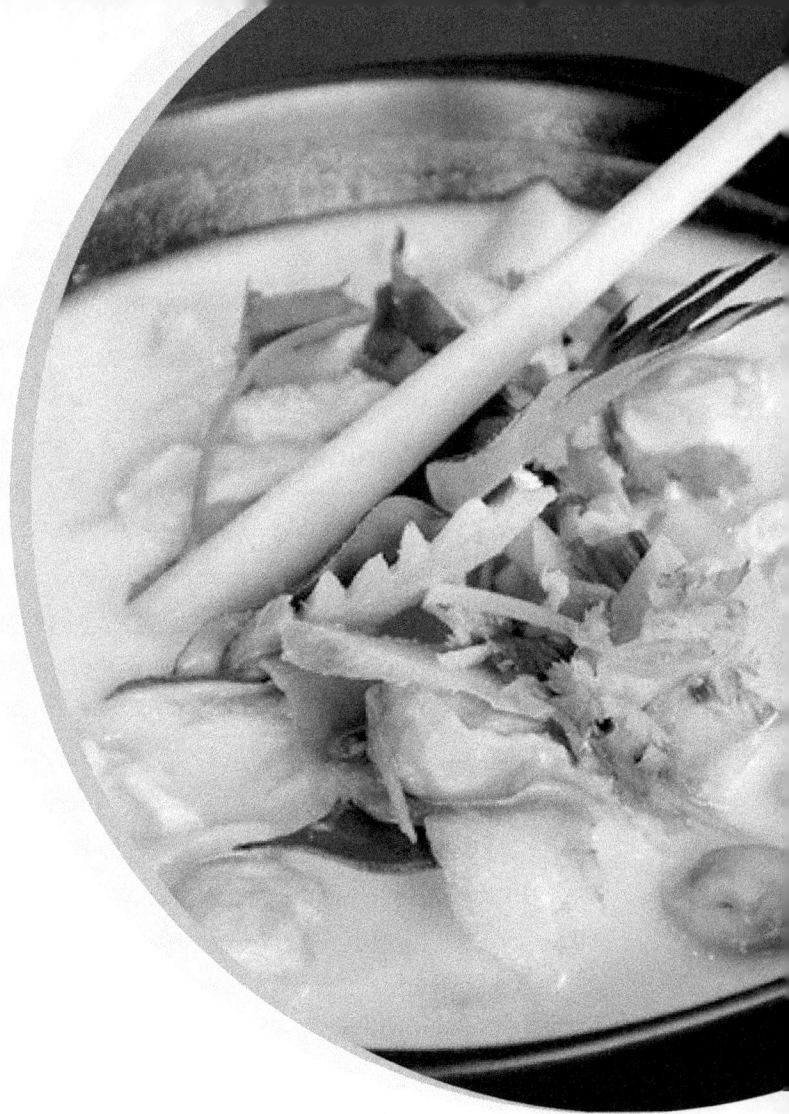

Calories: 191
Fat: 14g
Carbs: 12g
Protein: 8g
Sodium: 1000mg
Potassium: 343mg
Phosphorus: 141mg

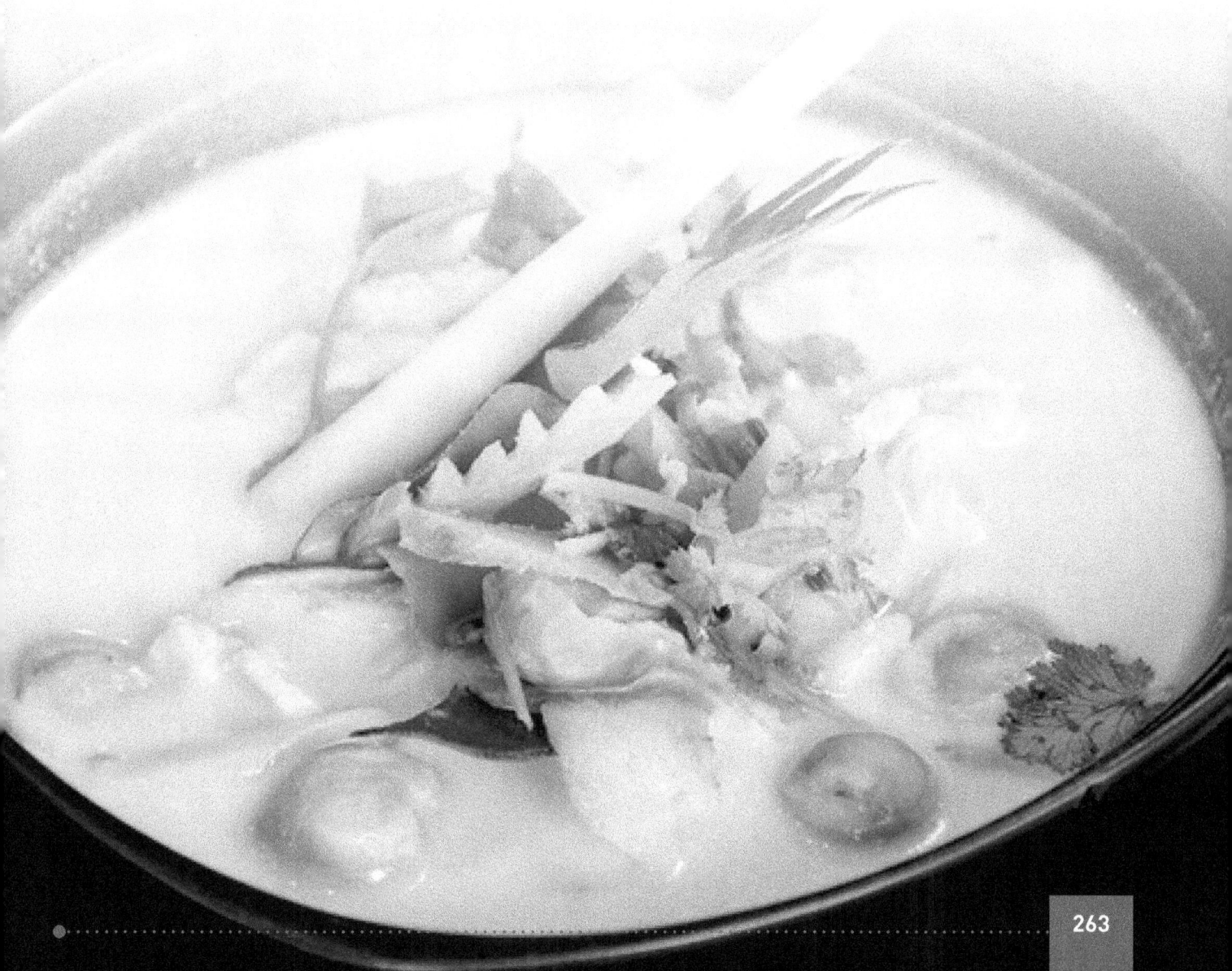

156 MEATLOAF SANDWICHES

Preparation Time: 25 minutes

Cooking Time: 50 minutes

Servings: 12

INGREDIENTS:

For Meatloaf
- 20 squares Unsalted saltine-type crackers
- 2 Tbsp. Onion finely chopped
-
  1 pound (10% fat) Lean ground beef
- 1 large Egg
- 2 Tbsp. low fat milk
- ¼ tsp. Black pepper grounded
- 1/3 cup Catsup
- 1 Tbsp. Brown sugar
- ½ tsp. Apple cider vinegar
- 1 tsp. Water

For Sandwiches
- 12 slices White bread slices
- 1 cup Lettuce chopped
- 1 large Onion sliced

DIRECTIONS:

1. Preheat oven to 375 F.
2. Take a large zip lock plastic bag, place crackers in it and crush them with a rolling pin.
3. In a mixing bowl, combine crushed crackers, ground beef, finely chopped onion, milk, egg, and black pepper.
4. Add this mixture to loaf pan and place it in oven.
5. Bake it for 40 minutes.

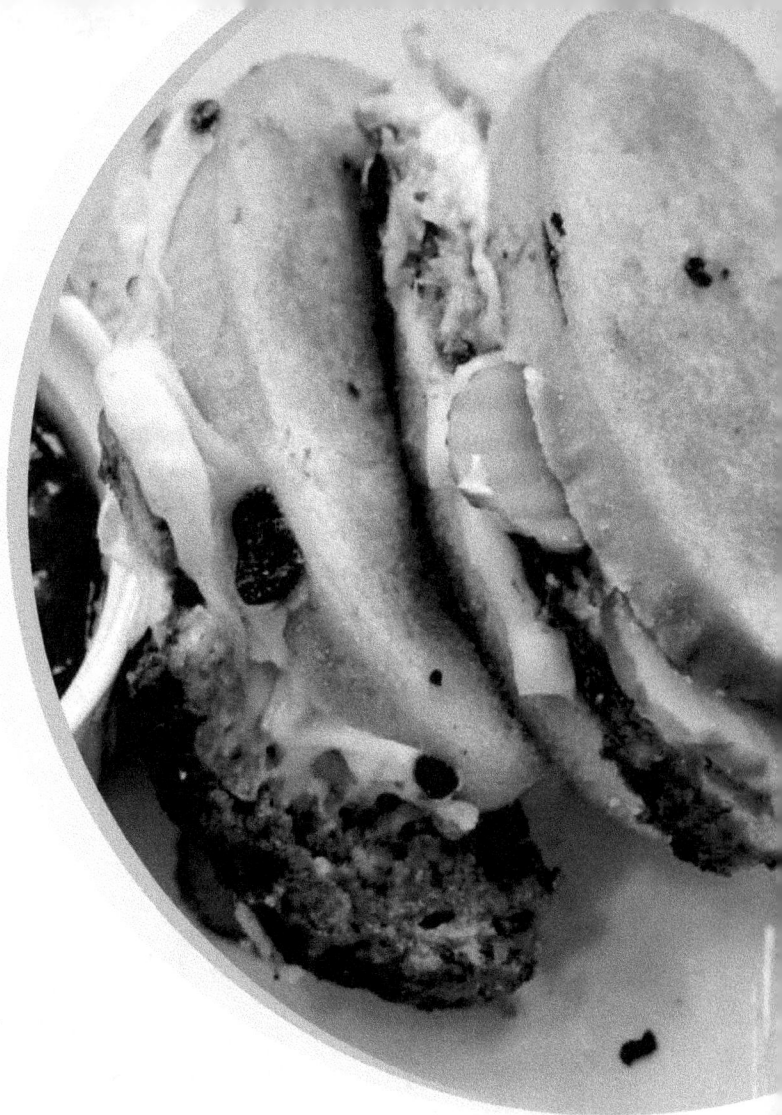

6. Mix catsup, vinegar, brown sugar, and water in a small bowl to make topping sauce.
7. Remove meatloaf after 40 minutes from the oven and cover with sauce.
8. Return meatloaf pan to the oven and bake for 10 minutes more.
9. Slice into six thick portions.
10. Take a bread slice, and place meatloaf slice on it.
11. Top it with lettuce and sliced onion, and cover with another slice.

NUTRITION:

Calories: 520
Fat: 35g
Carbs: 40g
Protein: 35g
Sodium: 370mg
Potassium: 450mg
Phosphorus: 40mg

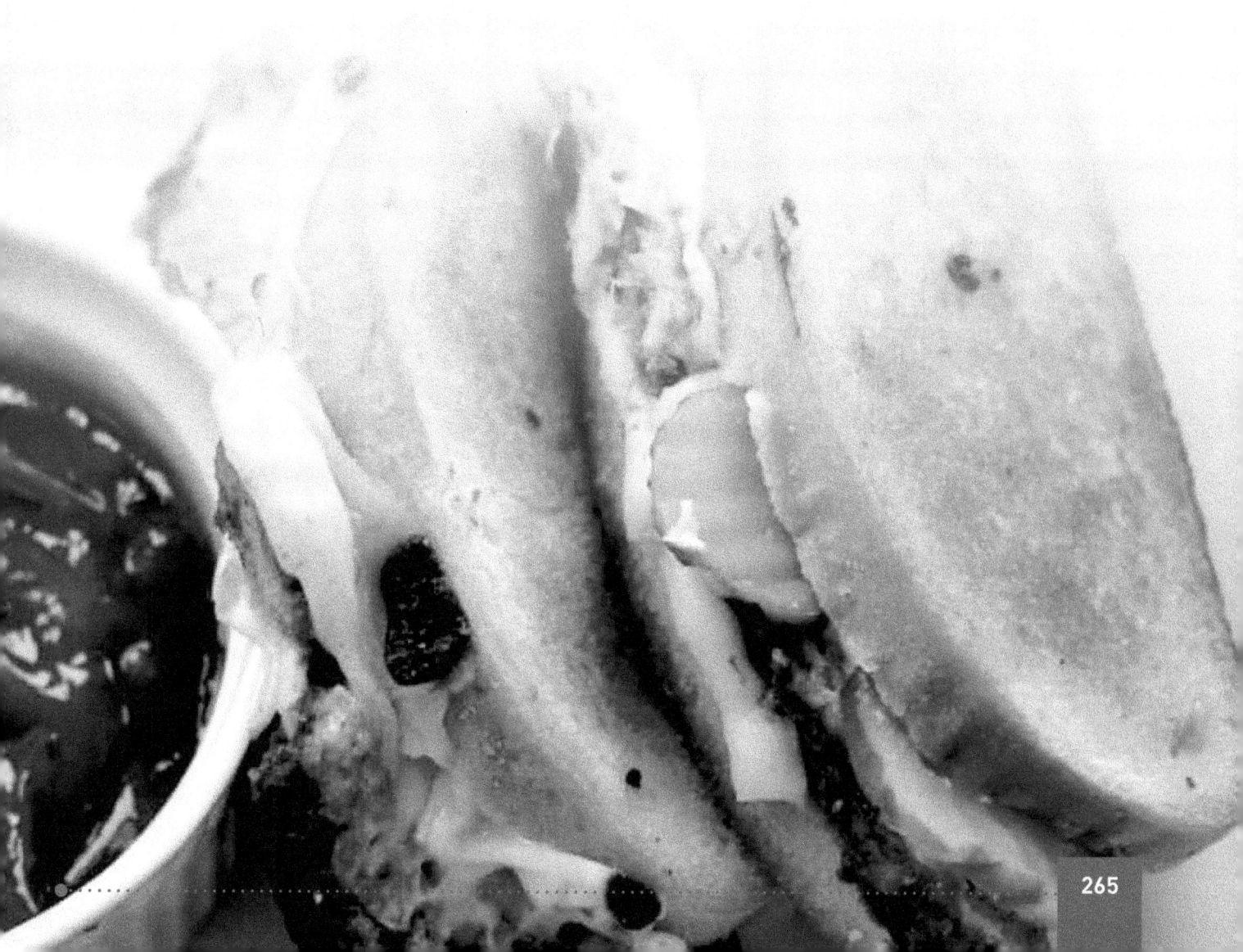

157 ZUCCHINI AND CORN PANCAKES WITH CHILI LIME DIP

Preparation Time: 15 minutes

Cooking Time: 35 minutes

Servings: 4

INGREDIENTS:

For pancakes:
- 2 medium Zucchini shredded
- 1 cup Corn
- 3 Eggs
- 1 Tbsp. White sugar
- 2 tsp. Vegetable oil
- ½ cup Milk
- 1 cup All-purpose flour
- 1 tsp. Baking soda
- 2 Tbsp. Chopped cilantro
- ½ tsp. Black pepper powder
- ½ tsp. Ground cumin

For chili lime dip
- ½ cup Silken tofu
- 2 Tbsp. Mayonnaise
- ½ cup Roasted red pepper
- 1 tsp. Chili powder
- 1 tsp. Onion powder
- 1 ½ Tbsp. Lime juice
- 3 Tbsp. cilantros chopped

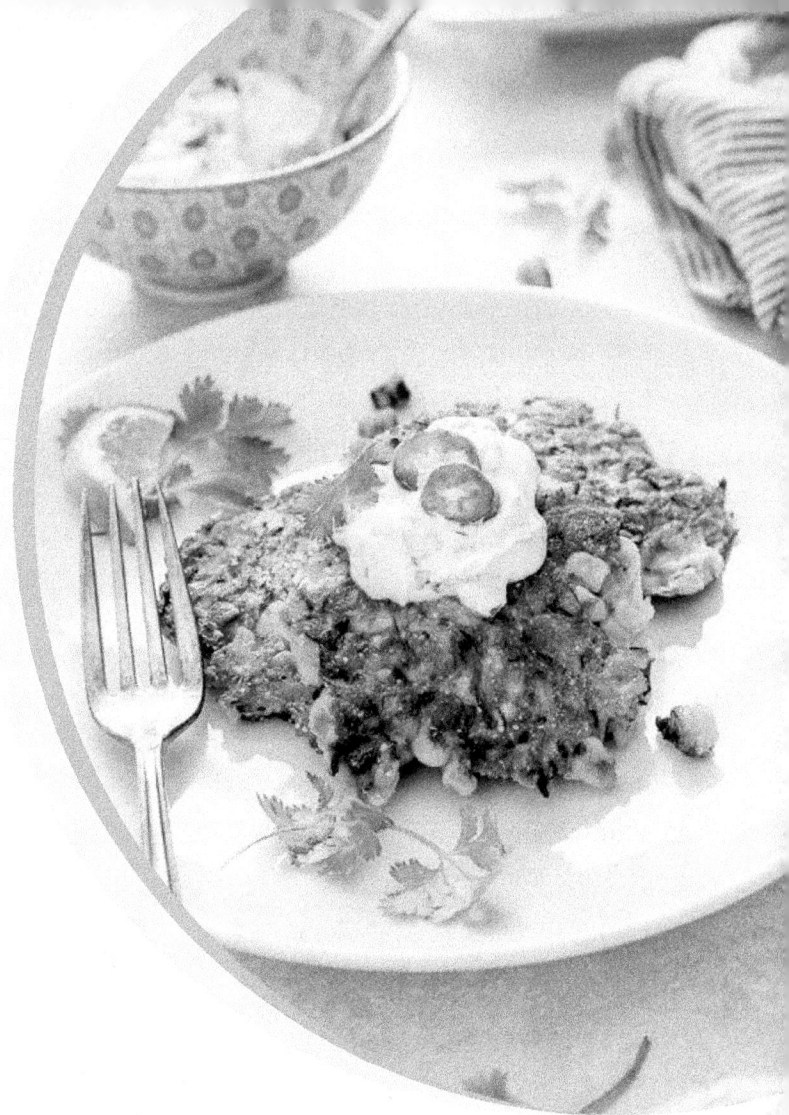

For Pancakes:

1. Whisk eggs, and then add milk, sugar, flour, vegetable oil, and baking soda in a large bowl.
2. Fold in cumin, black pepper, cilantro, corn, and zucchini.
3. Warm a fry pan over medium heat.
4. Spoon ¼ cup batter into fry pan.
5. Flip only one time, cook until golden on both sides.
6. Serve hot with chili lime dip.

For Chili lime dip:

1. Blend all ingredients for 30 seconds or until smooth.
2. Transfer dip and refrigerate for 30 minutes.

NUTRITION:

Calories: 115
Fat: 4g
Carbs: 17g
Protein: 3g
Sodium: 180mg
Potassium: 130mg
Phosphorus: 67mg

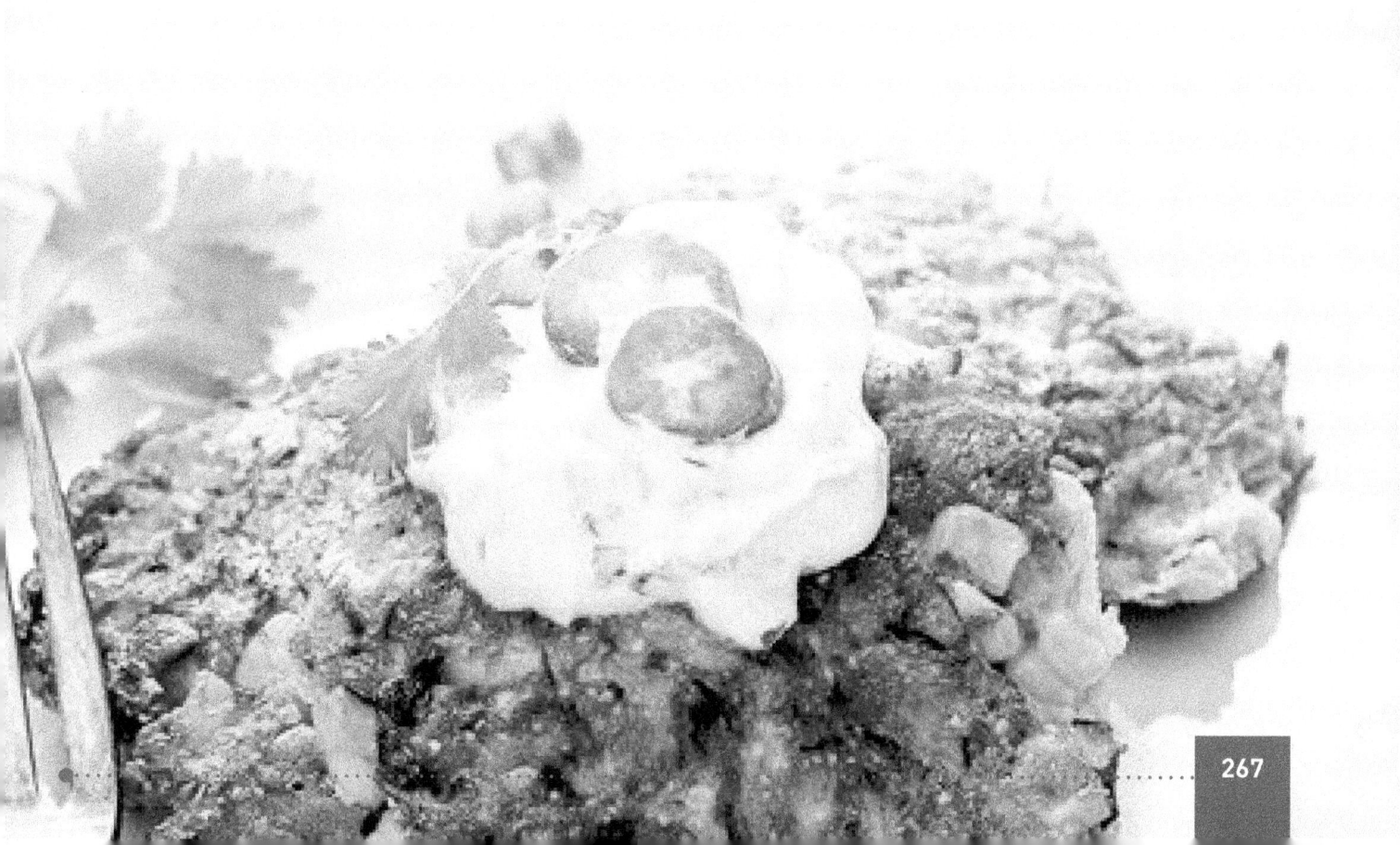

158 CHICKEN WITH PINEAPPLE AND HONEY

Preparation Time: 10 minutes

Cooking Time: 40 minutes

Servings: 3

INGREDIENTS:

- 20 ounces Pineapple slices canned
- 1-pound Chicken breast skinless boneless
- 2 cloves Minced garlic
- 1 tsp. Ground thyme
- ¼ tsp. Black pepper powder
- 1 Tbsp. Vegetable oil
- 1 Tbsp. Corn starch
- 3 Tbsp. Honey
- 3 Tbsp. Dijon mustard
- 2 Tbsp. Water

DIRECTIONS:

1. Drain pineapples from juice and reserve the juice.
2. Rub thyme and garlic on chicken and sprinkle black pepper.
3. Add chicken in heated skillet and cook until brown from both sides.
4. Add Dijon mustard, pineapple juice, and honey.
5. Spoon sauce over chicken.
6. Cover and simmer for 10 minutes.
7. Put water with corn starch in a bowl. Add chicken and sauce.
8. Put pineapple slices. Cook until the sauce boil and thickens.
9. Serve with rice.

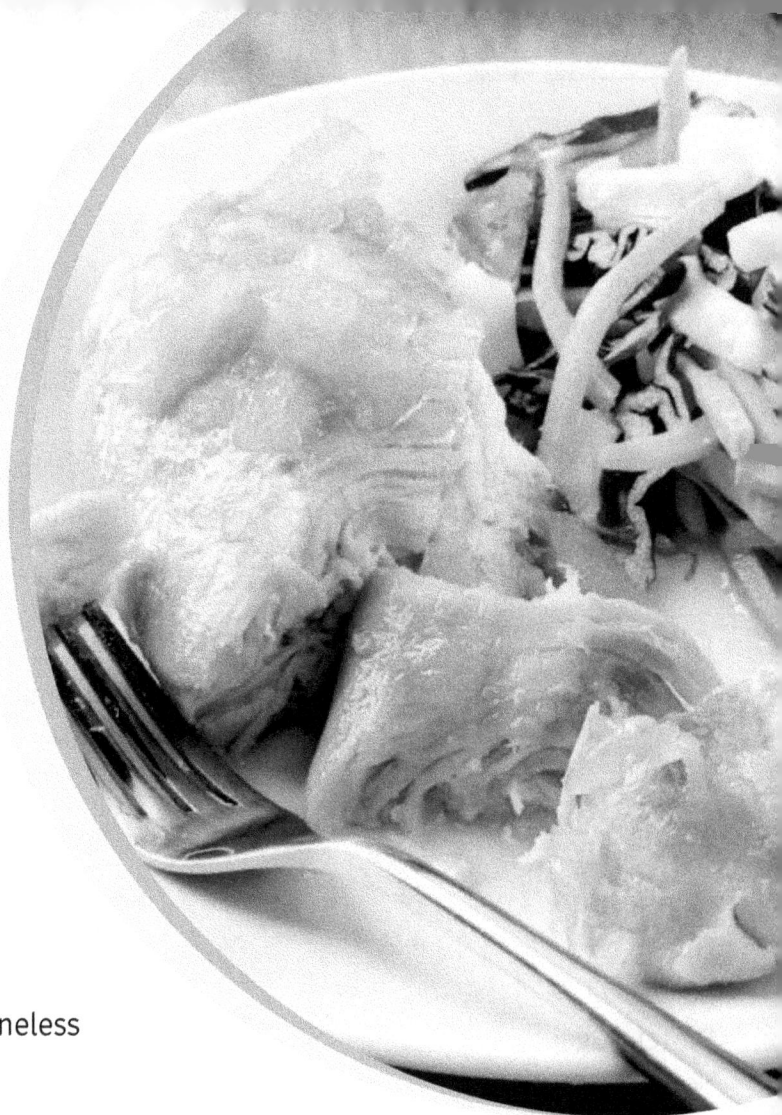

Calories: 192
Fat: 3.2g
Carbs: 13g
Protein: 26g
Sodium: 217mg
Potassium: 358mg
Phosphorus: 224mg

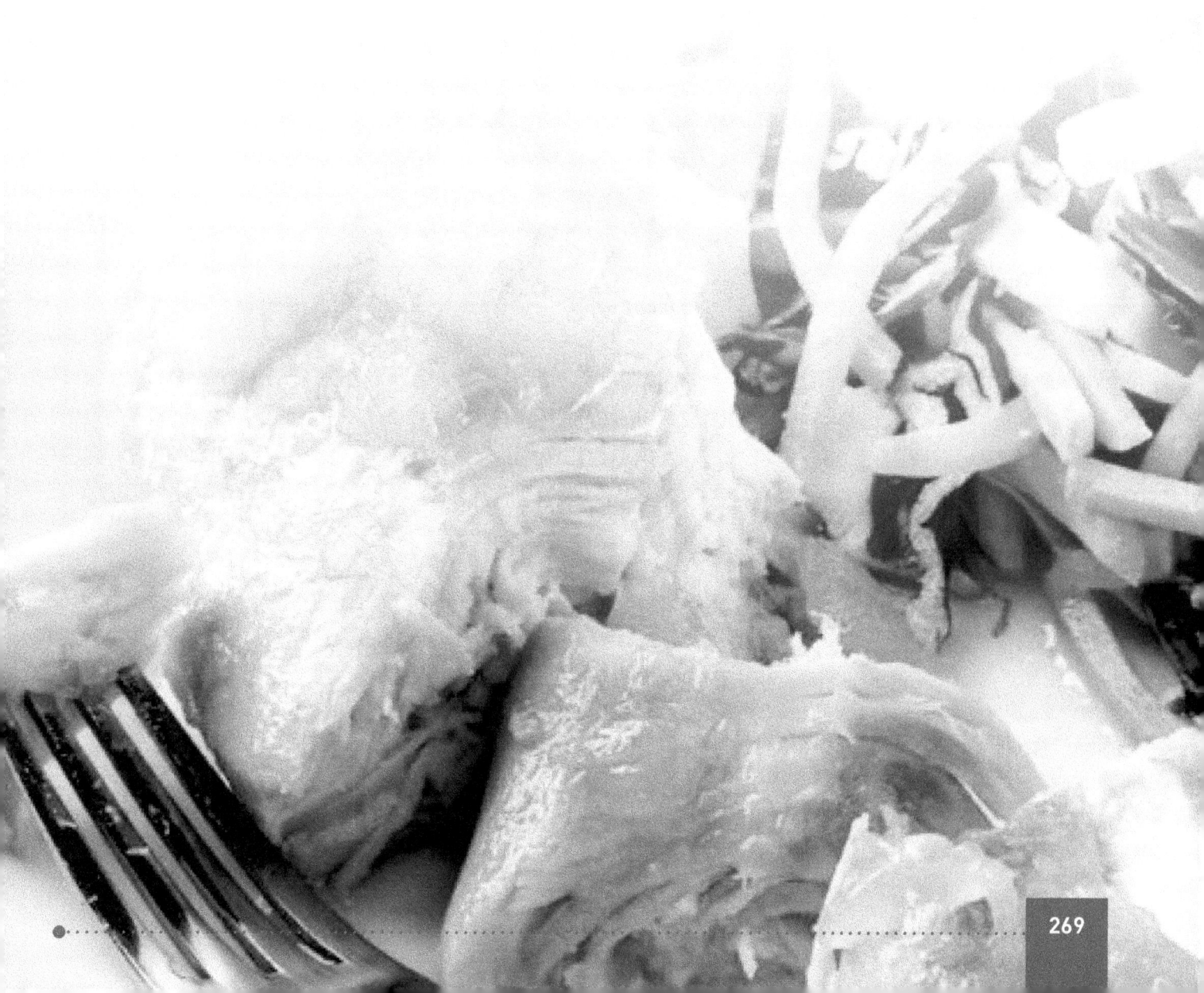

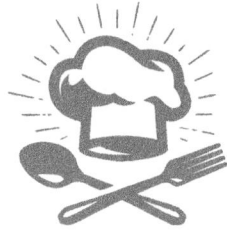

CHAPTER 21

SNACK RECIPES

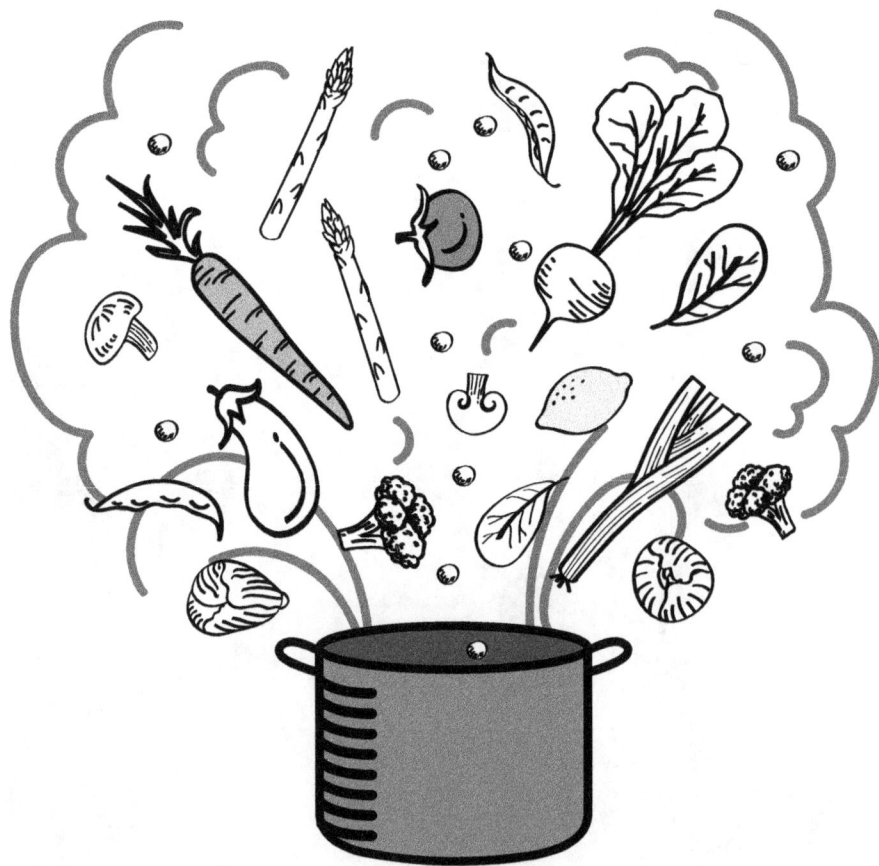

159 SESAME CRACKERS

Preparation Time: 15 minutes

Cooking Time: 12 minutes

Servings: 1

INGREDIENTS:

- 1 cup sesame seeds
- 2 tbsp. grapeseed oil
- 2 large eggs, beaten
- 1 ½ tsp. sea salt
- 3 cups almond flour

DIRECTIONS:

1. Mix well the sesame seeds, almond flour, oil, eggs, and salt in a bowl.
2. Divide the dough into two portions.
3. Place each into two baking sheets lined with parchment papers and cover with parchment paper.
4. Spread the dough between the papers to cover the entire baking sheet and remove the top paper.
5. Cut the dough into 2-inch squares and bake at 350°F until golden brown, for about 12 minutes.
6. Cool before serving.

NUTRITION:

Calories: 178
Fat: 15.6 g
Carbs: 6 g
Protein: 6.1 g

Sodium: 184 mg
Potassium: 468mg
Phosphorus: 0mg

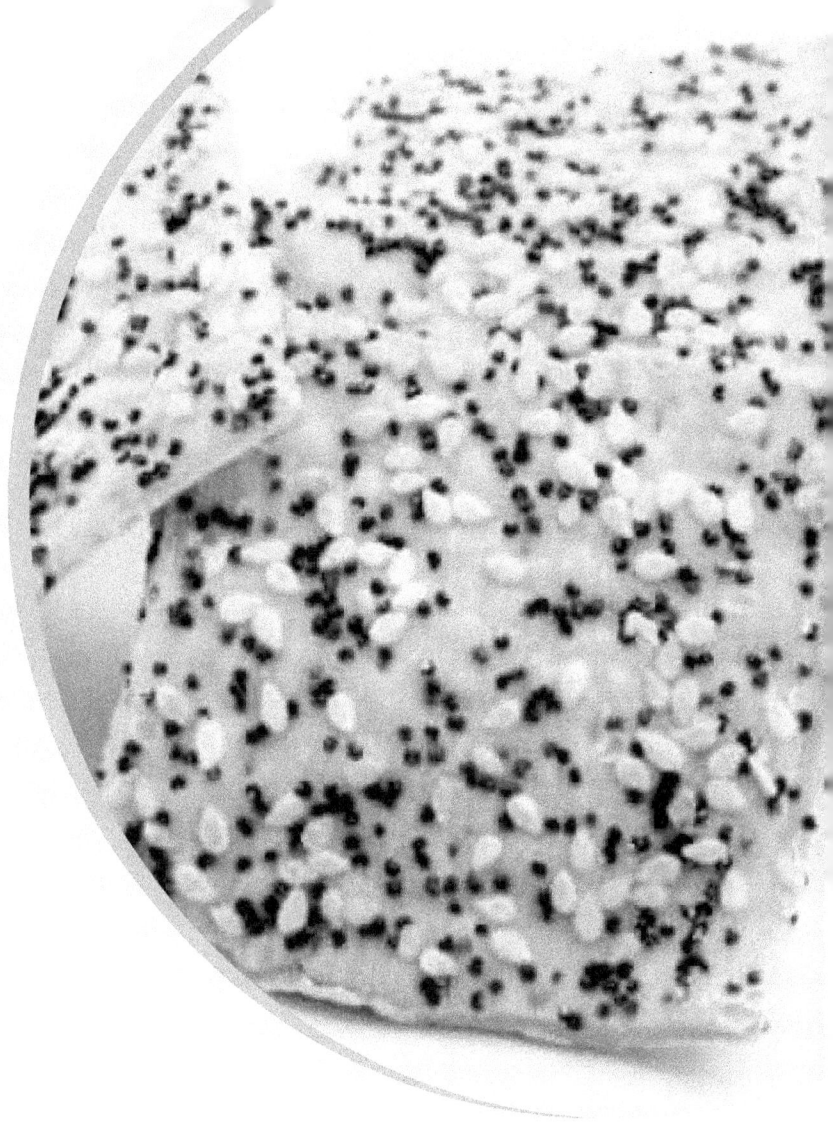

160 VEGGIE SNACK

Preparation Time: 5 minutes

Cooking Time: 10 minutes

Servings: 1

INGREDIENTS:

- 1 large yellow pepper
- 5 carrots
- 5 stalks celery

DIRECTIONS:

1. Clean the carrots and rinse under running water.
2. Rinse celery and yellow pepper. Remove seeds of pepper and chop the veggies into small sticks.
3. Put in a bowl and serve.

NUTRITION:

Calories: 189
Fat: 0.5 g
Carbs: 44.3 g
Protein: 5 g
Sodium: 282 mg
Potassium: 0mg
Phosphorus: 0mg

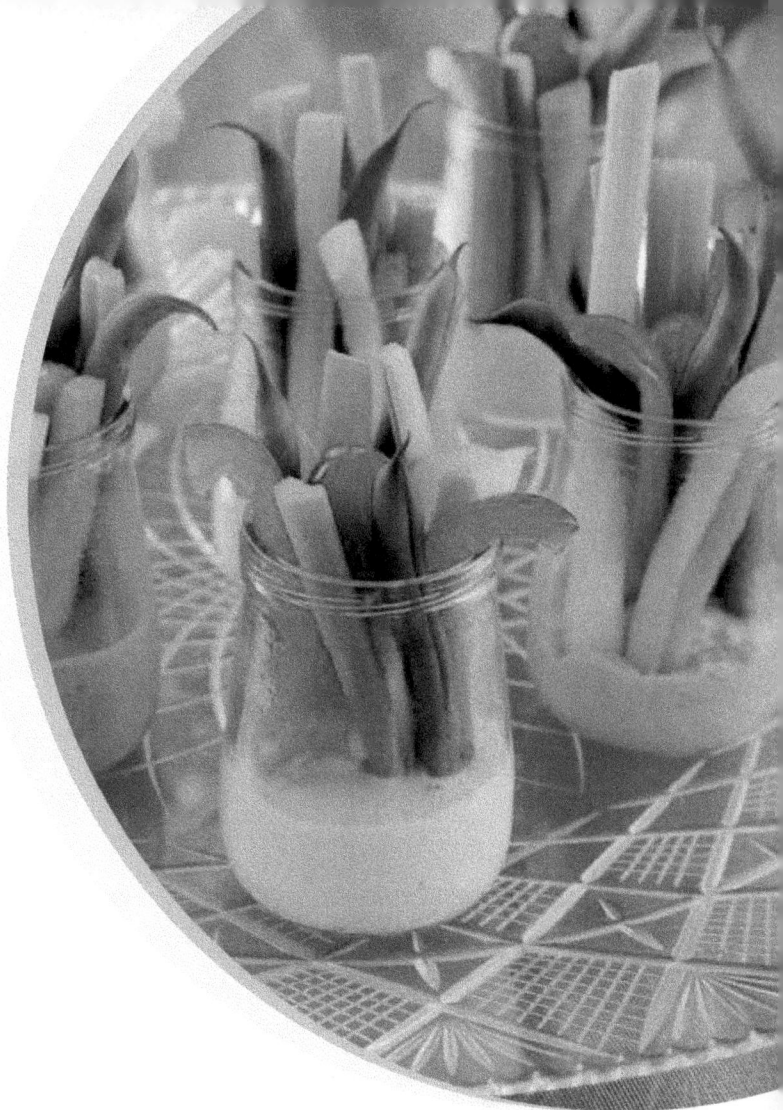

161 HEALTHY SPICED NUTS

Preparation Time: 10 minutes

Cooking Time: 10 minutes

Servings: 4

INGREDIENTS:

- 1 tbsp. extra virgin olive oil
- ¼ cup walnuts
- ¼ cup pecans
- ¼ cup almonds
- ½ tsp. sea salt
- ½ tsp. cumin
- ½ tsp. pepper
- 1 tsp. chili powder

DIRECTIONS:

1. Put the skillet on medium heat and toast the nuts until lightly browned.
2. Prepare the spice mixture and add black pepper, cumin, chili, and salt.
3. Put extra virgin olive oil and sprinkle with spice mixture to the toasted nuts before serving.

NUTRITION:

Calories: 88
Fat: 8g
Carbs: 4g
Protein: 2.5g
Sodium: 51mg
Potassium: 88mg
Phosphorus: 6.3mg

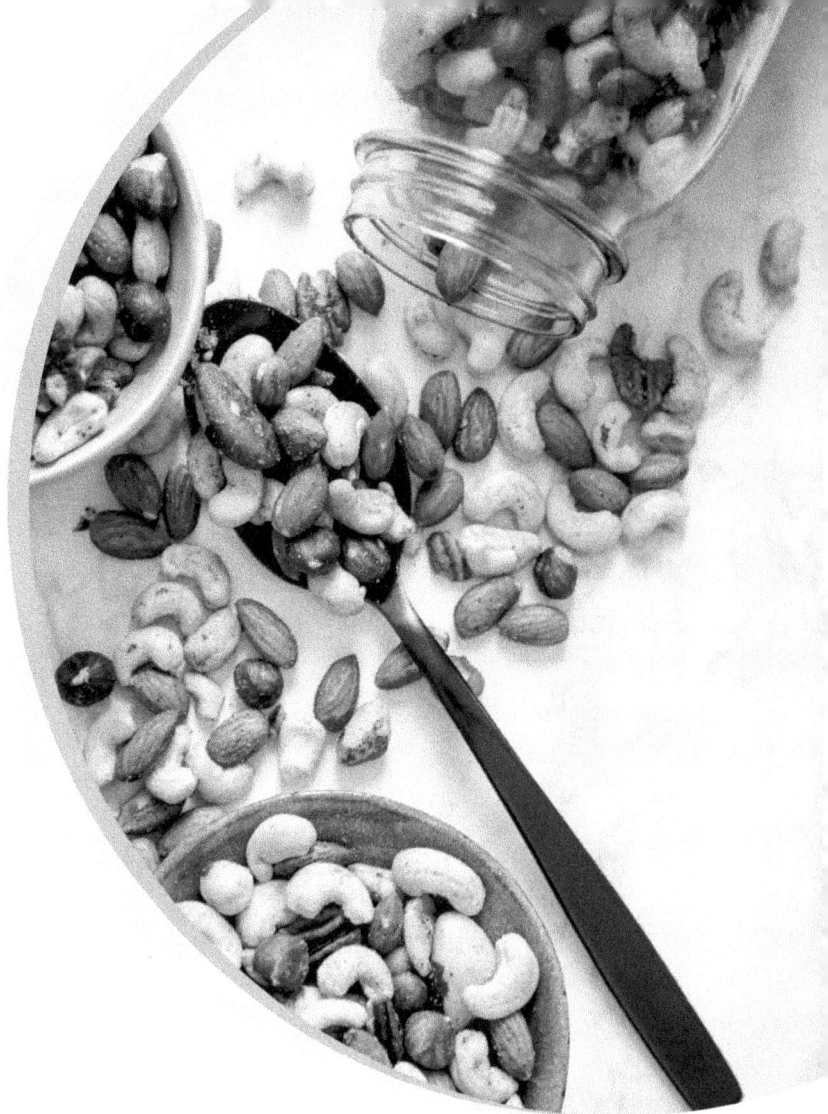

162 ROASTED ASPARAGUS

Preparation Time: 5 minutes

Cooking Time: 10 minutes

Servings: 4

INGREDIENTS:

- 1 tbsp. extra virgin olive oil
- 1-pound fresh asparagus
- 1 medium lemon, zested
- 1/2 tsp. freshly grated nutmeg
- 1/2 tsp. kosher salt
- ½ tsp. black pepper

DIRECTIONS:

1. Preheat your oven to 500 degrees F.
2. Put asparagus on an aluminum foil and add extra virgin olive oil.
3. Prepare asparagus in a single layer and fold the edges of the foil.
4. Cook in the oven for 5 minutes. Continue roasting until browned.
5. Add the roasted asparagus with nutmeg, salt, zest, and pepper before serving.

NUTRITION:

Calories: 55
Fat: 3.8 g
Carbs: 4.7 g
Protein: 2.5 g
Sodium: 98mg
Potassium: 172mg
Phosphorus: 35mg

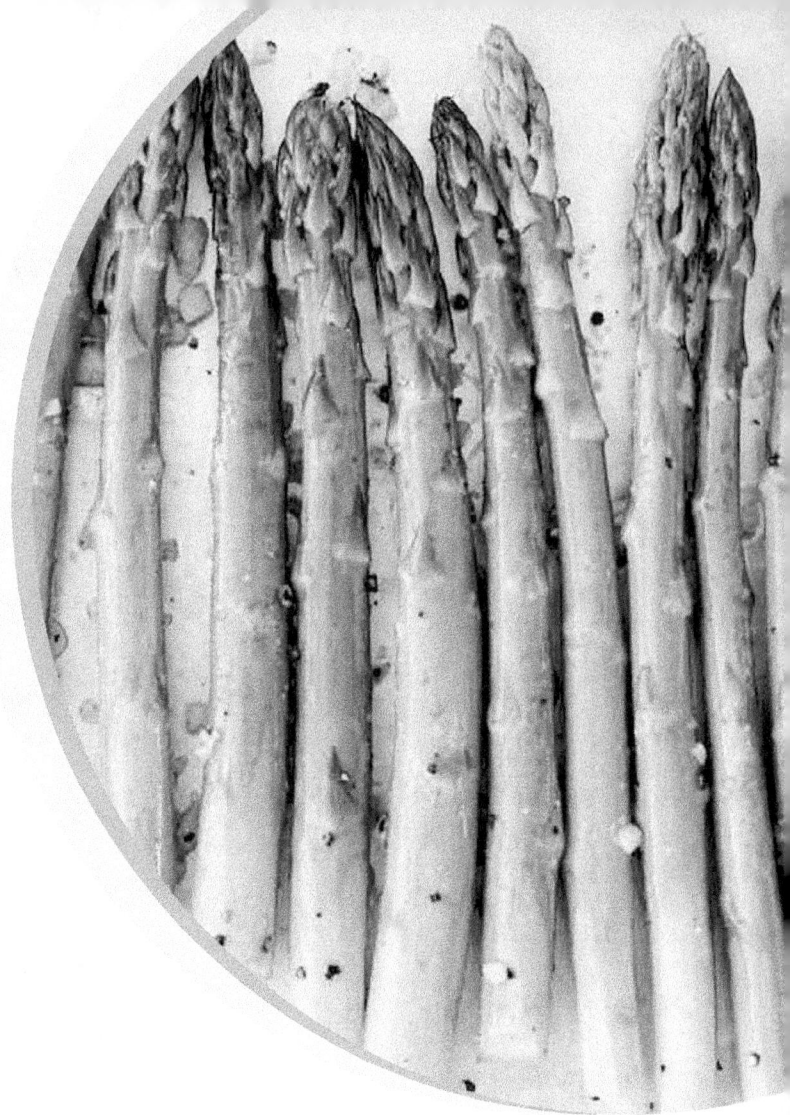

163 WARM LEMON ROSEMARY OLIVES

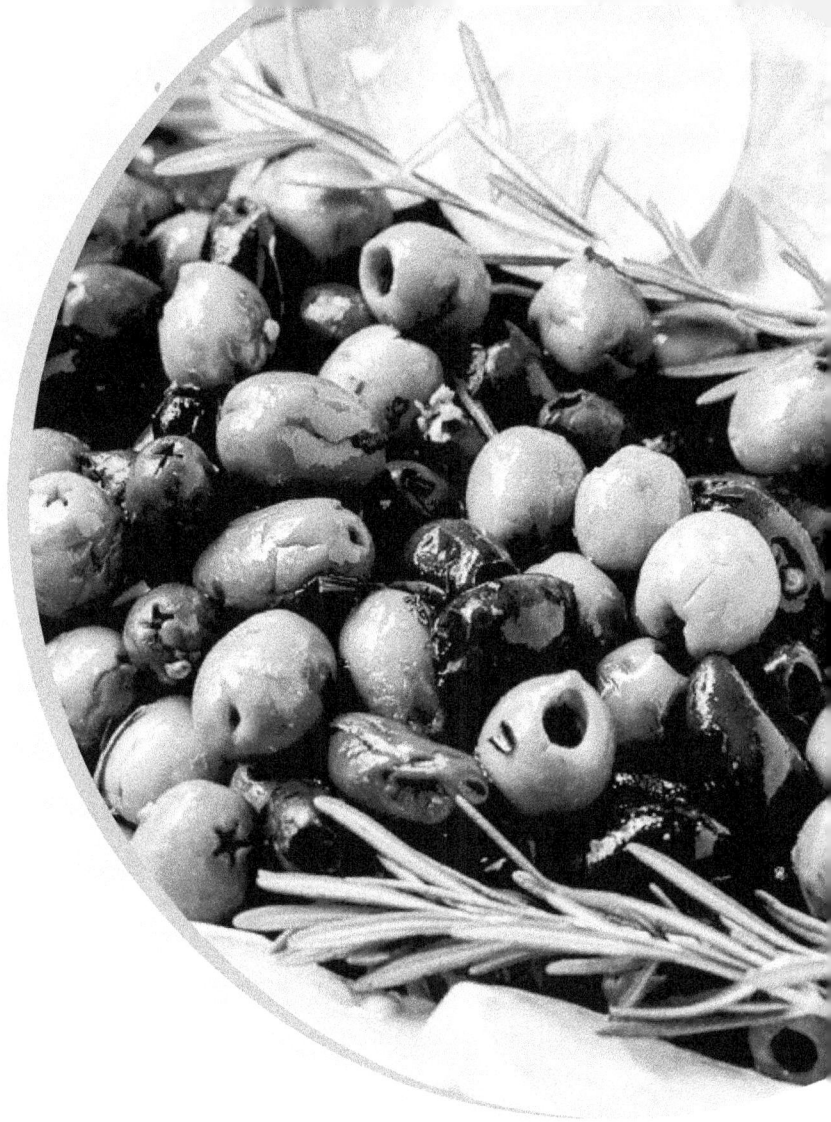

Preparation Time: 5 minutes

Cooking Time: 20 minutes

Servings: 12

INGREDIENTS:

- 1 teaspoon extra-virgin olive oil
- 1 teaspoon grated lemon peel
- 1 teaspoon crushed red pepper flakes
- 2 sprigs fresh rosemary
- 3 cups mixed olives
- Lemon twists, optional

DIRECTIONS:

1. Preheat your oven to 400°F. Place pepper flakes, rosemary, olives, and grated lemon peel onto a large sheet of foil; drizzle with oil and fold the foil.
2. Pinch the edges of the sheet to seal tightly.
3. Bake in the preheated oven for about 30 minutes.
4. Remove from the sheet and place the mixture in the serving dish.
5. Serve warm garnished with lemon twists.

NUTRITION:

Calories: 43
Fat: 4 g
Carbs: 2.2 g
Protein: 0.3 g

Sodium: 250mg
Potassium: 6.4mg
Phosphorus: 2.2mg

164 LOW-FAT MANGO SALSA

Preparation Time: 10 minutes

Cooking Time: 10 minutes

Servings: 4

INGREDIENTS:

- 1 cup cucumber, chopped
- 2 cups mango, diced
- ½ cup cilantro, minced
- 2 tablespoons fresh lime juice
- 1 tablespoon scallions, minced
- ¼ teaspoon chipotle powder
- ¼ teaspoon sea salt

DIRECTIONS

1. Mix the ingredients in a bowl and serve or refrigerate.

NUTRITION:

Calories: 155
Fat: 0.6 g
Carbs: 38.2 g
Protein: 1.4 g
Sodium: 3.2 mg
Potassium: 221mg
Phosphorus: 27mg

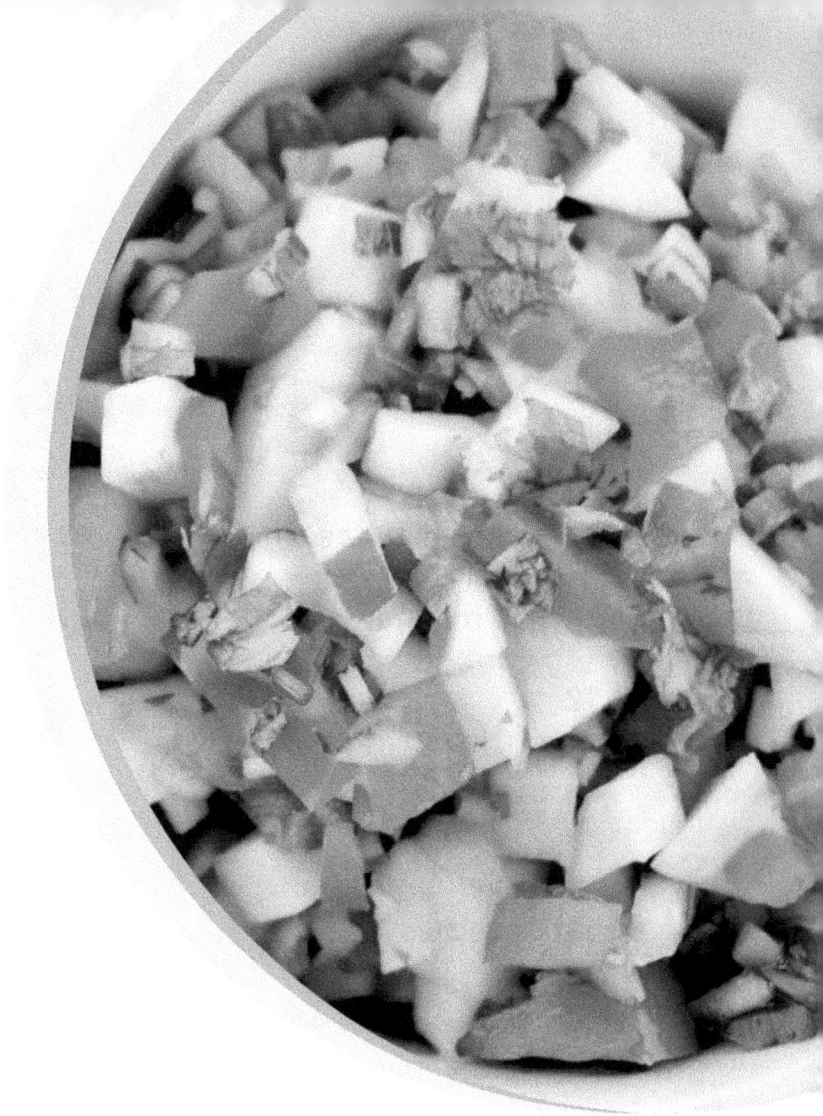

165 VINEGAR & SALT KALE CHIPS

Preparation Time: 10 minutes

Cooking Time: 12 minutes

Servings: 2

INGREDIENTS:

- 1 head kale, chopped
- 1 teaspoon extra virgin olive oil
- 1 tablespoon apple cider vinegar
- ½ teaspoon of sea salt

DIRECTIONS:

1. Prepare kale in a bowl and put vinegar and extra virgin olive oil.
2. Sprinkle with salt and massage the ingredients with hands.
3. Spread the kale out onto two paper-lined baking sheets and bake at 375°F for about 12 minutes or until crispy.
4. Let cool for about 10 minutes before serving.

NUTRITION:

Calories: 152
Fat: 8.2 g
Carbs: 15.2 g
Protein: 4 g
Sodium: 170mg
Potassium: 304mg
Phosphorus: 37mg

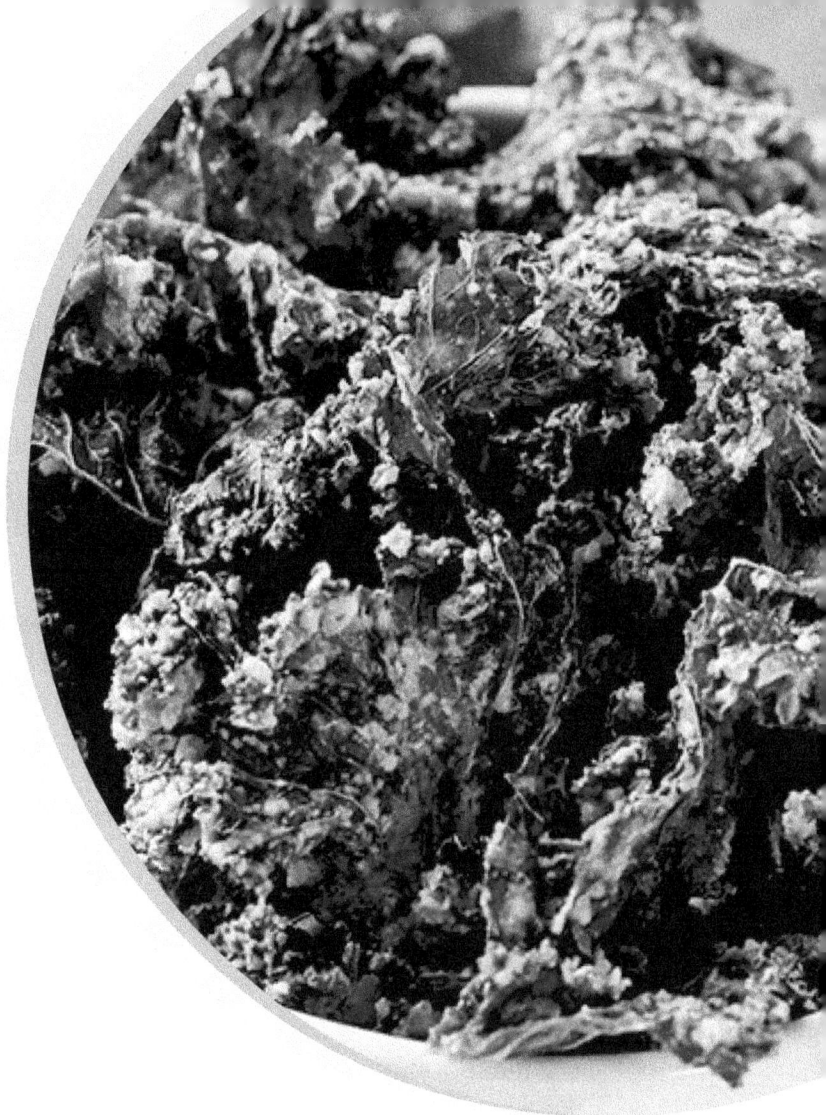

166 CARROT AND PARSNIPS FRENCH FRIES

Preparation Time: 15 minutes

Cooking Time: 20 minutes

Servings: 2

INGREDIENTS:

- 6 large carrots
- 6 large parsnips
- 2 tablespoons extra virgin olive oil
- ½ teaspoon of sea salt

DIRECTIONS:

1. Chop the carrots and parsnips into 2-inch slices and then cut each into thin sticks.
2. Toss together the carrots and parsnip sticks with extra virgin olive oil and salt in a bowl and spread into a baking sheet lined with parchment paper.
3. Bake the sticks at 425° for about 20 minutes or until browned.

NUTRITION:

Calories: 179
Fat: 4g
Carbs: 14g
Protein: 11g
Sodium: 27.3mg
Potassium: 625mg
Phosphorus: 116mg

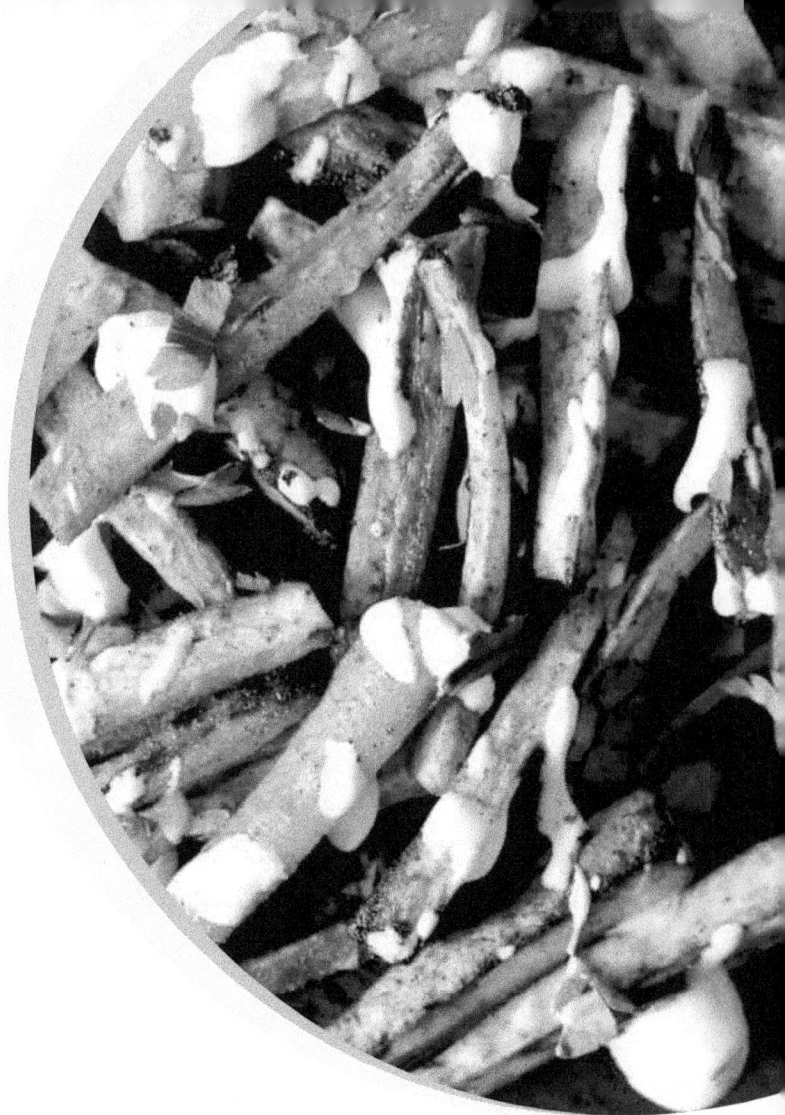

167 APPLE & STRAWBERRY SNACK

Preparation Time: 5 minutes

Cooking Time: 2 minutes

Servings: 1

INGREDIENTS:

- ½ apple, cored and sliced
- 2-3 strawberries
- dash of ground cinnamon
- 2-3 drops stevia 2-3 drops

DIRECTIONS:

1. In a bowl, mix strawberries and apples and sprinkle with stevia and cinnamon.
2. Microwave for about 1-2 minutes. Serve warm.

NUTRITION:

Calories: 145
Fat: 0.8 g
Carbs: 34.2 g
Protein: 1.6 g
Sodium: 20 mg
Potassium: 0mg
Phosphorus: 0mg

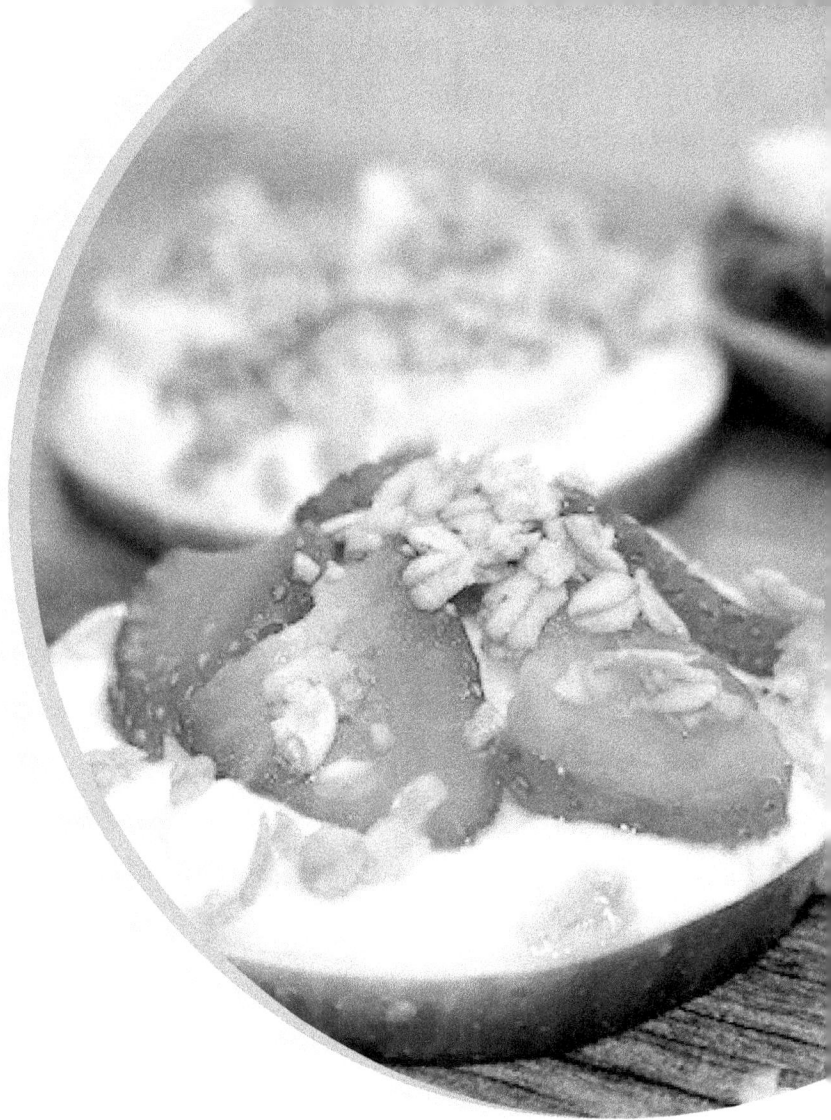

168 CANDIED MACADAMIA NUTS

Preparation Time: 5 minutes

Cooking Time: 15 minutes

Servings: 2

INGREDIENTS:

- 2 cups macadamia nuts
- 1 tablespoon extra-virgin olive oil
- 2 tablespoons honey

DIRECTIONS:

1. Toss ingredients in bowl and spread into a baking dish.
2. Bake for 15 minutes at 350°F.
3. Let cool before serving.

NUTRITION:

Calories: 200
Fat: 18 g
Carbs: 10g
Protein: 1g
Sodium: 5 mg
Potassium: 55mg
Phosphorus: 10mg

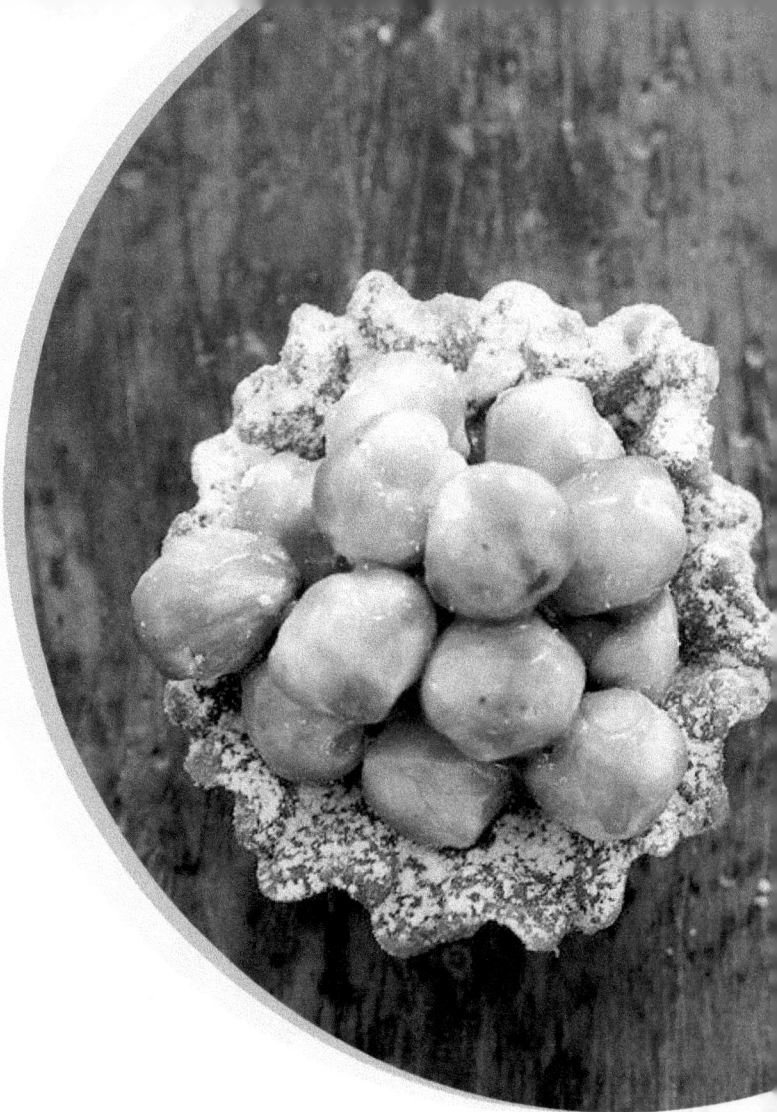

169 CINNAMON APPLE CHIPS

Preparation Time: 5 minutes

Cooking Time: 15 minutes

Servings: 1

INGREDIENTS:

- 1 apple, sliced thinly
- Dash of cinnamon
- Stevia

DIRECTIONS:

1. Coat apple slices with cinnamon and stevia.
2. Bake for 15 minutes or until tender and crispy at 325 degrees F.

NUTRITION:

Calories: 146
Fat: 0.7 g
Carbs: 36.4 g
Protein: 1.6 g
Sodium: 10 mg
Potassium: 100mg
Phosphorus: 0mg

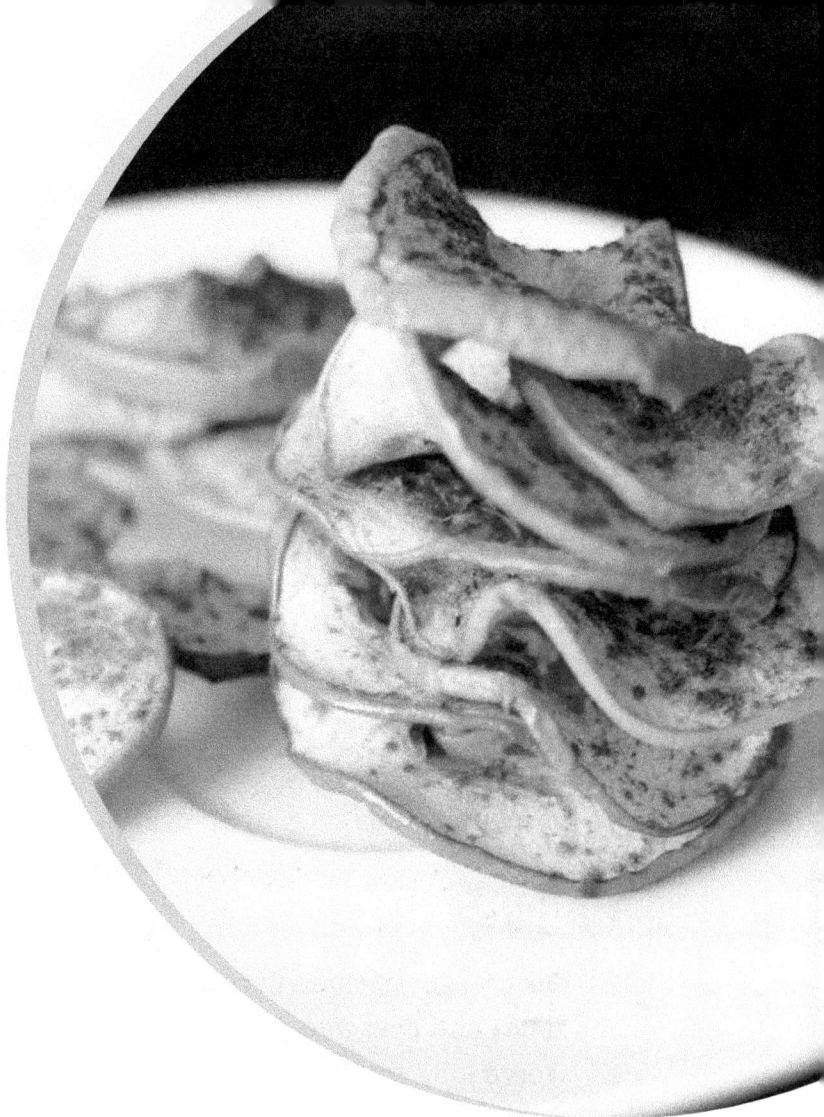

170 LEMON POPS

Preparation Time: 5 minutes

Cooking Time: 5 minutes

Servings: 1

INGREDIENTS:

- 4 tablespoons fresh lemon juice
- Powdered stevia

DIRECTIONS:

1. Mix orange or lemon juice and stevia and pour into molds.
2. Freeze until firm.

NUTRITION:

Calories: 46
Fat: 0.2g
Carbs: 16g
Protein: 0.9g
Sodium: 3.7mg
Potassium: 104mg
Phosphorus: 11mg

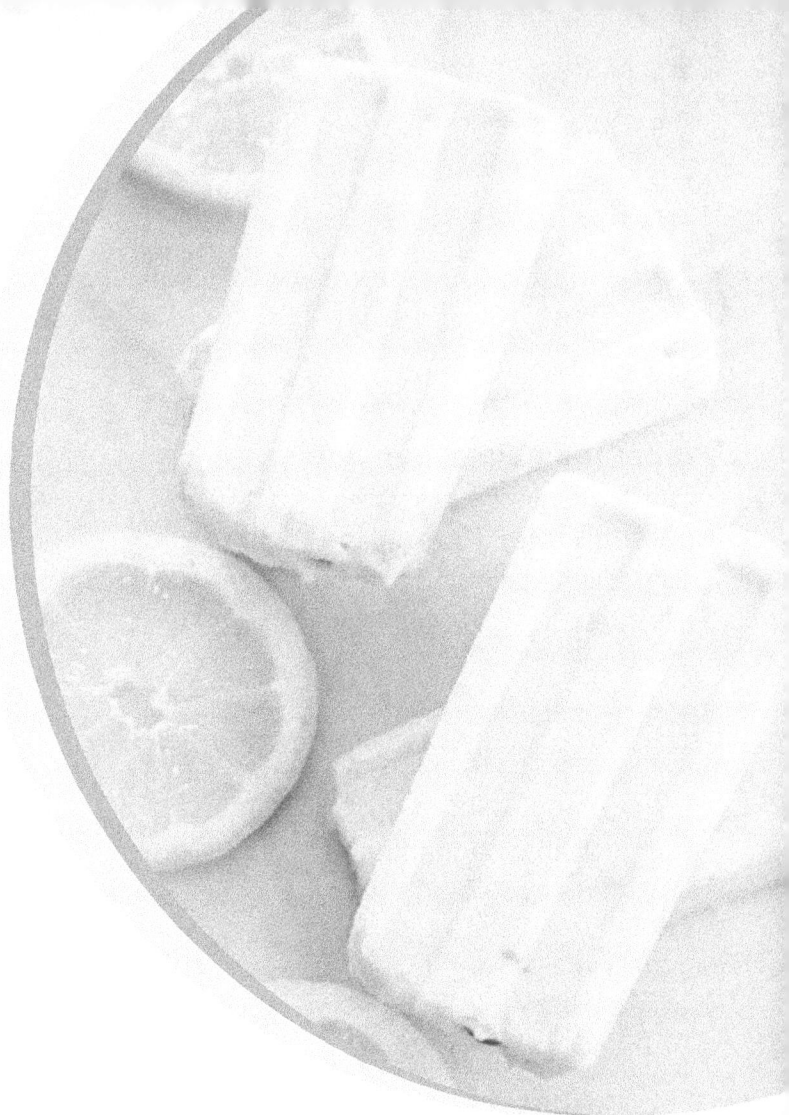

171 EASY NO-BAKE COCONUT COOKIES

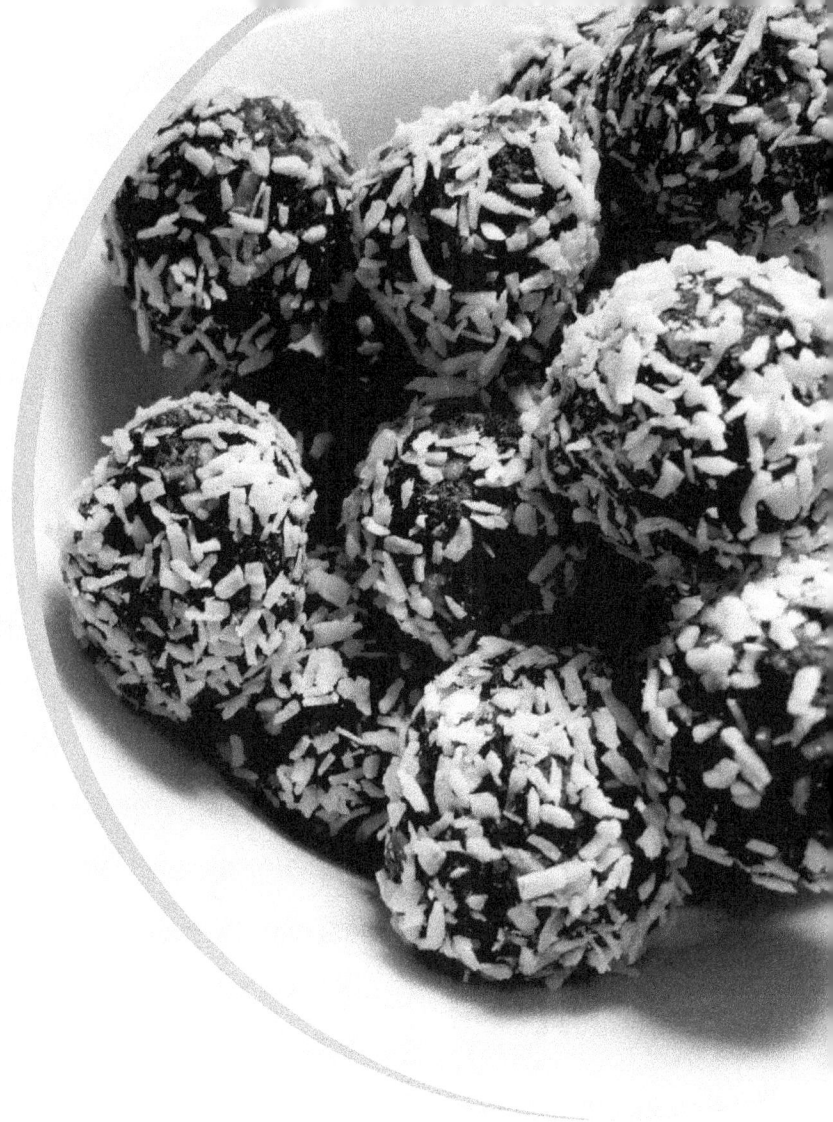

Preparation Time: 5 minutes

Cooking Time: 10 minutes

Servings: 20

INGREDIENTS:

- 3 cups finely shredded coconut flakes
- 1 cup melted coconut oil
- 1 teaspoon liquid stevia

DIRECTIONS:

1. Prepare all ingredients in a large bowl; stir until well blended.
2. Form the mixture into small balls and arrange them on a paper-lined baking tray.
3. Press each cookie down with a fork and refrigerate until firm. Enjoy!

NUTRITION:

Calories: 99
Fat: 10 g
Carbs: 2 g
Protein: 3 g
Sodium: 7 mg
Potassium: 105mg
Phosphorus: 11mg

172 ROASTED CHILI-VINEGAR PEANUTS

Preparation Time: 5 minutes

Cooking Time: 10 minutes

Servings: 4

INGREDIENTS:

- 1 tablespoon coconut oil
- 2 cups raw peanuts, unsalted
- 2 teaspoon sea salt
- 2 tablespoon apple cider vinegar
- 1 teaspoon chili powder
- 1 teaspoon fresh lime zest

DIRECTIONS:

1. Preheat oven to 350° F.
2. In a large bowl, toss together coconut oil, peanuts, and salt until well coated.
3. Transfer to a rimmed baking sheet and roast in the oven for about 15 minutes or until fragrant.
4. Transfer the roasted peanuts to a bowl and add vinegar, chili powder, and lime zest.
5. Toss to coat well and serve.

NUTRITION:

Calories: 447
Fat: 39.5g
Carbs: 12.3 g
Protein: 18.9 g
Sodium: 160 mg
Potassium: 200mg
Phosphorus: 0mg

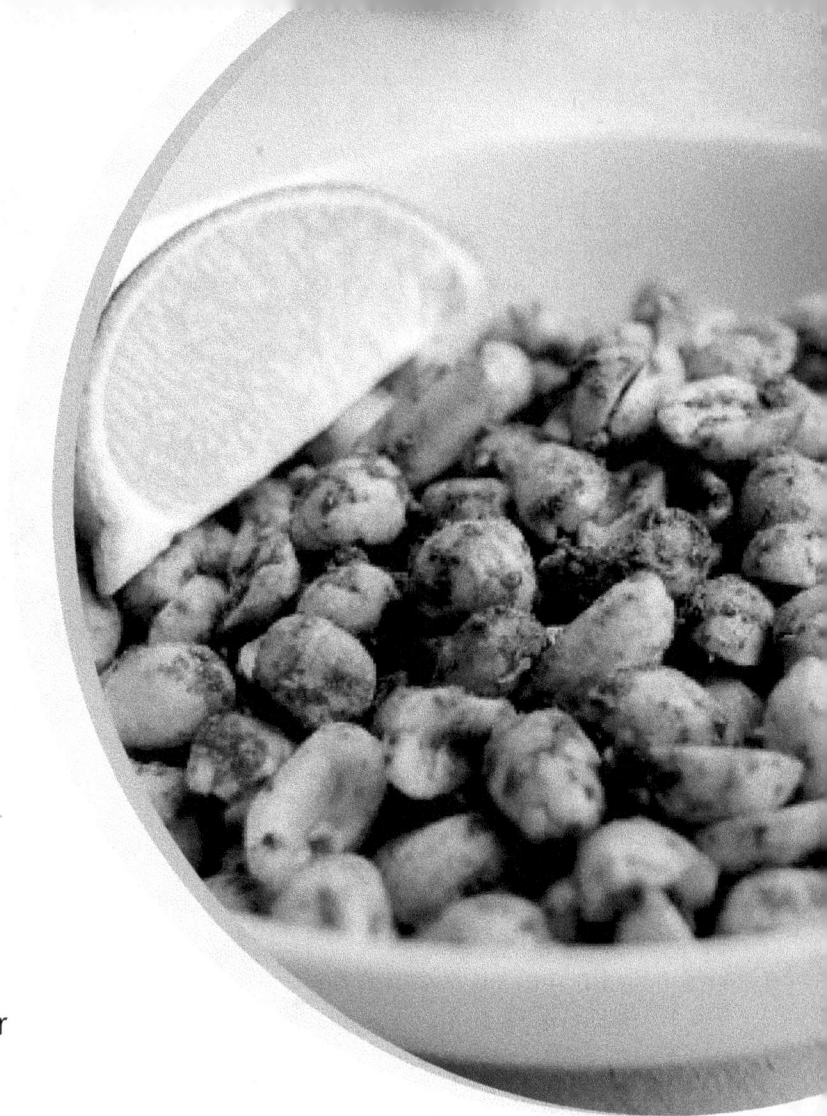

173 POPCORN WITH SUGAR AND SPICE

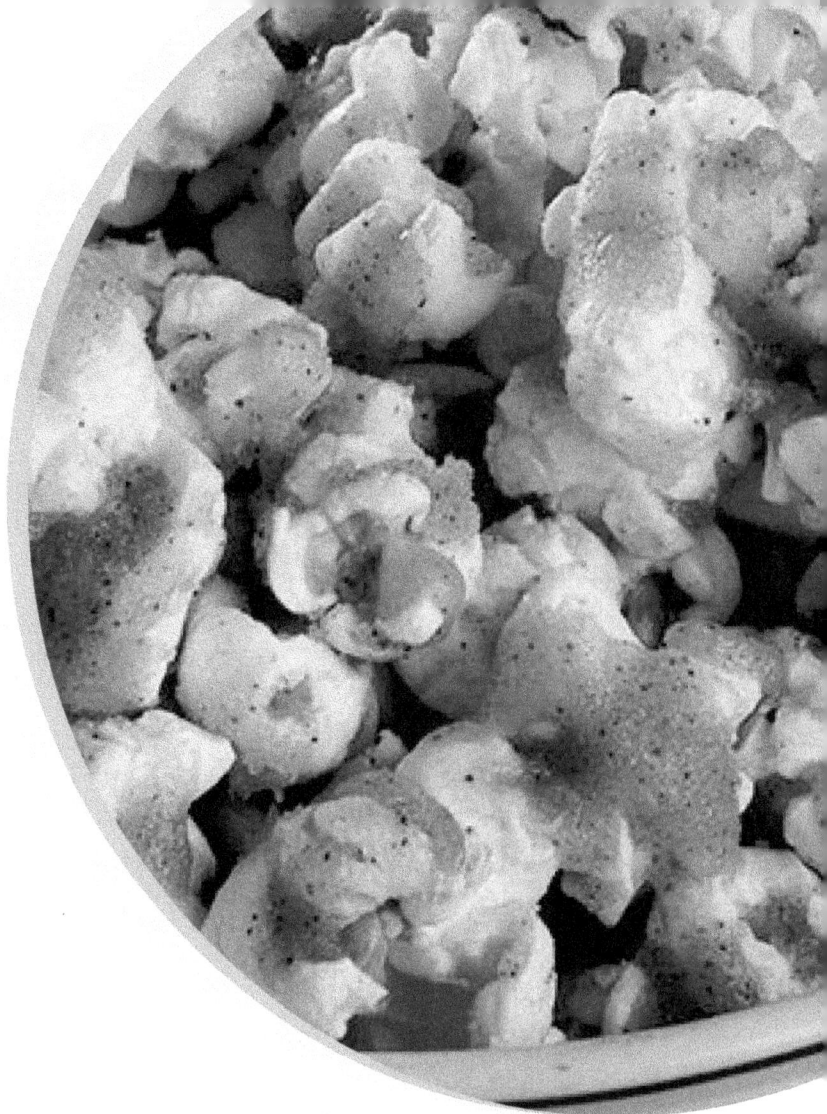

Preparation Time: 10 minutes

Cooking Time: 10 minutes

Servings: 2

INGREDIENTS:

- 8 cups hot popcorn
- 2 tablespoons unsalted butter
- 2 tablespoons sugar
- 1/2 teaspoon cinnamon
- 1/4 teaspoon nutmeg

DIRECTIONS:

1. Popping the corn; put aside.
2. Heat the butter, sugar, cinnamon, and nutmeg in the microwave or saucepan over a range fire until the butter is melted, and the sugar dissolved.
3. Sprinkle the corn with the spicy butter, mix well.
4. Serve immediately for optimal flavor.

NUTRITION:

Calories: 120
Fat: 7g
Carbs: 12g
Protein: 2g
Sodium: 2mg
Potassium: 56mg
Phosphorus: 60mg

174 EGGPLANT AND CHICKPEA BITES

Preparation Time: 15 minutes

Cooking Time: 50 minutes

Servings: 6

INGREDIENTS:

- 3 large aubergine cut in half (make a few cuts in the flesh with a knife)
- 2 large cloves garlic, peeled and deglazed
- 2 tbsp. coriander powder
- 2 tbsp. cumin seeds
- 400 g canned chickpeas, rinsed and drained
- 2 Tbsp. chickpea flour
- Zest and juice of 1/2 lemon
- 1/2 lemon quartered for serving
- 3 tbsp. tablespoon of polenta

DIRECTIONS:

1. Heat the oven to 200ºC. Spray the eggplant halves generously with oil and place them on the meat side up on a baking sheet.
2. Sprinkle with coriander and cumin seeds, and then place the cloves of garlic on the plate.
3. Season and roast for 40 minutes until the flesh of eggplant is completely tender. Reserve and let cool a little.
4. Scrape the flesh of the eggplant in a bowl with a spatula and throw the skins in the compost. Thoroughly scrape and make sure to incorporate spices and crushed roasted garlic.
5. Add chickpeas, chickpea flour, zest, and lemon juice. Crush roughly and mix well.
6. Check to season. Do not worry if the mixture seems a bit soft - it will firm up in the fridge.

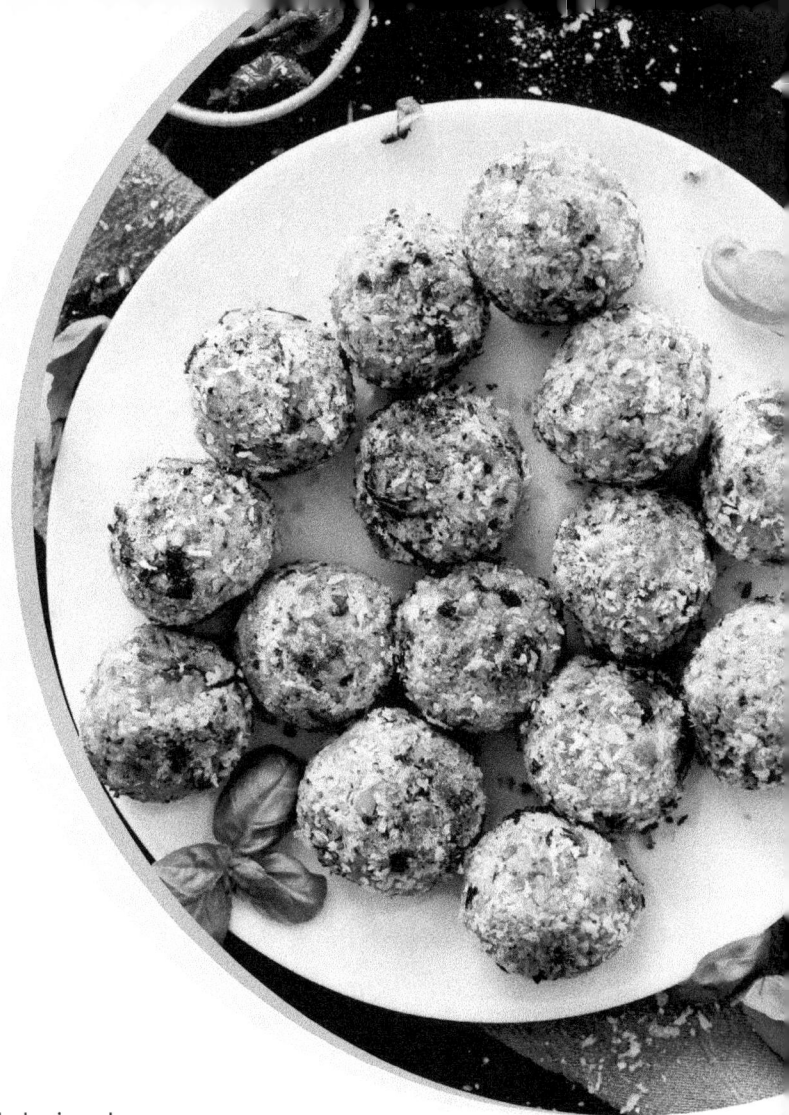

7. Form about twenty pellets and place them on a baking sheet covered with parchment paper. Refrigerate for at least 30 minutes.
8. Preheat oven to 180ºC. Remove the meatballs from the fridge and coat them by rolling them in the polenta.
9. Place them back on the baking sheet and spray a little oil on each. Roast for 20 minutes until golden and crisp.
10. Serve with lemon wedges. You can also serve these dumplings with a spicy yogurt dip.

NUTRITION:

Calories: 72
Fat: 1g
Carbs: 18g
Protein: 3g
Sodium: 63mg
Potassium: 162mg
Phosphorus: 36mg

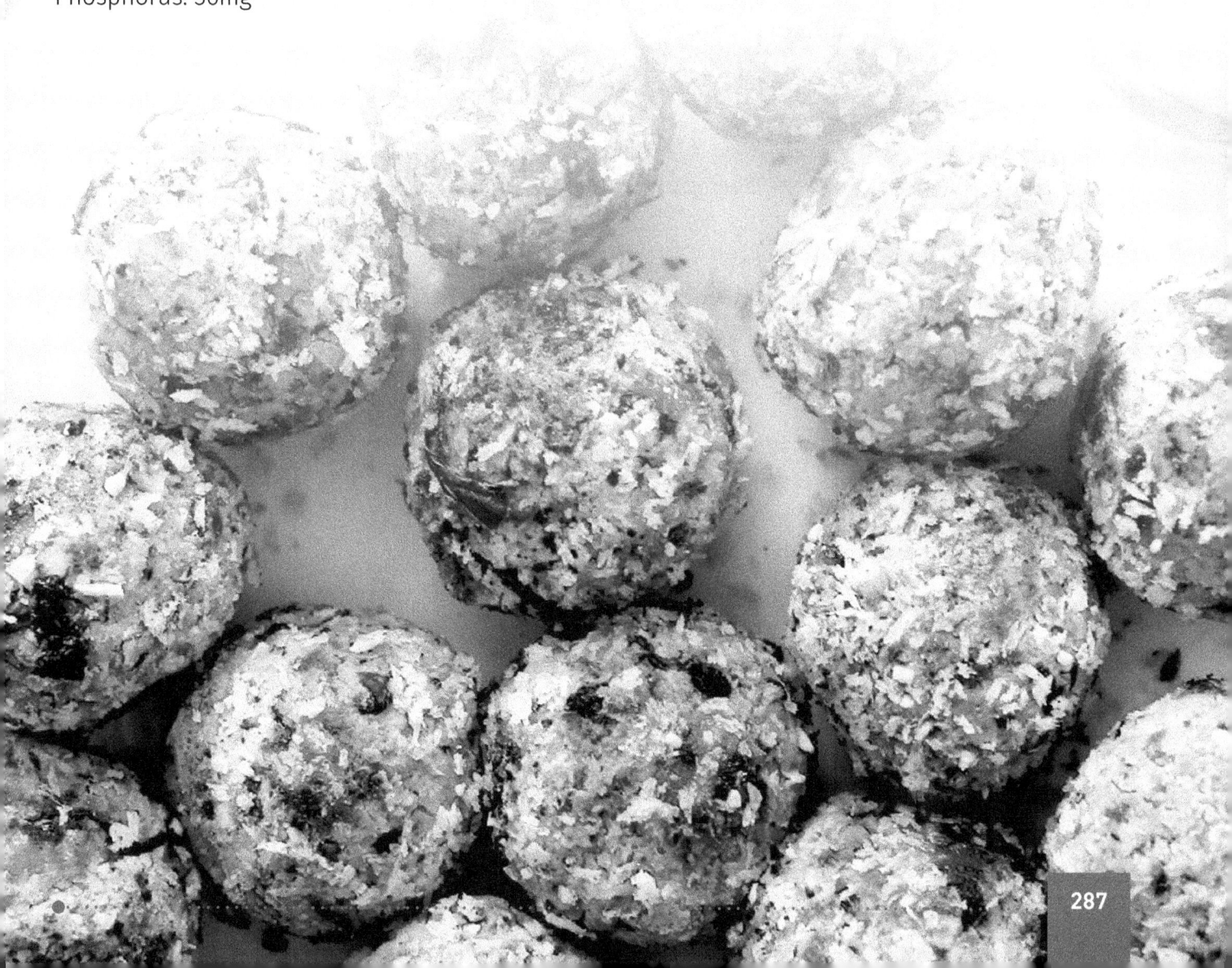

175 BABA GHANOUJ

Preparation Time: 10 minutes

Cooking Time: 1 hour and 20 minutes

Servings: 1

INGREDIENTS:

- 1 large aubergine, cut in half lengthwise
- 1 head of garlic, unpeeled
- 30 ml (2 tablespoons) of olive oil
- Lemon juice to taste

DIRECTIONS:

1. Preheat the oven to 350 degrees F.
2. Place the eggplant on the plate, skin side up. Roast until the meat is very tender and detaches easily from the skin, about 1 hour depending on the eggplant's size. Let cool.
3. Meanwhile, cut the tip of the garlic cloves. Put garlic cloves in a square aluminum foil. Fold the edges of the sheet and fold together to form a tightly wrapped foil.
4. Roast with the eggplant until tender, about 20 minutes. Let cool. Purée the pods with a garlic press.
5. With a spoon, scoop out the eggplant's flesh and place it in the bowl of a food processor. Add the garlic puree, the oil, and the lemon juice. Stir until purée is smooth and pepper.
6. Serve with mini pita bread.

NUTRITION:

Calories: 110
Fat: 12g
Carbs: 5g
Protein: 1g

Sodium: 180mg
Potassium: 207mg
Phosphorus: 81mg

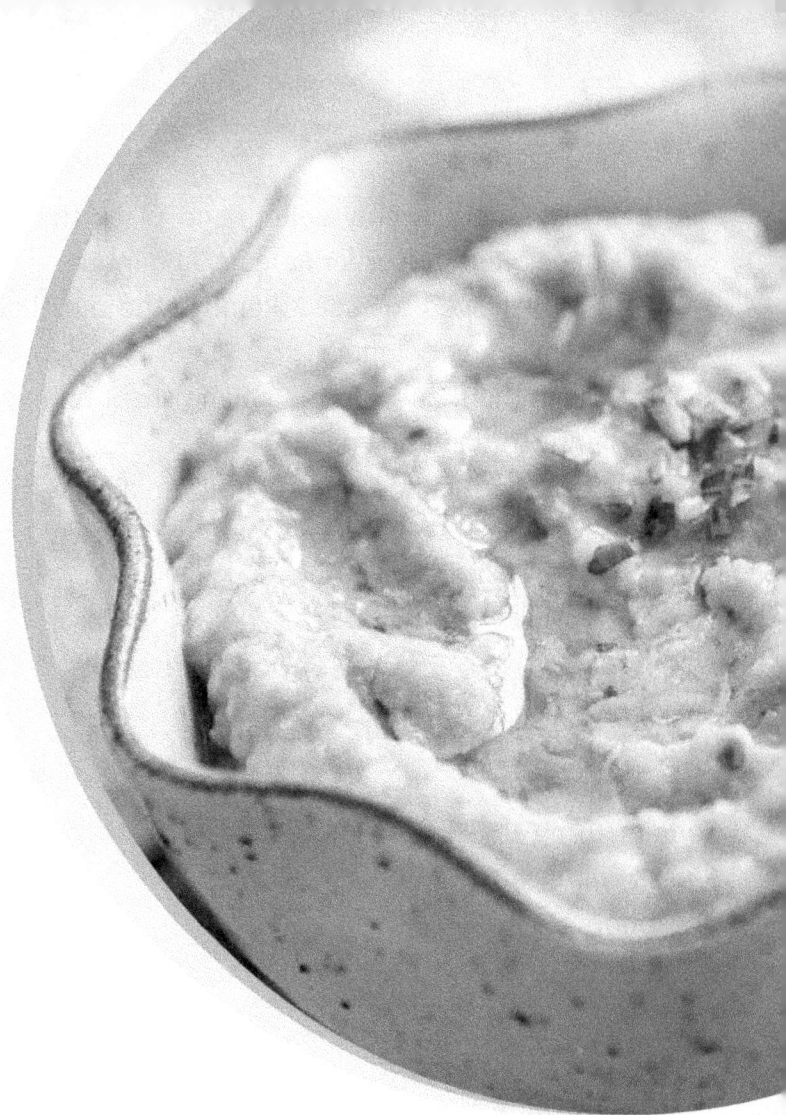

176 | BAKED PITA CHIPS

Preparation Time: 5 minutes

Cooking Time: 15 minutes

Servings: 6

INGREDIENTS:

- 3 pita loaves (6 inches)
- 3 tablespoons olive oil
- Chili powder

DIRECTIONS:

1. Separate each bread in half with scissors to obtain 6 round pieces.
2. Cut each piece into eight points. Brush each with olive oil and sprinkle with chili powder.
3. Bake at 350 degrees F for about 15 minutes until crisp.

NUTRITION:

Calories: 120
Fat: 2.5g
Carbs: 22g
Protein: 3g
Sodium: 70mg
Potassium: 0mg
Phosphorus: 0mg

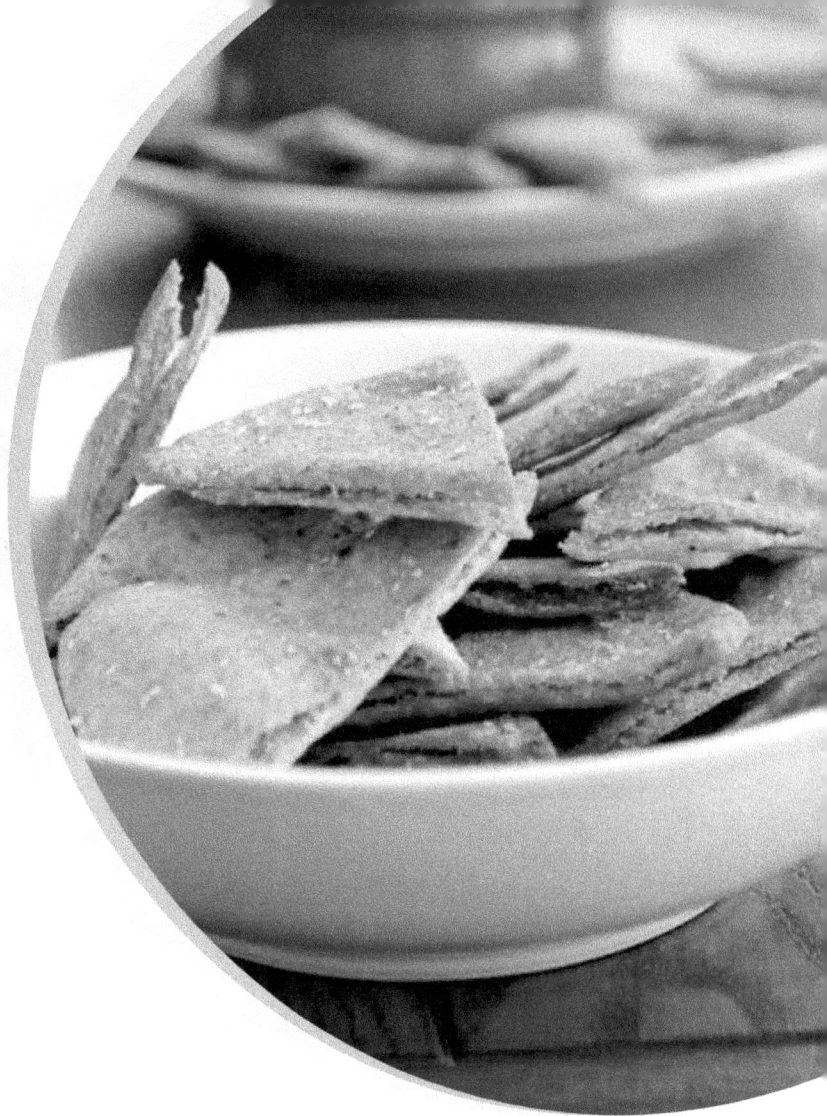

177 HERBAL CREAM CHEESE TARTINES

Preparation Time: 15 minutes

Cooking Time: 15 minutes

Servings: 2

INGREDIENTS:

- 20 regular round melba crackers
- 1 clove garlic, halved
- 1 cup cream cheese spread
- ¼ cup chopped herbs such as chives, dill, parsley, tarragon, or thyme
- 2 tbsp. minced French shallot or onion
- ½ tsp. black pepper
- 2 tbsp. tablespoons water

DIRECTIONS:

1. In a medium-sized bowl, combine the cream cheese, herbs, shallot, pepper, and water with a hand blender.
2. Rub the crackers with the cut side of the garlic clove.
3. Serve the cream cheese with the rusks.

NUTRITION:

Calories: 476
Fat: 9g
Carbs: 75g
Protein: 23g

Sodium: 885mg
Potassium: 312mg
Phosphorus: 165mg

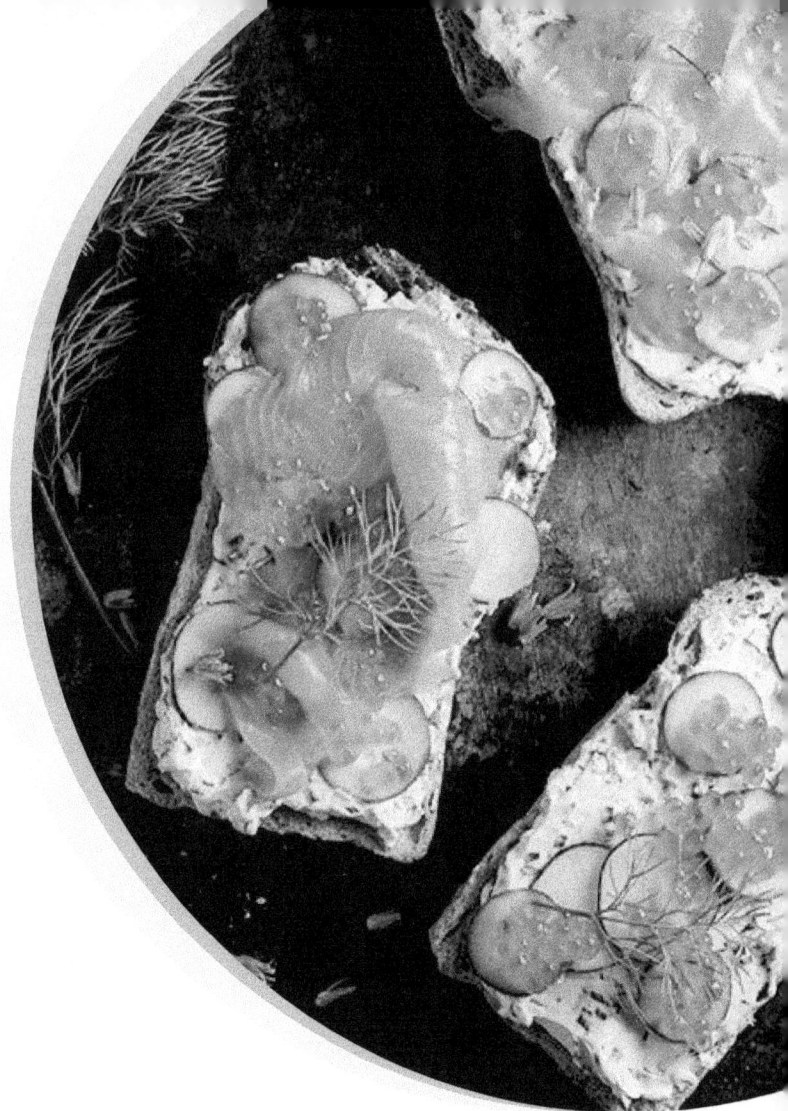

MIXES OF SNACKS

Preparation Time: 15 minutes

Cooking Time: 1 hour

Servings: 1

INGREDIENTS:

- 6 c. margarine
- 2 tbsp. Worcestershire sauce
- 1 ½ tbsp. spice salt
- ¾ c. garlic powder
- ½ tsp. onion powder
- 3 cups Cheerios
- 3 cups corn flakes
- 1 cup pretzel
- 1 cup broken bagel chip into 1-inch pieces

DIRECTIONS:

1. Preheat the oven to 250F (120C)
2. Melt the margarine in a large roasting pan. Stir in the seasoning. Gradually add the ingredients remaining by mixing so that the coating is uniform.
3. Cook 1 hour, stirring every 15 minutes.
4. Spread on paper towels to let cool. Store in a tightly closed container.

NUTRITION:

Calories: 150
Fat: 6g
Carbs: 20g
Protein: 3g
Sodium: 300mg
Potassium: 93mg
Phosphorus: 70mg

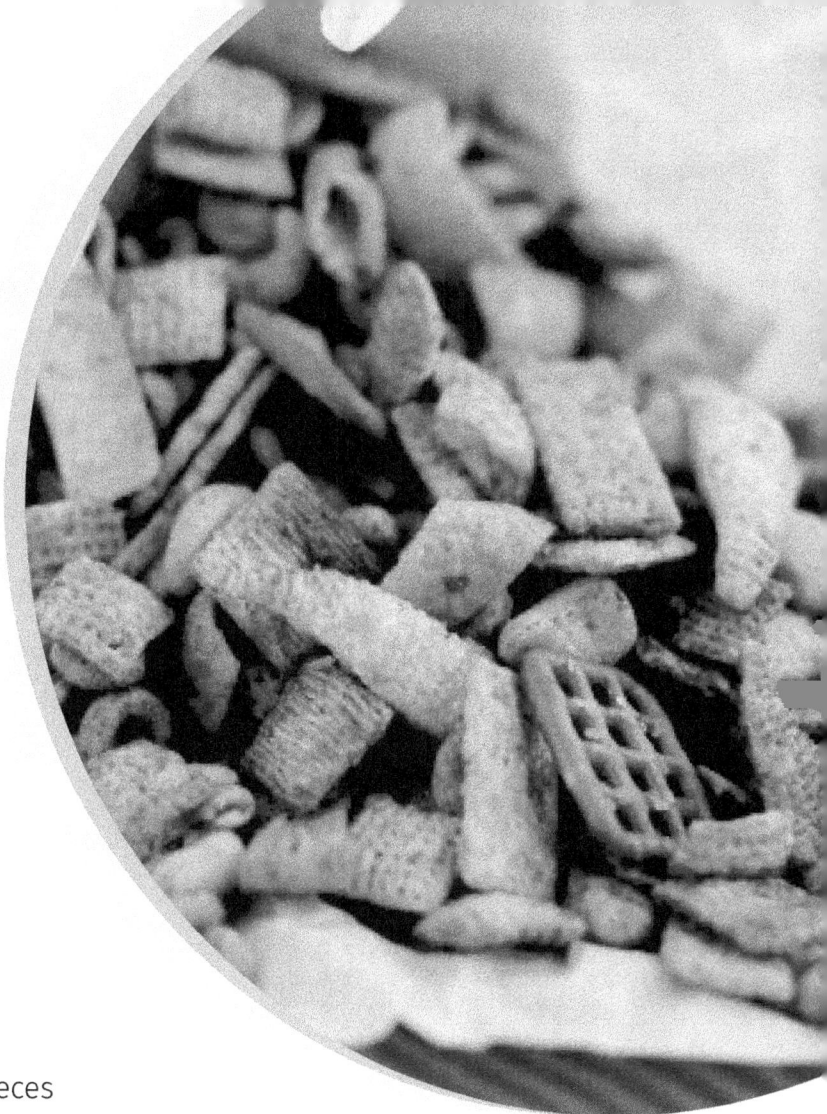

179 SPICY CRAB DIP

Preparation Time: 10 minutes

Cooking Time: 20 minutes

Servings: 1

INGREDIENTS:

- 1 can of 8 oz softened cream cheese
- 1 tbsp. finely chopped onions
- 1 tbsp. lemon juice
- 2 tbsp. Worcestershire sauce
- 1/8 tsp. black pepper Cayenne pepper to taste
- 2 tbsp. to s. of milk or non-fortified rice drink
- 1 can of 6 oz of crabmeat

DIRECTIONS:

1. Preheat the oven to 375 degrees F.
2. Pour the cheese cream into a bowl. Add the onions, lemon juice, Worcestershire sauce, black pepper, and cayenne pepper. Mix well. Stir in the milk/rice drink.
3. Add the crabmeat and mix until you obtain a homogeneous mixture.
4. Pour the mixture into a baking dish. Cook without covering for 15 minutes or until bubbles appear. Serve hot with low-sodium crackers or triangle cut pita bread.
5. Microwave until bubbles appear, about 4 minutes, stirring every 1 to 2 minutes.

NUTRITION:

Calories: 42
Fat: 0.5g
Carbs: 2g
Protein: 7g

Sodium: 167mg
Potassium: 130mg
Phosphorus: 139mg

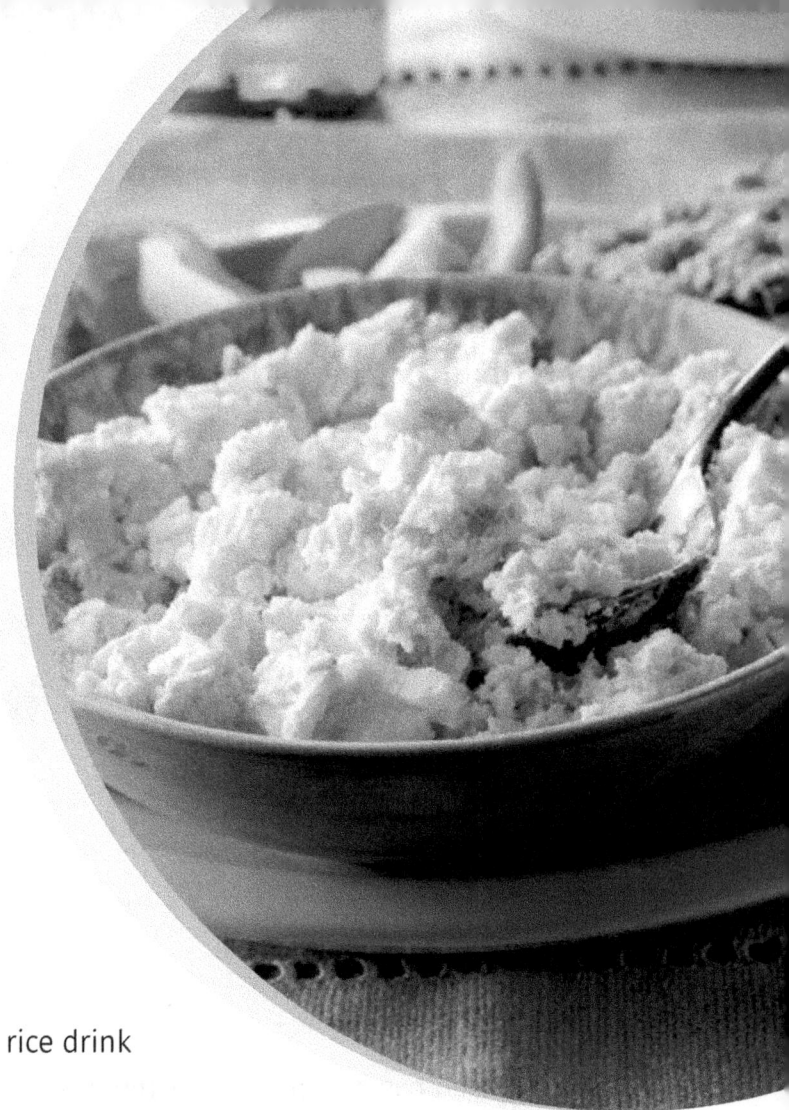

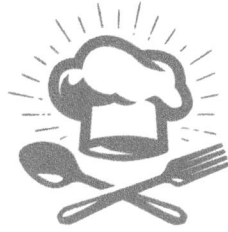

CHAPTER 22

DESSERT RECIPES

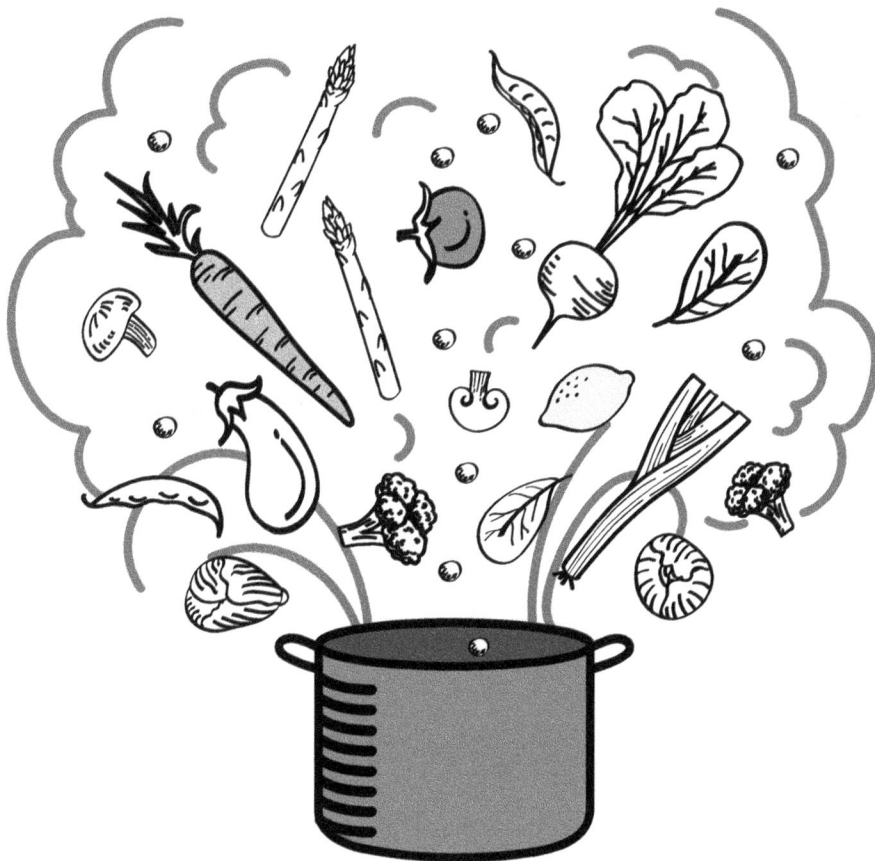

180 APPLE CHUNKS PIE

Preparation Time: 20 minutes

Cooking Time: 40 minutes

Servings: 1

INGREDIENTS:

- 2 apples
- 1 cup of unsalted butter
- 1 cup of brown sugar
- 1 cup of sour cream
- 1 teaspoon vanilla extract
- 1 teaspoon baking soda
- ½ spoon of salt
- 2 cups of flour
- 1 teaspoon of cinnamon
- ½ glass of milk
- 1 cup of powdered sugar

DIRECTIONS:

1. Preheat the oven (350°F or 200°C)
2. Cut the apples, put together a half cup of butter with granulated sugar and brown sugar.
3. Add vanilla, sour cream, baking soda, salt, and flour. Mix and add the apples.
4. Put everything in a pan (9"x 13") and then in the oven. In a small container, mix 2 little spoons of butter, brown sugar, and cinnamon.
5. Spread on the top of the prepared batter and bake for 40 minutes. Let the pan cool and make icing.
6. Add some butter, milk substitute, and sugar on top, cutting the dessert into 18 or even 20 small chunks.

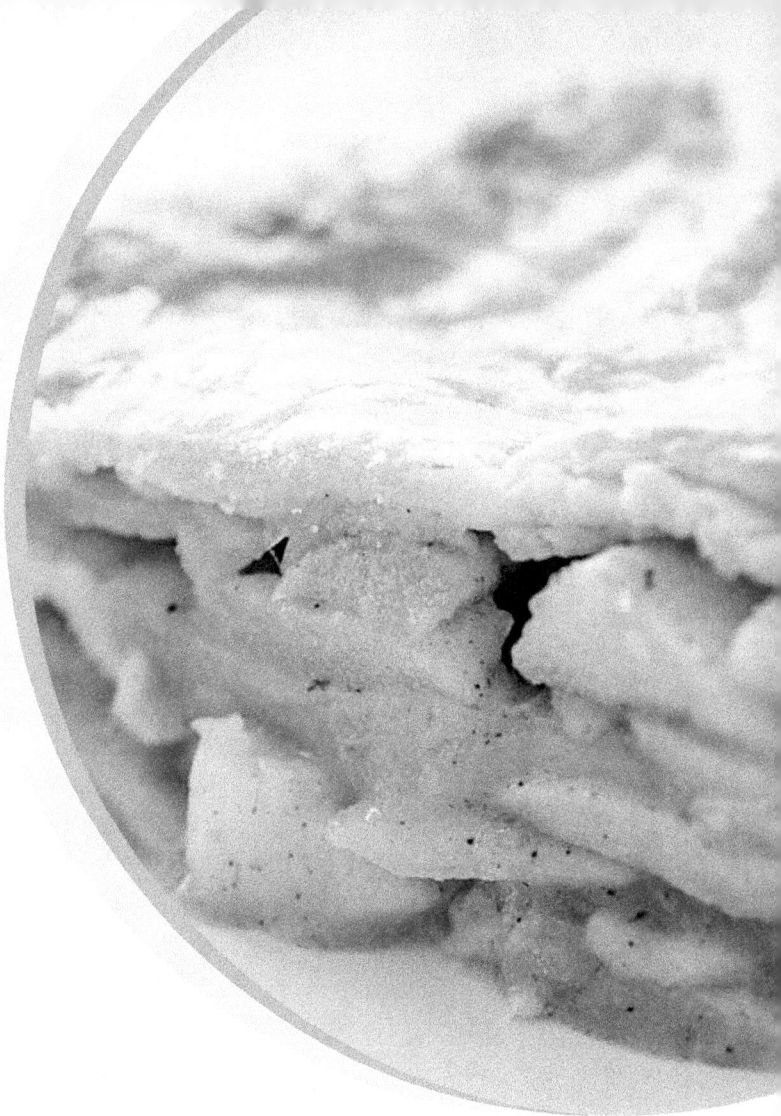

Calories 245
Protein 2g
Carbohydrates 35g
Fat 10g
Sodium 140mg
Potassium 70mg
Phosphorus 25mg

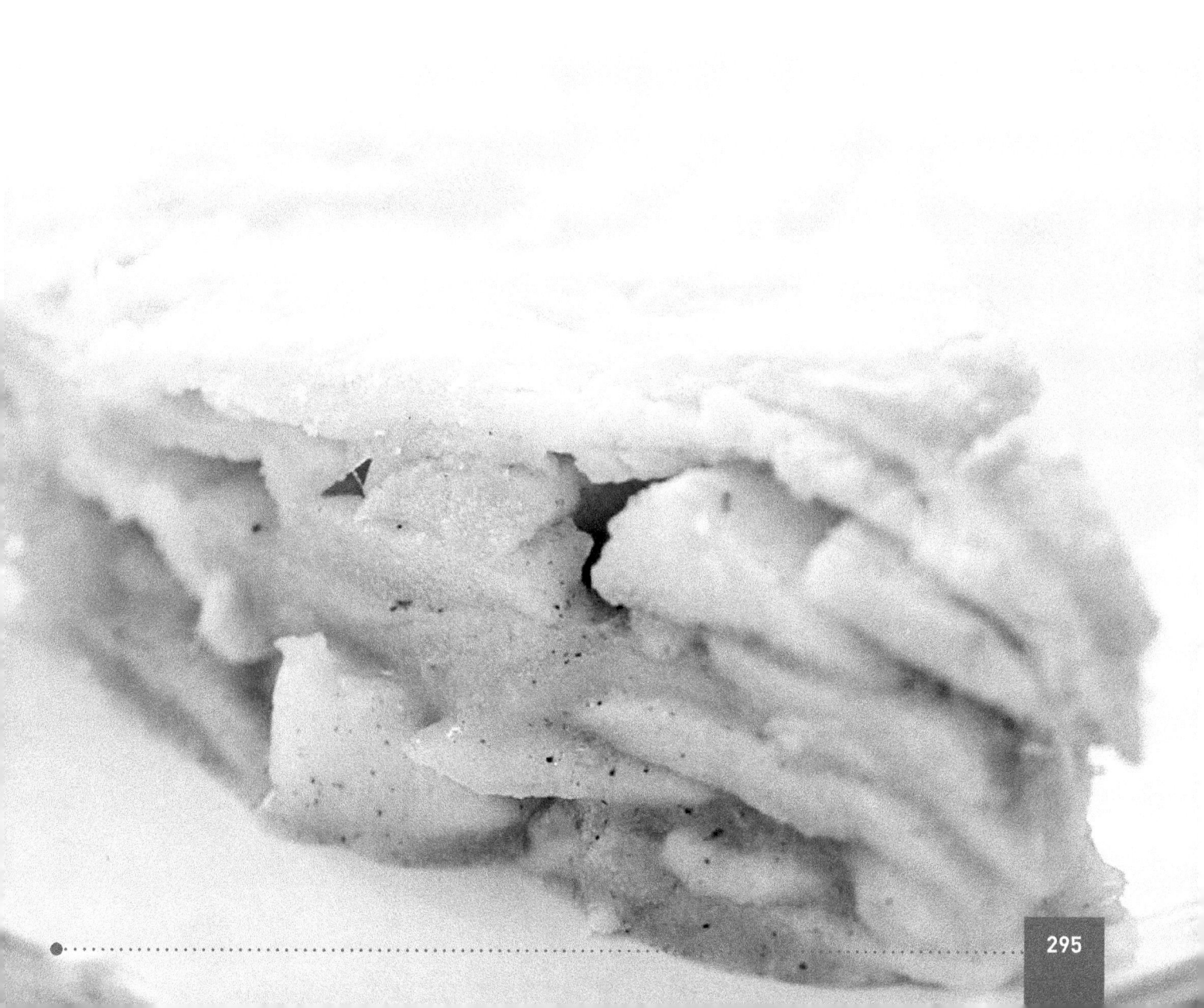

181 APPLE OATMEAL CRUNCHY

Preparation Time: 10 minutes

Cooking Time: 35 minutes

Servings: 1

INGREDIENTS:

- 5 Green apples
- 1 bowl of oatmeal
- A small cup of brown sugar
- 1/2 cup of flour
- 1 teaspoon of cinnamon
- ½ bowl of butter

DIRECTIONS:

1. Prepare apples by cutting them into tiny slices and preheat the oven at 350°F.
2. In a cup, mix oatmeal, flour, cinnamon, and brown sugar. Put butter in the batter and place sliced apple in a baking pan (9" x 13").
3. Spread oatmeal mixture over the apples and bake for 35 minutes.

NUTRITION:

Calories 295

Protein 3 g

Carbohydrates 40 g

Fat 12 g

Sodium 95 mg

Potassium 190 mg

Phosphorus 73 mg

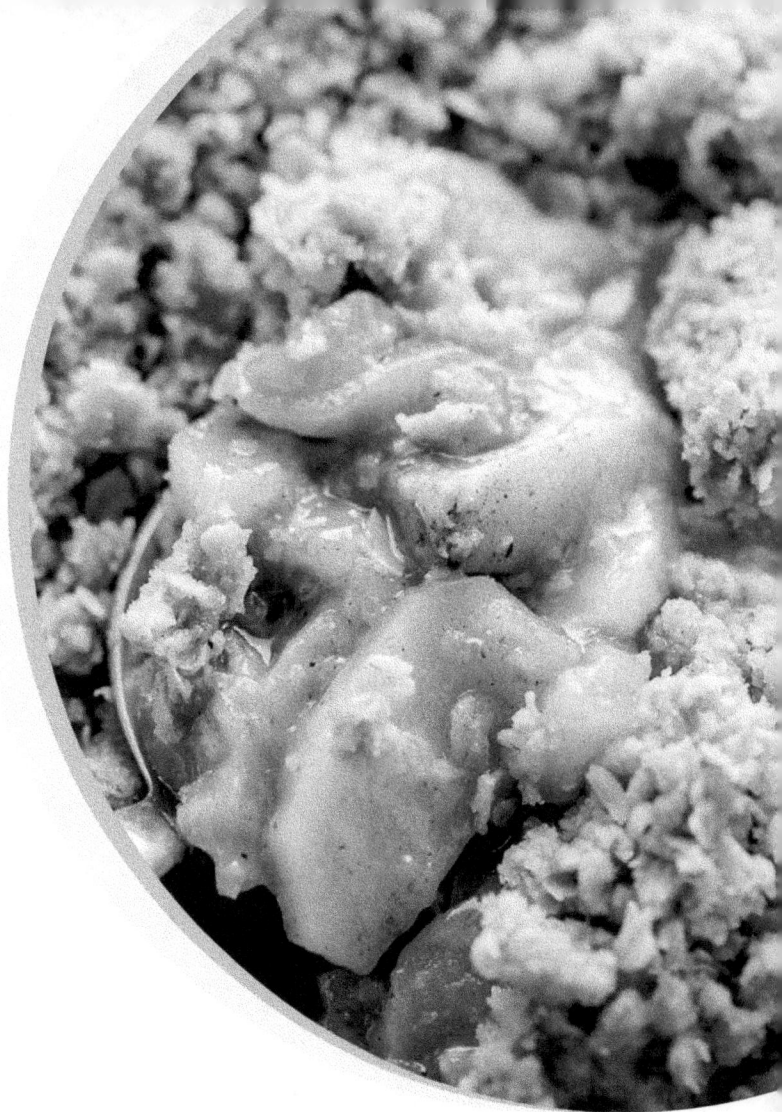

182 BERRY ICE CREAM

Preparation Time: 10 minutes

Cooking Time: 1 hour

Servings: 1

INGREDIENTS:

- 6 ice cream cones
- 1 cup of whipped topping
- 1 cup of fresh blueberries
- 4 ounces cream cheese
- ¼ cup of blueberry jam

DIRECTIONS:

1. Put the cream cheese in a large cup and beat it with a mixer until it is fluffy.
2. Mix with fruit and jam and whipped topping.
3. Put the mixture on the small ice cream cones and refrigerate them in the freezer for 1 hour or more until they are ready to serve.

NUTRITION:

Calories 175
Protein 3 g
Carbohydrates 20 g
Fat 9 g
Sodium 95 mg
Potassium 80 mg
Phosphorus 40 mg

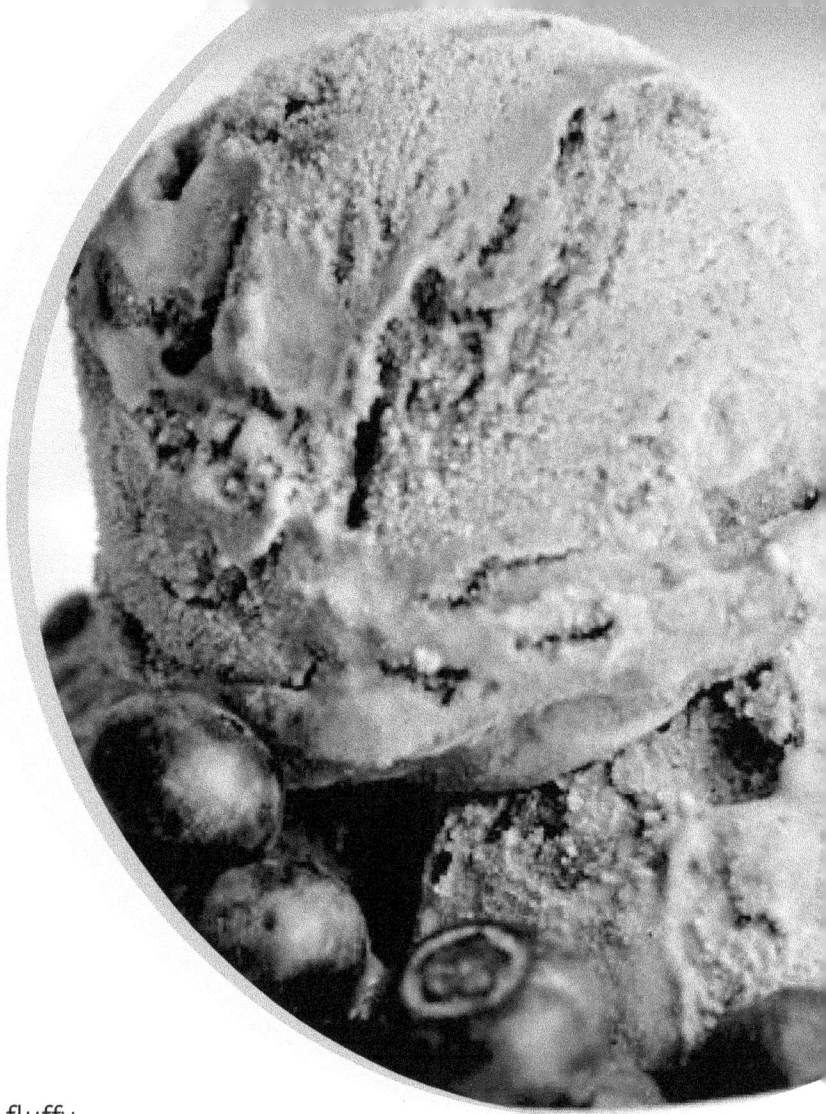

183 BUTTERMILK CAKE

Preparation Time: 15 minutes

Cooking Time: 1 hour

Servings: 1

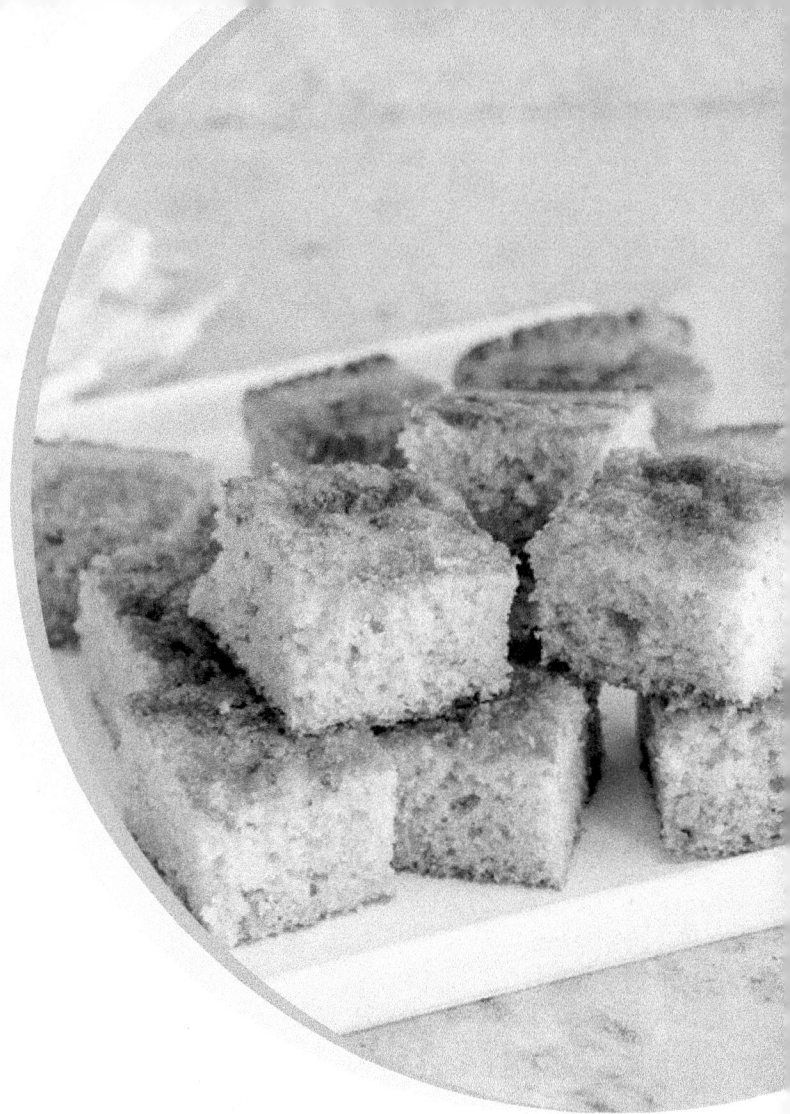

INGREDIENTS:

- 1 buttermilk cup
- 1 deep dish of 9" pie crust
- 2 small spoons of lemon juice
- 2 eggs
- ¼ buttercup
- 1 small spoon of almond extract
- 1 teaspoon of vanilla extract
- ½ cup of sugar
- 4 small spoons of flour

DIRECTIONS:

1. Mix the eggs, softened butter (pre-cooked and softened at 375°F), buttermilk, almond vanilla extract, sugar, and flour in a large bowl.
2. Put the mixture in a dish for the pie crust and bake it for one hour.
3. Leave it aside to cool, and then serve it in slices.

NUTRITION:

Calories 373

Protein 4 g

Carbohydrates 45 g

Fat 18 g

Sodium 145 mg

Potassium 90 mg

Phosphorus 65 mg

184 CARAMEL PIE WITH APPLES

Preparation Time: 10 minutes

Cooking Time: 1 hour

Servings: 1

INGREDIENTS:

- 3 big apples
- 8 ounces of frozen dessert topping
- 2 caramel nut blast gold bars

DIRECTIONS:

1. Cut apples into small pieces and also cut caramel bars into small pieces.
2. Prepare whipped cream out of the fridge and mix it with caramel bar and apple pieces in a large bowl.
3. Cool it for one hour before eating it.

NUTRITION:

Calories 200
Protein 5 g
Carbohydrates 25 g
Fat 10 g
Sodium 45 mg
Potassium 115 mg
Phosphorus 45 mg

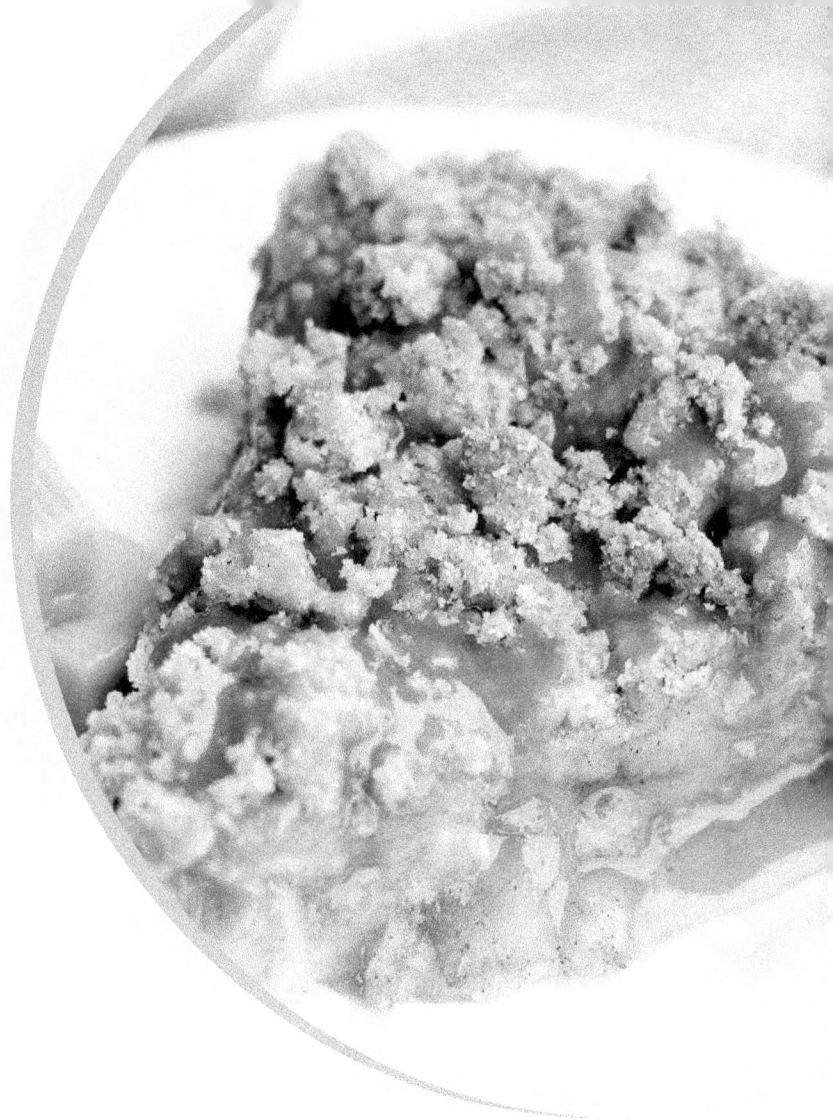

185 CHERRY PIE

Preparation Time: 15 minutes

Cooking Time: 40 – 45 minutes

Servings: 1

INGREDIENTS:

- 2 eggs
- 1 small cup of granulated sugar
- Some sour cream
- 1 vanilla teaspoon
- 1/2 cup of unsalted butter
- 2 spoons of white flour
- 1 teaspoon of baking powder
- 1 teaspoon of baking soda
- 20 ounces of cherry pie filling or
- 10 cherries to be beaten and put in the cake

DIRECTIONS:

1. Use a mixer and make softened butter, sugar, eggs, vanilla, and sour cream.
2. Preheat the oven to 350°F (or 200°C). in another bowl, put together flour, baking powder, and baking soda.
3. Mix all together both dry and soft ingredients and pour the batter into a cooking dish for the oven. You can disperse cherry pie filling or/and the cherries on the batter.
4. Bake in the oven for 40 - 45 minutes.

NUTRITION:

Calories 390
Protein 3 g
Carbohydrates 59 g
Fat 16 g

Sodium 369 mg
Potassium 115 mg
Phosphorus 70 mg

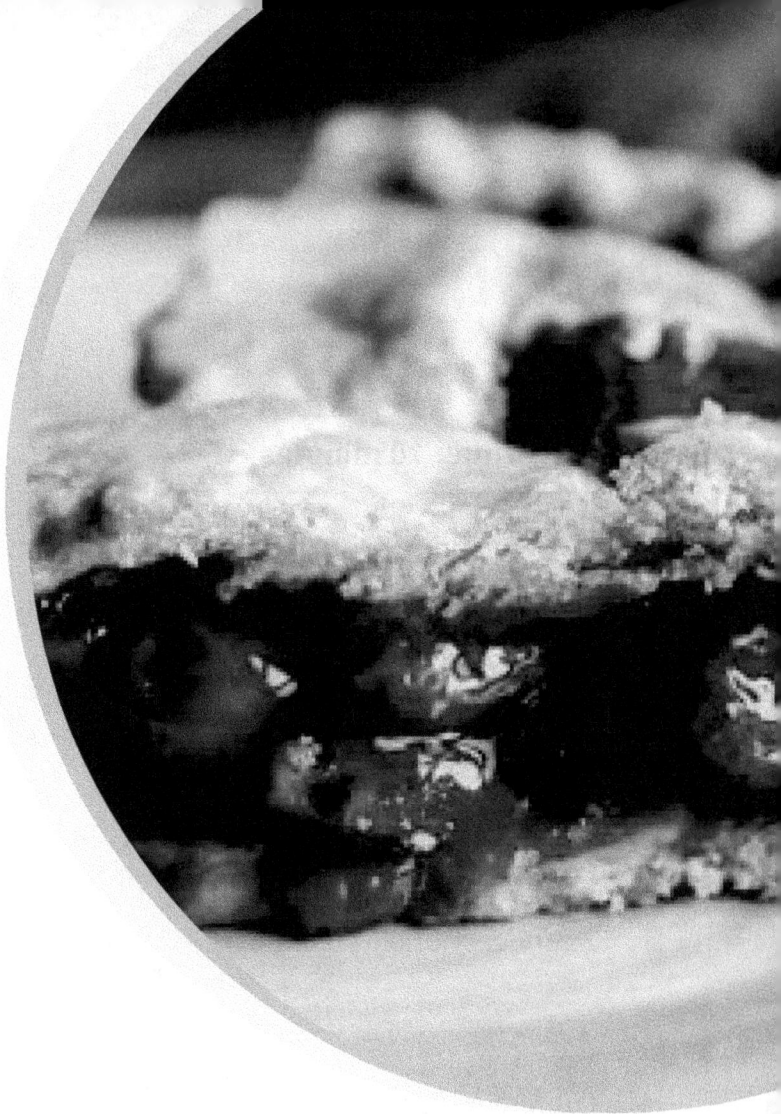

186 CRANBERRY DESSERT

Preparation Time: 10 minutes

Cooking Time: 15 minutes

Servings: 1

INGREDIENTS:

- Cherry gelatin mix
- Boiling water
- 12 ounces of cranberries
- ½ glass of sugar
- 12 ounces canned jelly cranberry sauce
- 12 ounces free whipped topping

DIRECTIONS:

1. Put the gelatin mix in the boiled water and set aside, letting it cool down. Put sugar in another boiling water.
2. Then add the cranberries and boil for 5 minutes. When hot, remove the cranberries and add jellied cranberry sauce.
3. Blend all together and break the jelly sauce into little chunks.
4. Add cool gelatin and whipped topping.
5. Distribute topping throughout and removing it from the heat, cool it for one hour. Serve it cold.

NUTRITION:

Calories 195
Protein 1 g
Carbohydrates 35 g
Fat 5 g

Sodium 35 mg
Potassium 30 mg
Phosphorus 10 mg

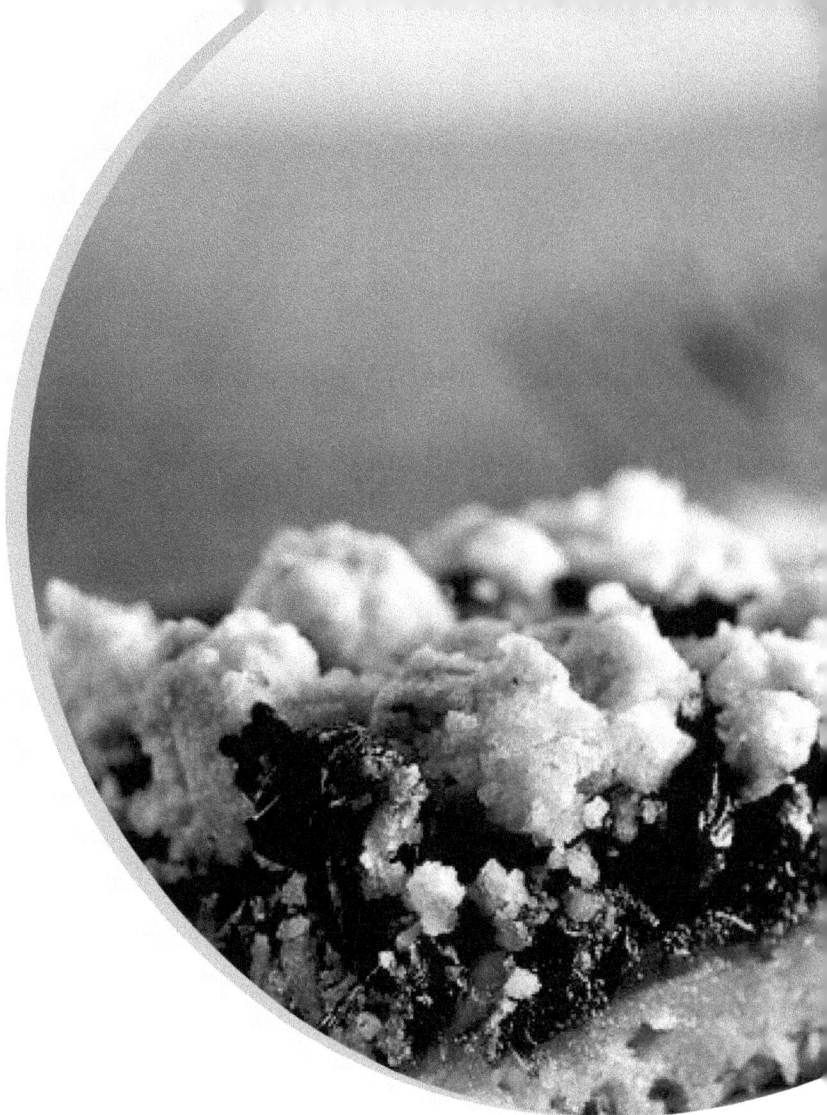

187 LIME DESSERT

Preparation Time: 10 minutes

Cooking Time: 15 minutes

Servings: 1

INGREDIENTS:

- 5 tablespoons extra virgin olive oil
- 1 and ¼ bowl of cracker crumbs
- ¼ glass granulated sugar
- Lime juice
- 14 ounces canned sweetened condensed milk
- 1 small cup of heavy whipping cream

DIRECTIONS:

1. Preheat oven at 350-degree F.
2. Blend olive oil, cracker crumbs, and sugar, mix and save a pair of spoons to sprinkle in the end on top of the dessert.
3. Press the ingredients already mixed up in a 9" pie shell and bake for 5 minutes and cool it. Meanwhile, add lime juice and mix with milk.
4. Use a chilled bowl and whip the heavy cream to a stiff peak. Blend the cream with the condensed milk mixture.
5. Blend leftover crumb mixture on the dessert/pie. Chill and serve.

NUTRITION:

Calories 425
Protein 5 g
Carbohydrates 45 g
Fat 24 g

Sodium 148 mg
Potassium 240 mg
Phosphorus 160 mg

188 ORANGE AND ANISE COOKIES

Preparation Time: 10 minutes

Cooking Time: 45 minutes

Servings: 1

INGREDIENTS:

- White flour (2 cups)
- 2 teaspoons of baking powder
- 2 teaspoons of anise seed
- 1 teaspoon of grated orange peel
- ½ small cup of sugar
- 1 egg
- 2 tablespoons of canola oil
- 1 teaspoon orange extract

DIRECTIONS:

1. Preheat oven at 350°F (or 200 ° C). Line a large baking tray with baking paper.
2. Mix the dry ingredients in a large cup and blend, then place oil, egg and extract in a bowl and smooth, doing it either with a whisk or electric mixer for about 30 seconds.
3. Add the liquid and the dry mixture with a wooden spoon and prepare the dough by shaping it into a ball.
4. Cut it in two parts and roll each half, then flatten it and place it on the cooking tray in the oven for about 20 minutes.
5. Remove it and cut it with a bread knife to get around 18-20 cookies. Place them again in the oven for about 5 minutes. Remove them from the oven and cool on a rack.

NUTRITION:

Calories 170
Protein 2 g
Carbohydrates 17 g

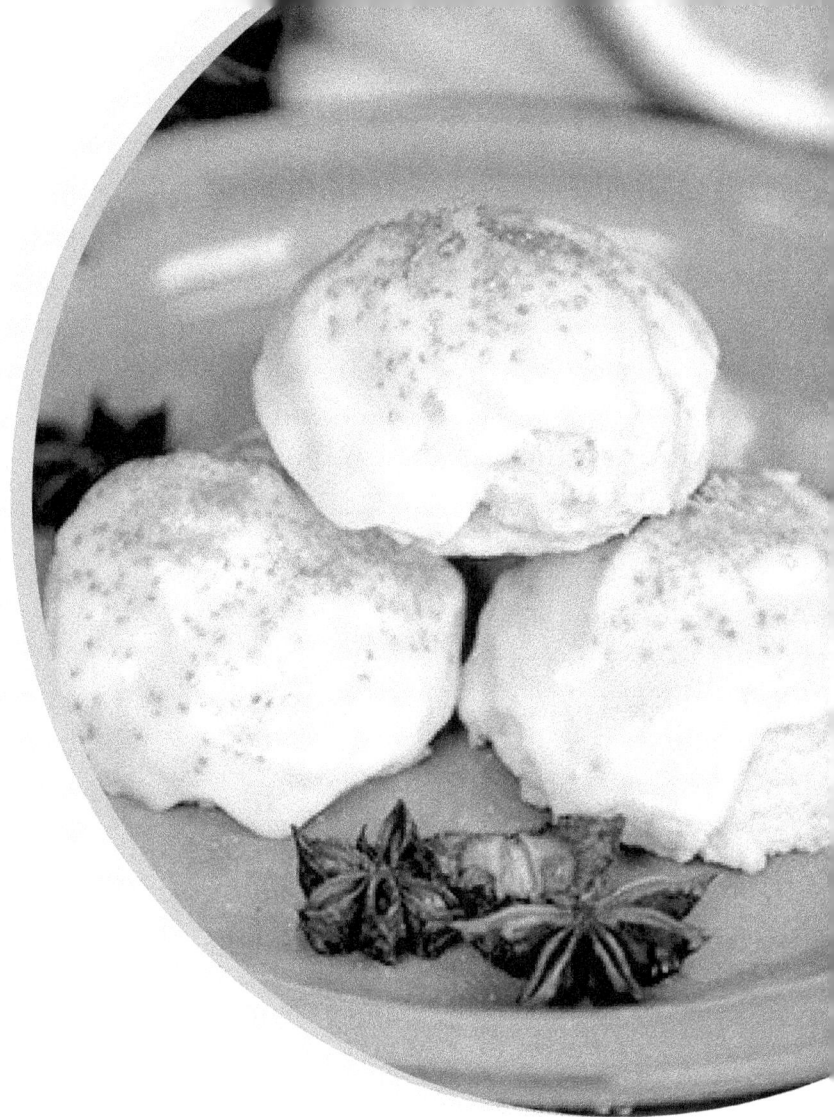

Fat 8 g
Sodium 45 mg

Potassium 25 mg
Phosphorus 75 mg

189 PUMPKIN CHEESECAKE

Preparation Time: 15 minutes

Cooking Time: 55 minutes

Servings: 8

INGREDIENTS:

- 1 egg white
- 1 wafer crumb 9" pie crust
- ½ small bowl of granulated sugar
- Vanilla extract (1 teaspoon)
- 1 teaspoon of pumpkin pie flavoring
- ½ small bowl of liquid egg substitute
- ½ bowl of pumpkin cream
- 8 tablespoons of frozen topping for desserts
- 16 ounces cream cheese

DIRECTIONS:

1. Brush pie crust with egg white and cook for 5 minutes in a preheated oven from 375° F from 375° F now down to 350° F.
2. Put together sugar, vanilla, and cream cheese in a large cup, beating with a mixer until smooth.
3. Beat the egg substitute and add pumpkin cream with pie flavoring: blend everything until softened.
4. Put the pumpkin mixture in a pie shell and bake for 50 minutes to set the center. Then let the pie cool down and then put it in the fridge.
5. When you wish to, serve it in 8 slices, putting some topping on it.

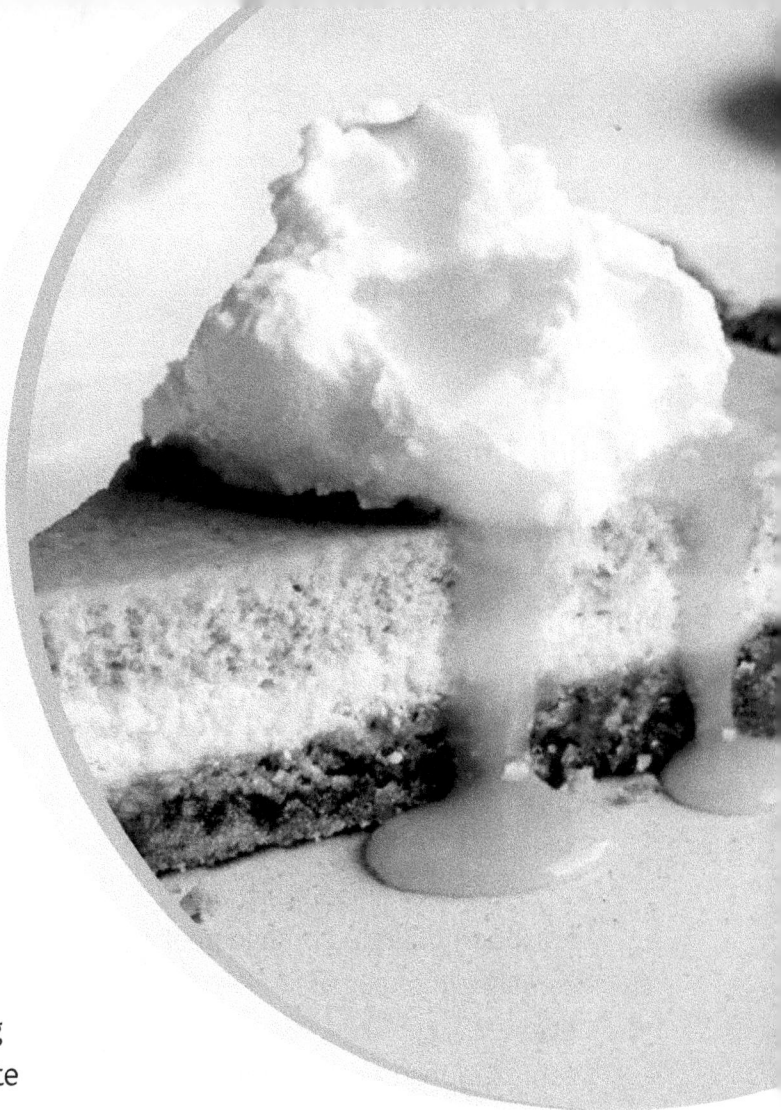

Calories 364
Protein 5 g
Carbohydrates 28 g
Fat 25 g
Sodium 245 mg
Potassium 125 mg
Phosphorus 65 mg

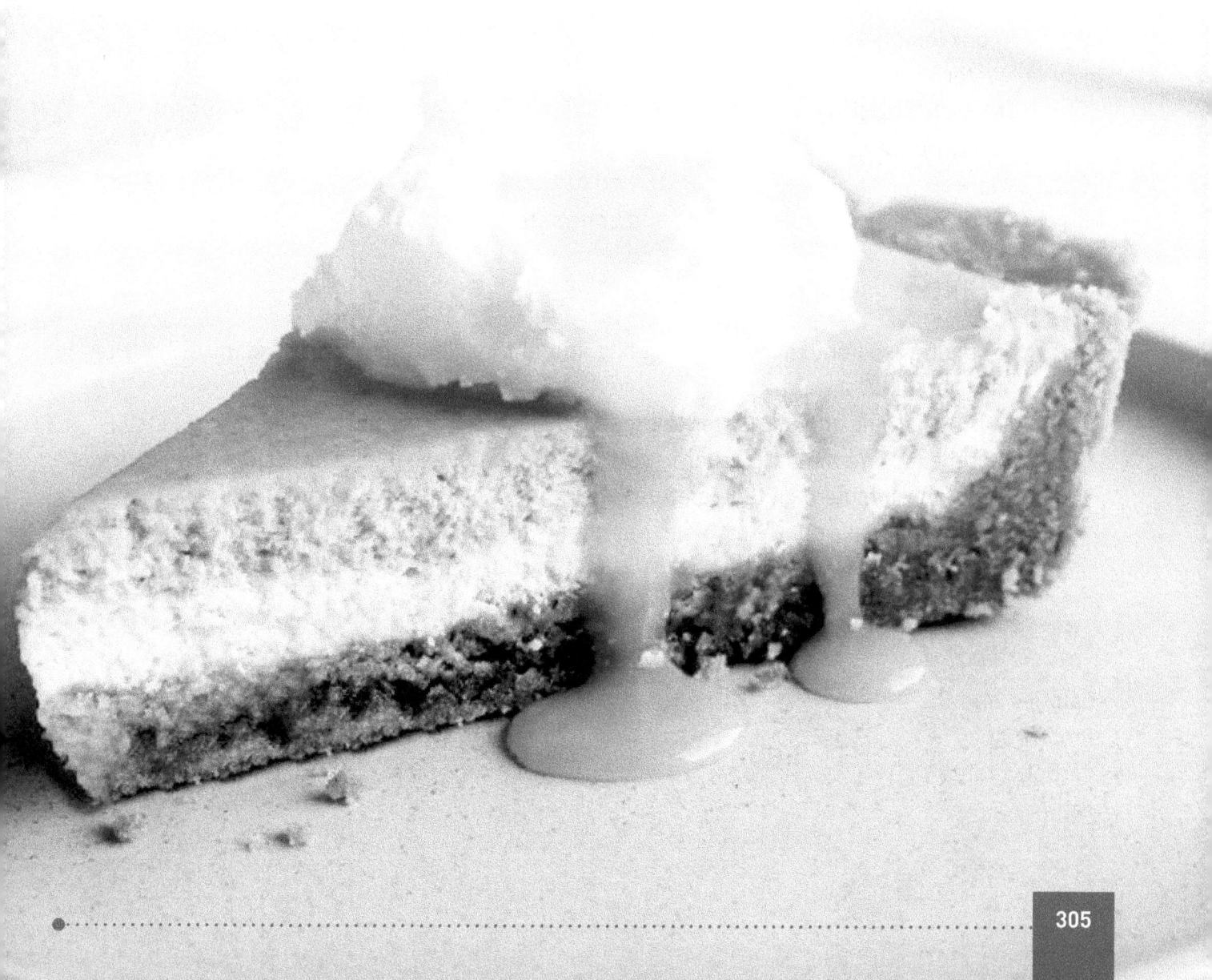

SMALL
CHOCOLATE
CAKES

Preparation Time: 10 minutes

Cooking Time: 5 minutes

Servings: 1

INGREDIENTS:

- 1 box angel food cake mix
- 1 box lemon cake mix
- Water
- Non-stick cooking spray or butter
- Dark Chocolate small squared chops and chocolate powder

DIRECTIONS:

1. Use a transparent kitchen cooking bag and put inside both lemon cake mixes, angel food mix, and chocolate chips.
2. Mix everything and add water to prepare a small cupcake.
3. Put the mix in a mold to prepare a cupcake containing the ingredients and put in microwave for a one-minute high temperature.
4. Slip the cupcake out of the mold, put it on a dish, let it cool, and put some more chocolate crumbs on it.

NUTRITION:

Calories 241
Protein 3g
Carbohydrates 41g
Fat 7g

Sodium 175 mg
Potassium 15 mg
Phosphorus 80 mg

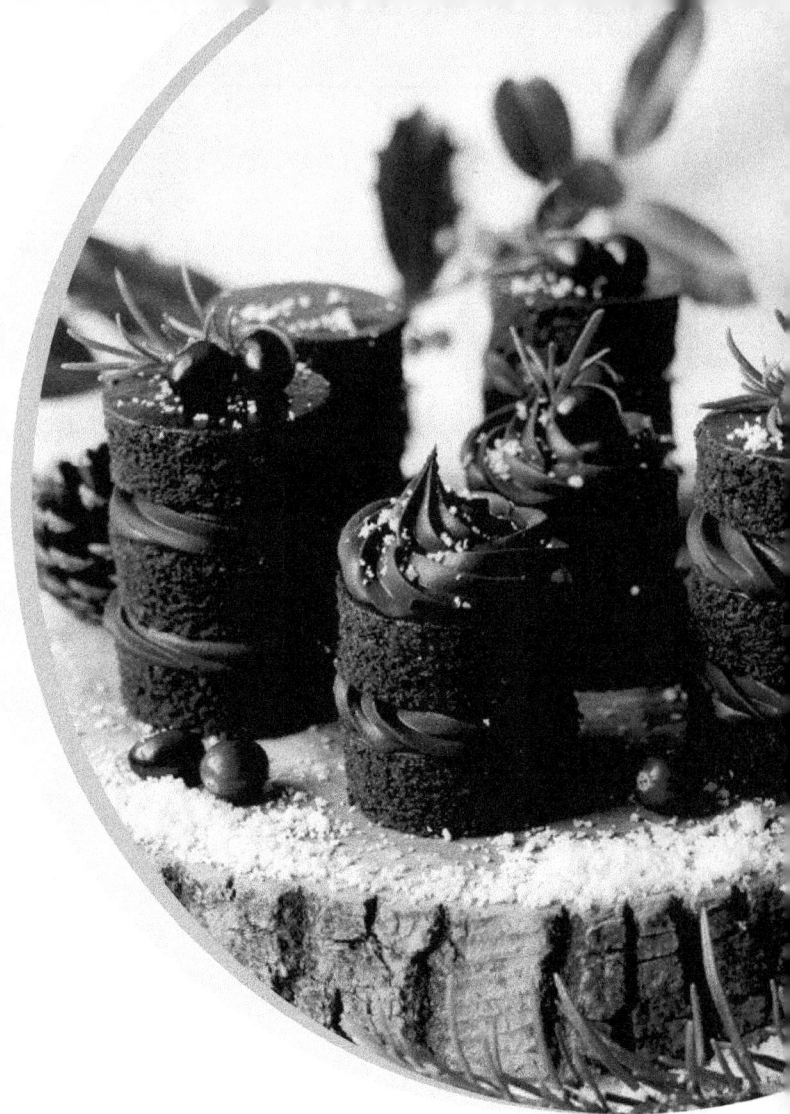

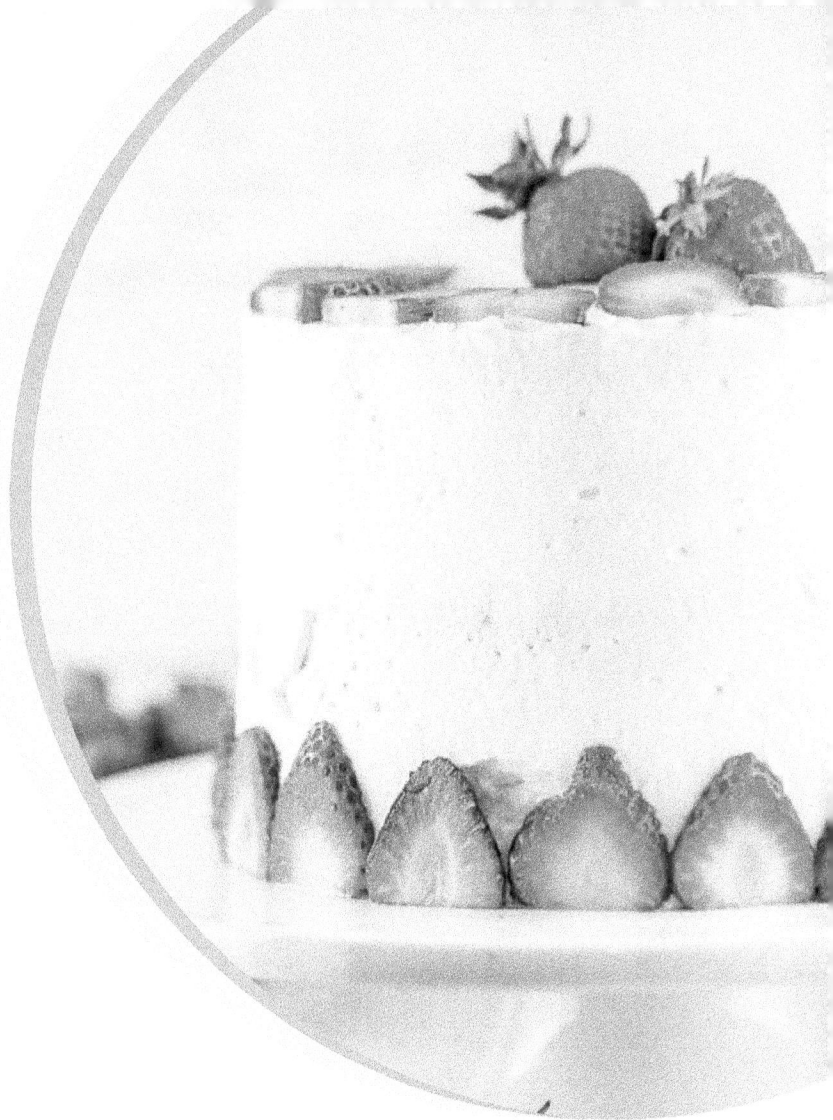

191 STRAWBERRY WHIPPED CREAM CAKE

Preparation Time: 15 minutes

Cooking Time: 24 hours

Servings: 1

INGREDIENTS:

- 1 pint of whipping cream
- 2 tablespoons of gelatin
- 1/2 a glass of cold water
- 1 glass of boiling water
- 3 tablespoons of lemon juice
- 1 orange glass juice
- 1 spoon of sugar
- ¾ cup of sliced strawberries
- 1 large angel food cake or light sponge cake

DIRECTIONS:

1. Put the gelatin in cold water, then add hot water and blend.
2. Add orange and lemon juice, also add some sugar and go on blending. Refrigerate and leave it there until you see it is starting to gel.
3. Whip half a portion of cream, add it to the mixture, strawberries, put wax paper in the bowl, and cut the cake into small pieces.
4. In between the pieces, add the whipped cream and put everything in the fridge for one night.
5. When you take out the cake, add some whipped cream on top and decorate some more fruit.

Calories 355
Protein 4 g
Carbohydrates 43 g
Fat 18 g
Sodium 275 mg
Potassium 145 mg
Phosphorus 145 mg

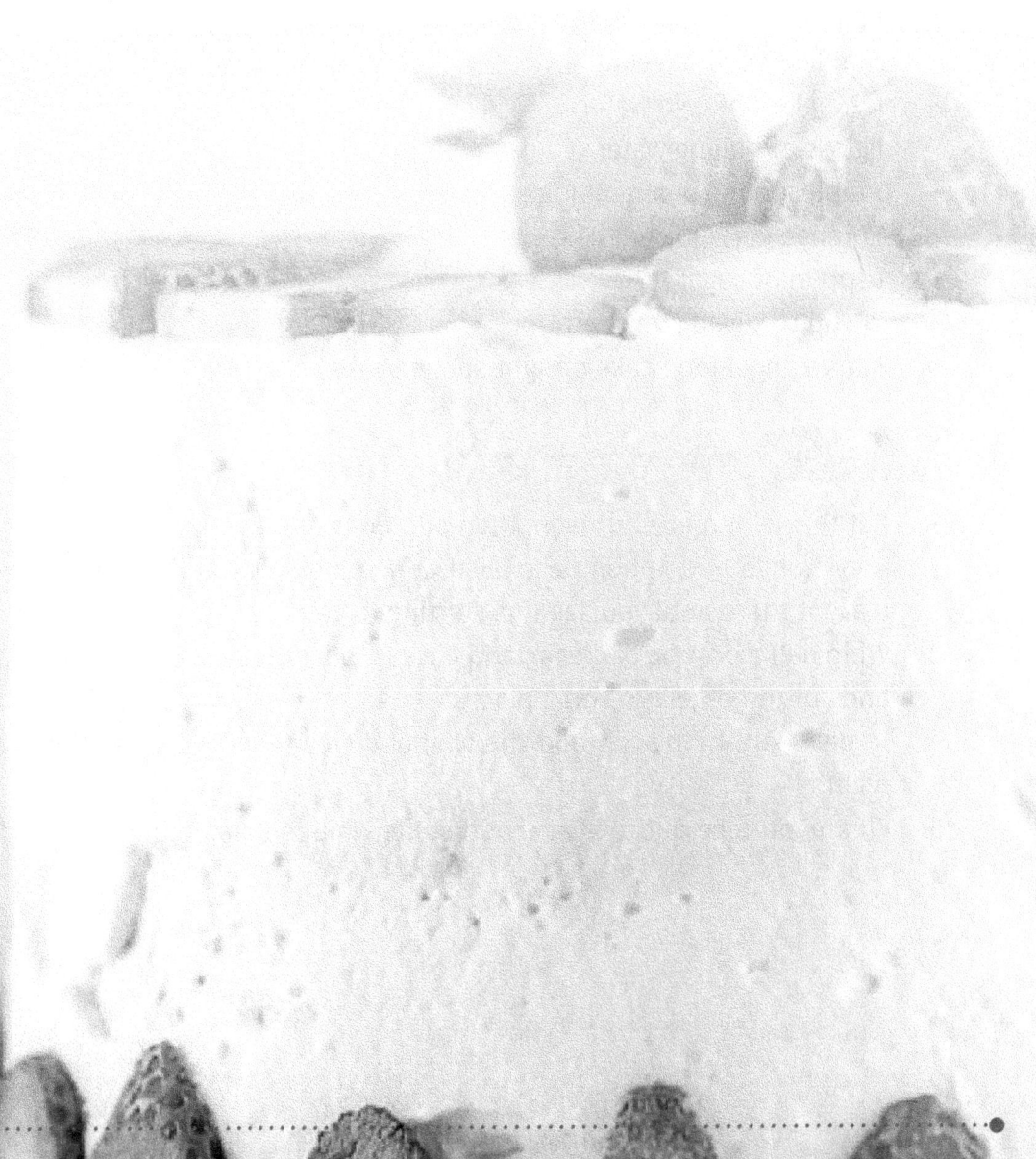

192 LEMON MERINGUE PIE

Preparation Time: 15 minutes

Cooking Time: 1 hour

Servings: 1

INGREDIENTS:

For Pie Filling

- 6 raw egg yolks
- 1/2 cup lemon juice
- 2 tablespoons lemon zest
- 1 1/4 tbsp unsalted butter
- 1/3 cup cornstarch
- 1 1/2 cups water
- 1 1/3 cup sugar or sugar replacement
- 1/4 tsp salt
- 1 store-bought pie shell

For Meringue

- 6 egg whites
- 2 1/2 tbsp sugar or sugar replacement
- 1 pinch cream of tartar

DIRECTIONS:

For Pie Filling

1. Preheat oven to 375 ° F.
2. Combine cornstarch, water, salt, and sugar in a medium saucepan. Combine by whisking and then turn the stove plate onto medium heat. When the mixture comes to a boil, stir frequently and allow it to boil for 2 minutes.
3. Put the egg yolks into a medium bowl and gradually add the hot mixture to the egg yolks and stir until combined and the mixture is smooth.

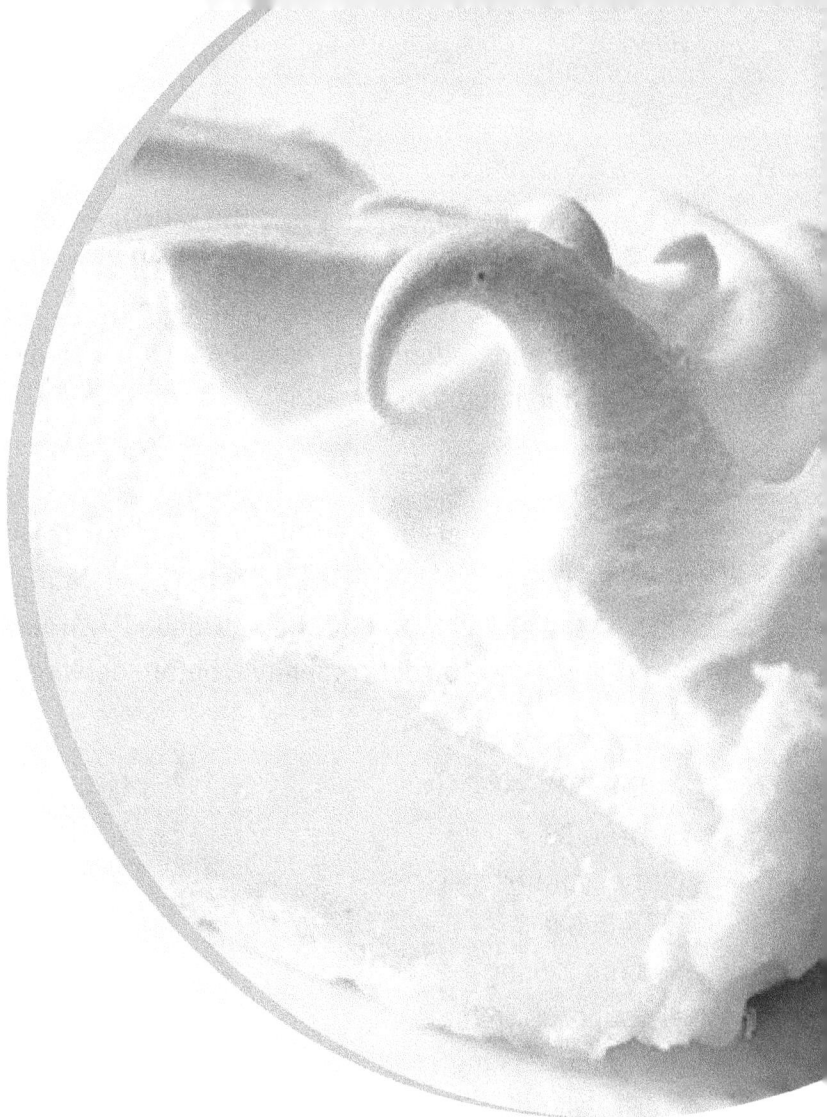

4. Put the mixture in the same saucepan and over low heat, cook for 2 more minutes, stirring continuously.
5. Remove from heat and stir in lemon zest, lemon juice, and butter. Continue stirring until all the ingredients are completely incorporated into a smooth mixture. Pour mixture into the pie shell and set aside.

For Meringue
1. 1.Beat egg whites and cream of tartar, then gradually add sugar and continue beating until stiff peaks form. Top your still-warm filling with the meringue mixture and bake the pie for 12 minutes or until the meringue is golden.
2. 2.Allow to cool completely before serving

NUTRITION:

Calories 28
Carbohydrates 44 g
Protein 6 g
Sodium 225 mg
Phosphorus 66 mg
Potassium 153 mg

193 FRESH FRUIT DESSERT CUPS

Preparation Time: 15 minutes

Cooking Time: 30 minutes

Servings: 1

INGREDIENTS:

- 4 sheets of 14-inch x 18-inch phyllo pastry dough
- Non-stick butter-flavored cooking spray
- 1 cup fresh strawberries
- 1 cup fresh raspberries
- 1 cup fresh blueberries
- 3 cups heavy whipped cream

DIRECTIONS:

1. Preheat oven to 400° F. Prepare a 12-cup muffin pan by spraying with butter-flavored non-stick cooking spray.
2. Pack the four sheets of phyllo dough on top of each other, lightly spraying with cooking spray between each layer. Cut dough into four 3 ½-inch squares.
3. Separate squares and place them into a muffin pan to form dessert cups and bake cups for 12 minutes or lightly browned. Allow cooling.
4. Fill each cup with equal amounts of berries and top with a small dollop of heavy whipped cream. Serve immediately

NUTRITION:

Calories 111
Carbohydrates 18 g
Protein 2 g

Sodium 51 mg
Phosphorus 14 mg
Potassium 83 mg

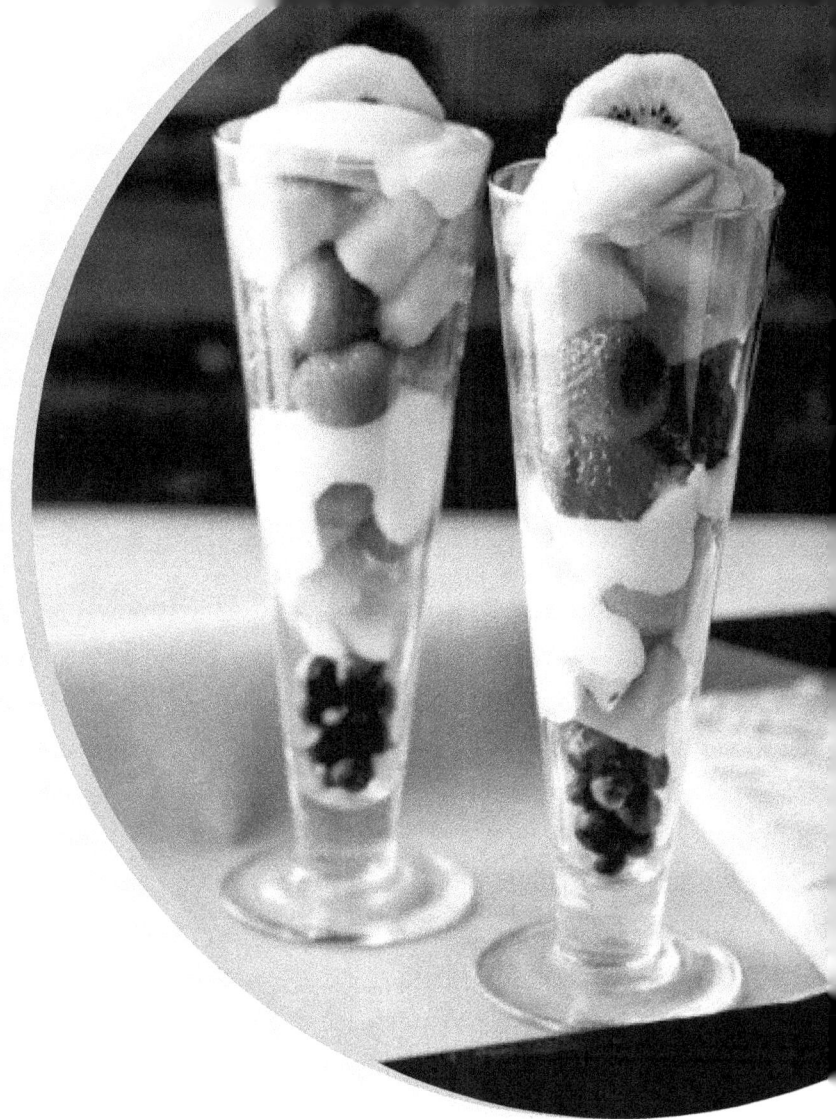

194 CARAMEL-CENTERED COOKIES

Preparation Time: 15 minutes

Cooking Time: 40 minutes

Servings: 1

INGREDIENTS:

- 1 ¾ cups all-purpose flour
- ½ cup unsalted margarine
- ½ tsp baking powder
- ½ tsp baking soda
- 1 ½ cups butterscotch chips
- ½ bag of caramel cubes
- 1 cup light brown sugar or sugar replacement
- 3 tbsp granulated sugar or sugar replacement
- 1 large egg
- 2 tsp vanilla extract

DIRECTIONS:

1. Preheat oven to 350°F. Using an electric mixer on a medium setting, cream the butter with the light brown sugar and granulated sugar until fluffy.
2. Whisk egg and vanilla extract for another 30 seconds.
3. Sift together dry ingredients in a mixing bowl and beat into the butter mixture at a low speed for about 15 seconds. Stir in butterscotch chips.
4. Using a scoop-shaped one tablespoon measure, drop dough onto a greased or lined cookie sheet about three inches apart.
5. Place one caramel square in the center of each scoop of dough and top with another tablespoon of dough. Roll in your hand until they are round.
6. Bake for 20 minutes or until browned on the edges.

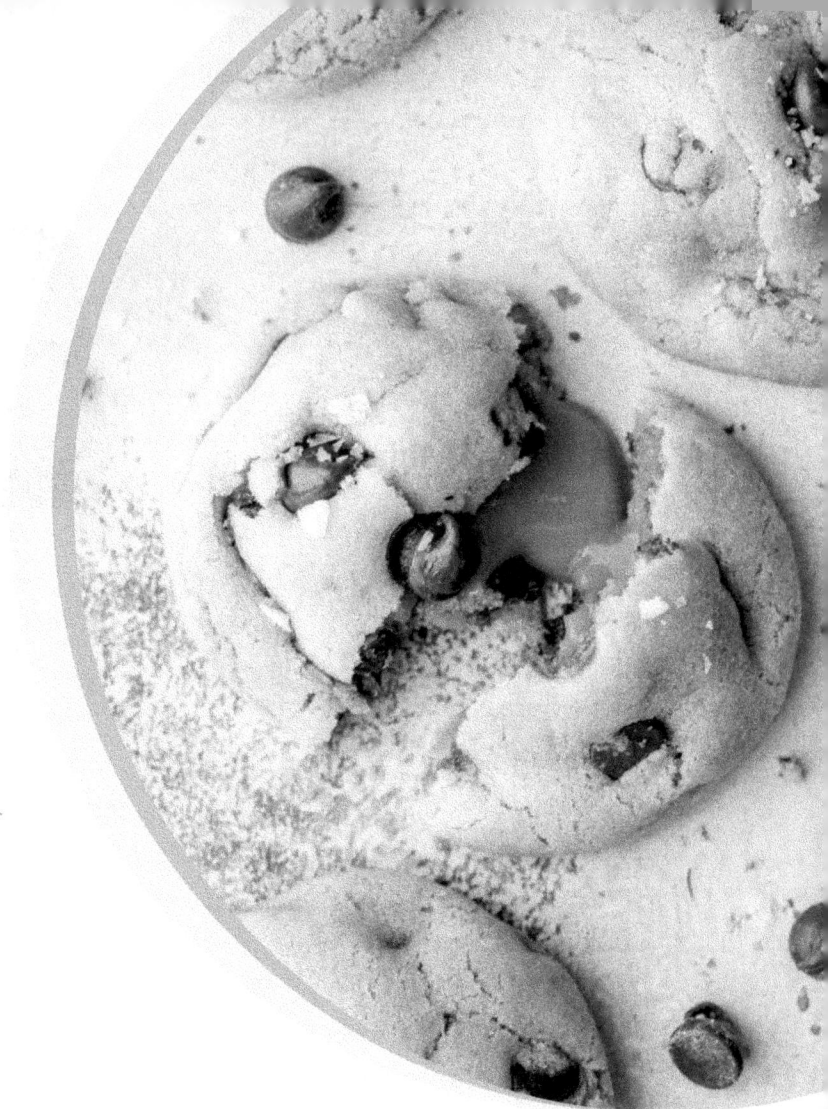

Calories 210
Carbohydrates 31 g
Protein 1.5 g
Sodium 67 mg
Phosphorus 35 mg
Potassium 82 mg

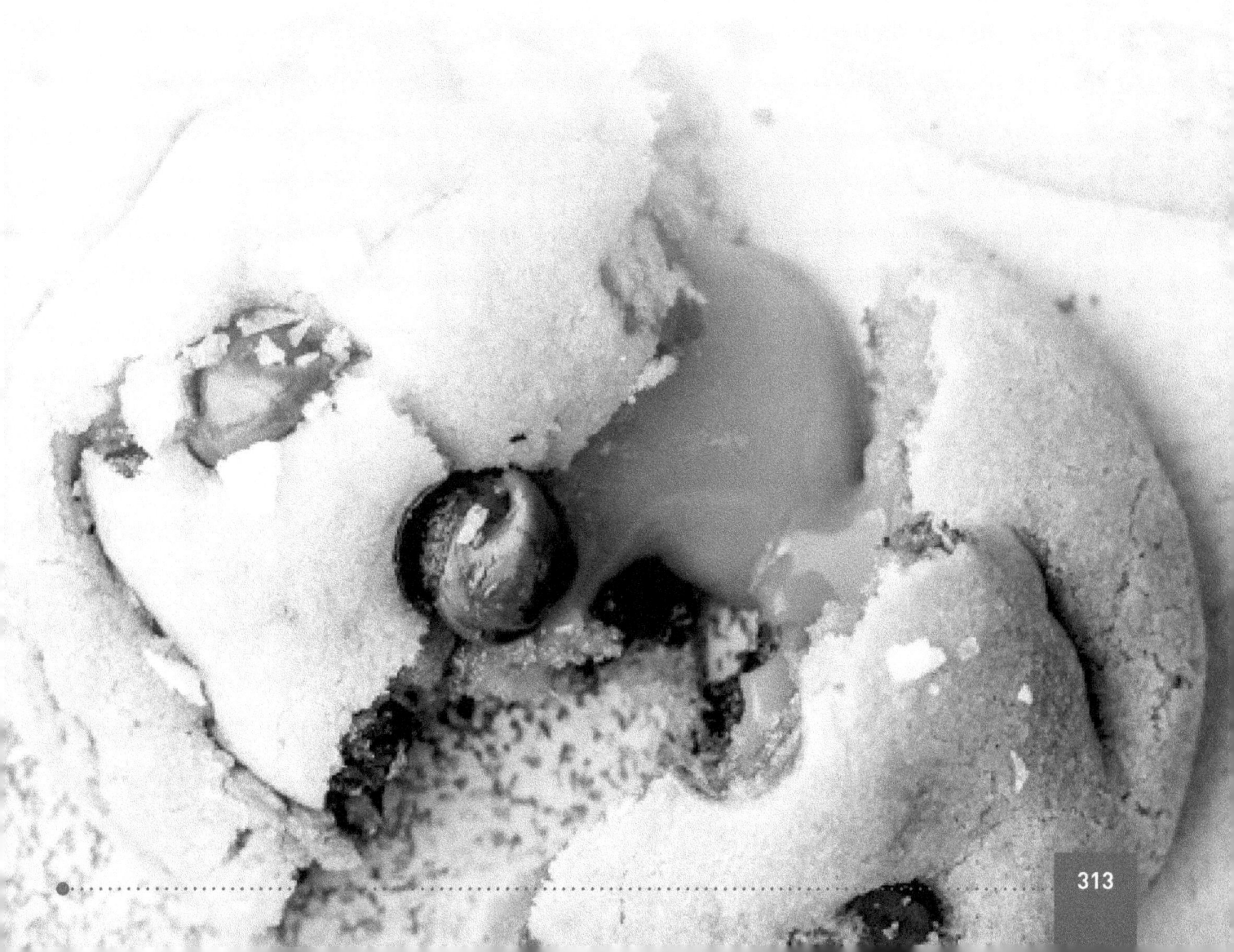

LOW-SODIUM POUND CAKE

Preparation Time: 10 minutes

Cooking Time: 30 minutes

Servings: 1

INGREDIENTS:

- 1 ¼ cup bread flour
- ¼ pound unsalted butter
- ¾ cup sugar or sugar replacement
- 2 large beaten eggs
- 3 oz non-fat milk or milk alternative

DIRECTIONS:

1. Preheat oven to 375° F. Prepare a pan by lining an 18-inch x 13-inch pan with baking paper.
2. Cream butter gradually adds sugar and beat until fluffy.
3. Add eggs, milk, and flour and mix well.
4. Pour mixture into the lined pan and bake at 375° F for approximately 30 minutes.

NUTRITION:

Calories 243
Carbohydrates 31 g
Protein 3.7 g
Sodium 18 mg
Phosphorus 45 mg
Potassium 47 mg

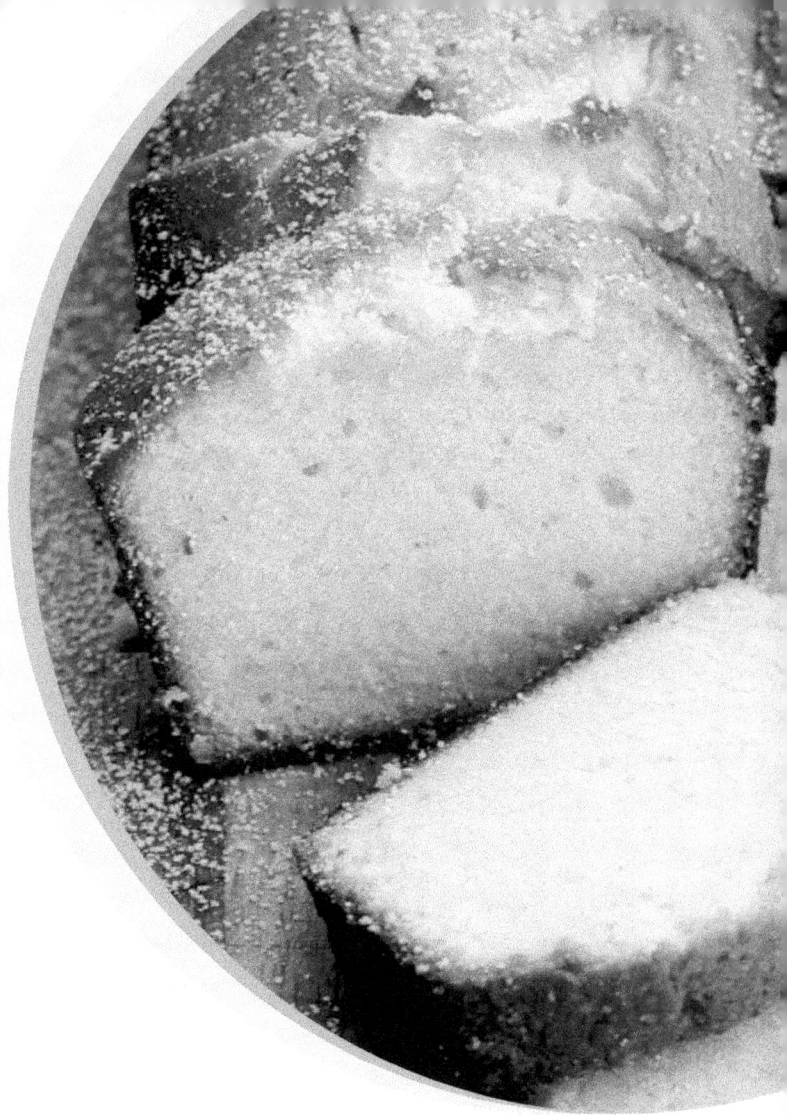

196 DESSERT PIZZA

Preparation Time: 10 minutes

Cooking Time: 15 minutes

Servings: 1

INGREDIENTS:

- 1 12-inch pre-cooked pizza base
- 2 cups fresh sliced strawberries
- 1 cup part-skim ricotta cheese
- ½ cup apricot jam or other light-colored jam
- 5 tbsp powdered sugar or sugar replacement
- 2 tbsp warm jelly or preserves
- ¼ cup chocolate chips

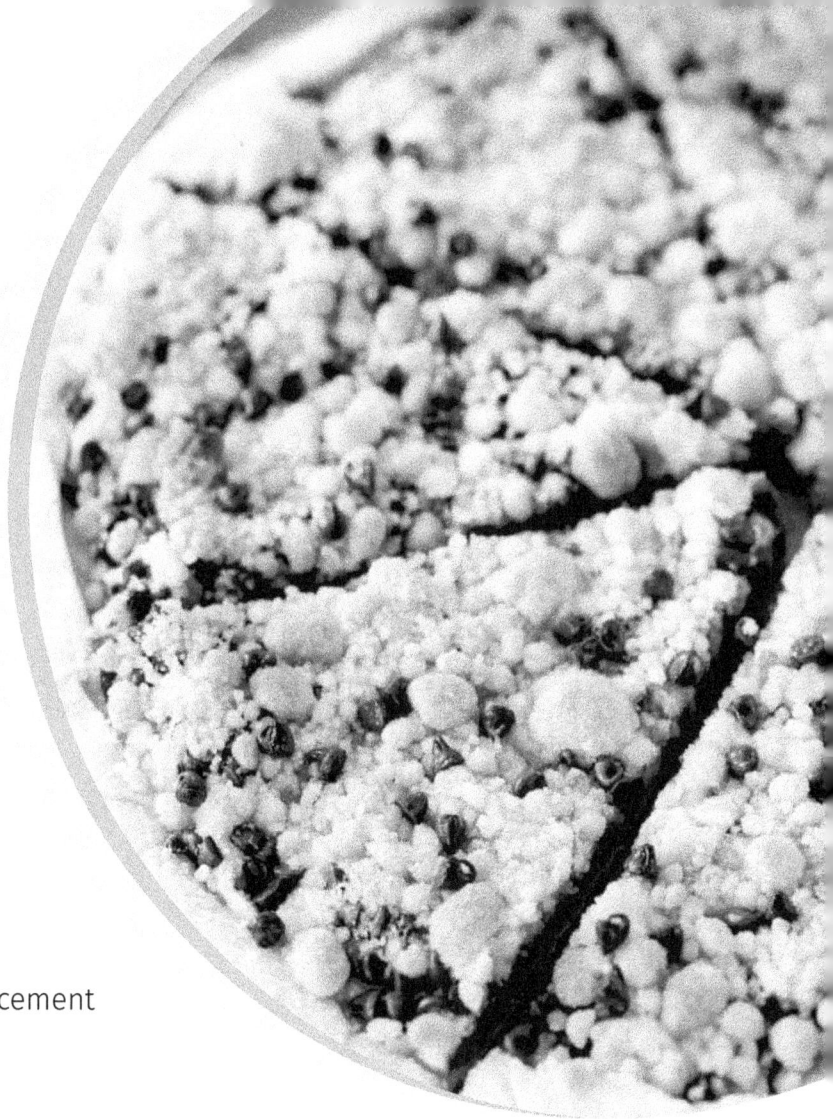

DIRECTIONS:

1. Preheat oven to 425° F.
2. Strain ricotta. Melt jam in microwave and brush jam on the pizza base.
3. Mix ricotta with three tablespoons of powdered sugar and spread on the pizza base.
4. Arrange strawberry slices on top of ricotta layer and sprinkle with remaining powdered sugar and chocolate chips.
5. Bake for 12 minutes, slice and serve.

NUTRITION:

Calories 288
Carbohydrates 49 g
Protein 8 g
Sodium 166 mg
Phosphorus 47 mg
Potassium 98 mg

197 LEMON BARS

Preparation Time: 20 minutes

Cooking Time: 45 minutes

Servings: 24

INGREDIENTS:

For Crust
- 2 cups all-purpose flour
- 1 cup unsalted butter
- ½ cup powdered sugar or sugar replacement

For Filling
- ¼ cup all-purpose flour
- ¼ tsp baking soda
- ½ tsp cream of tartar
- 4 eggs
- 1 ½ cups sugar or sugar replacement
- ¼ cup lemon juice

For Glaze
- 2 tbsp lemon juice
- 1 cup sifted powdered sugar or sugar replacement

DIRECTIONS:

For Crust
1. Preheat oven to 350° F. Mix flour, powdered sugar, and butter in a large bowl until crumbly.
2. Press mixture into a 9-inch x 13-inch baking pan.
3. Bake for about 20 minutes until lightly browned.

For Filling
1. Gently whisk eggs in a medium-sized bowl.
2. Mix flour, sugar, soda, and cream of tartar in a separate bowl and add these ingredients to the eggs. Whisk lemon juice into the egg mixture until slightly thickened.

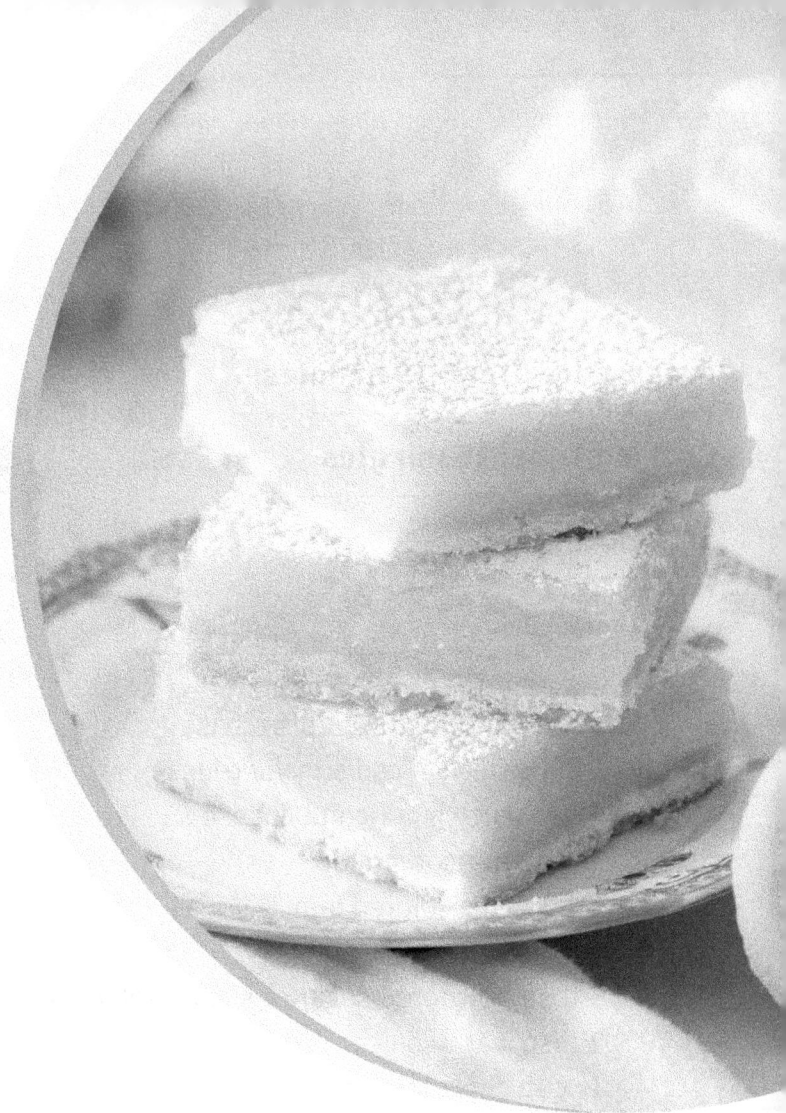

3. Pour over the warm crust and bake for another 20 minutes or until filling is set. Remove from the oven and allow to cool.

For Glaze
1. Slowly add the lemon juice into the sifted powdered sugar until spreadable.
2. Spread over cooled filling. Allow to set and then cut into 24 bars—store leftovers in the refrigerator.

NUTRITION:

Calories 200
Protein 2 g
Carbohydrates 28 g
Sodium 27 mg
Phosphorus 32 mg
Potassium 41 mg

198 BAKED PINEAPPLE

Preparation Time: 10 minutes

Cooking Time: 40 minutes

Servings: 1

INGREDIENTS:

- 20 oz canned, crushed pineapple with juice
- 2 large eggs or egg substitute
- 2 cups sugar or sugar replacement
- 3 tbsp tapioca
- 1/2 tsp cinnamon
- 1/8 tsp salt
- 3 tbsp unsalted butter

DIRECTIONS:

1. Preheat oven to 350°F.
2. Put the crushed pineapple with juice into a bowl.
3. Beat two eggs and add to crushed pineapple.
4. Put sugar, tapioca, and salt to pineapple egg mixture.
5. Pour mixture into 8-inch square baking dish.
6. Cut butter and place on top of pineapple mixture and sprinkle with cinnamon—Bake for 30 minutes.

NUTRITION:

Calories 270
Carbohydrates 54 g
Protein 2 g

Sodium 50 mg
Phosphorus 26 mg
Potassium 85 mg

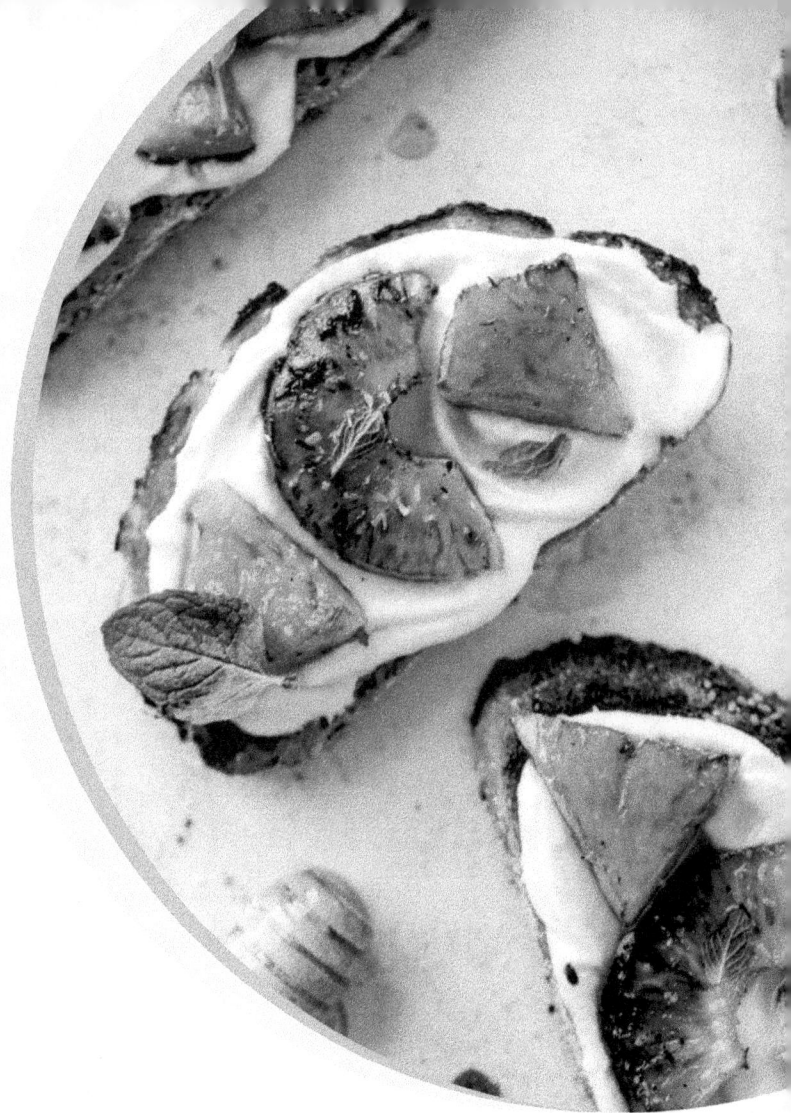

199 KIDNEY-FRIENDLY VANILLA ICE CREAM

Preparation Time: 15 minutes

Cooking Time: 1 hour

Servings: 1

INGREDIENTS:

- 1 cup low-cholesterol egg product
- ½ cup of sugar
- 2 cups liquid non-dairy creamer
- 1 tbsp vanilla extract
- Rock salt
- Ice

DIRECTIONS:

1. Beat egg and sugar in a large microwaveable bowl.
2. Stir in non-dairy creamer and microwave for one minute, or until mixture thickens. When cool, stir in vanilla.
3. Add the mixture into the center container of the ice cream machine and layer ice and rock salt around a container, alternating layers until the bucket is full.
4. Process according to manufacturer's instructions for your particular ice cream machine.

NUTRITION:

Calories 159
Carbohydrates 22 g
Protein 3 g
Sodium 64 mg
Phosphorus 36 mg
Potassium 87 mg

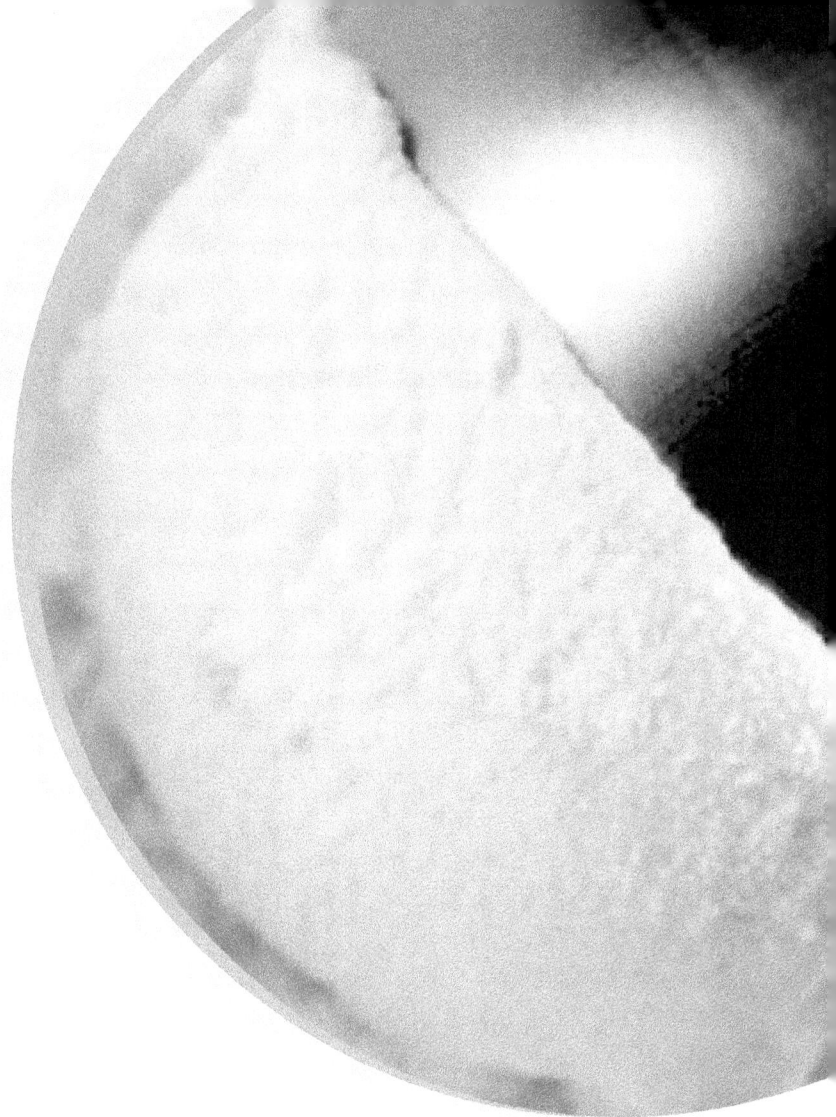

200 | QUICK CUPCAKES

Preparation Time: 10 minutes

Cooking Time: 10 minutes

Servings: 12

INGREDIENTS:

- 1 box angel food cake mix
- 1 box lemon cake mix
- 2 tsp water
- Non-stick cooking spray

DIRECTIONS:

1. In a large zip-lock bag, pour in angel food cake mix and lemon cake mix. Seal the plastic bag and shake to mix together.
2. Spray a small custard dish with non-stick cooking spray and add three tablespoons of dry cake mix to the dish. Add two tablespoons of water and mix with a fork.
3. Microwave on high for one minute. Slip muffin out of the dish and allow it to cool.
4. Repeat this process for as many cupcakes as you require.

NUTRITION:

Calories 97
Carbohydrates 21 g
Protein 1 g
Sodium 163 mg
Potassium 17 mg
Phosphorus 80 mg

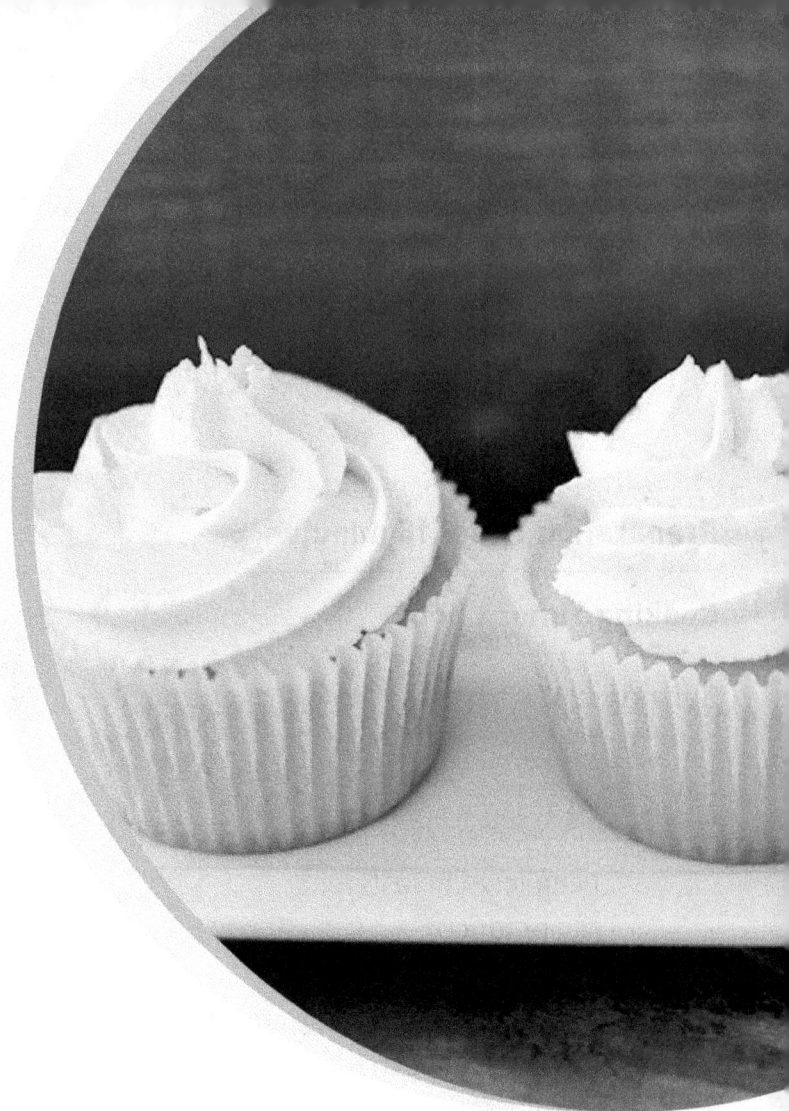

201 PEPPERMINT CRUNCH COOKIES

Preparation Time: 10 minutes

Cooking Time: 30 minutes

Servings: 18

INGREDIENTS:

- 18 peppermint candies
- ¼ tsp peppermint extract
- 1 ½ cups all-purpose flour
- 1 tsp baking powder
- ¼ tsp salt
- ¾ cup sugar or sugar replacement
- ½ cup soft unsalted butter
- 1 large egg or egg substitute

DIRECTIONS:

1. Put the 12 peppermint candies in a zip-lock bag and pound with a heavy pan until finely crushed.
2. Add sugar, butter, egg, and peppermint extract in a bowl. Beat ingredients at medium speed until creamy.
3. Mix flour, baking powder, and salt. Add flour mixture and beat until well-combined.
4. Stir in crushed peppermint candy by hand. Refrigerate for one hour.
5. Preheat the oven to 350 degrees F. Crushed the remaining peppermint candies in the same method as the first time. Line baking sheets.
6. Shape chilled dough into ¾-inch balls and place on baking sheets about 2 inches apart. Make an indentation in each cookie using your thumb, and top with about ½ teaspoon of crushed candy.
7. Bake until edges are lightly browned. Cool cookies completely and store them in a container between pieces of parchment or wax paper.

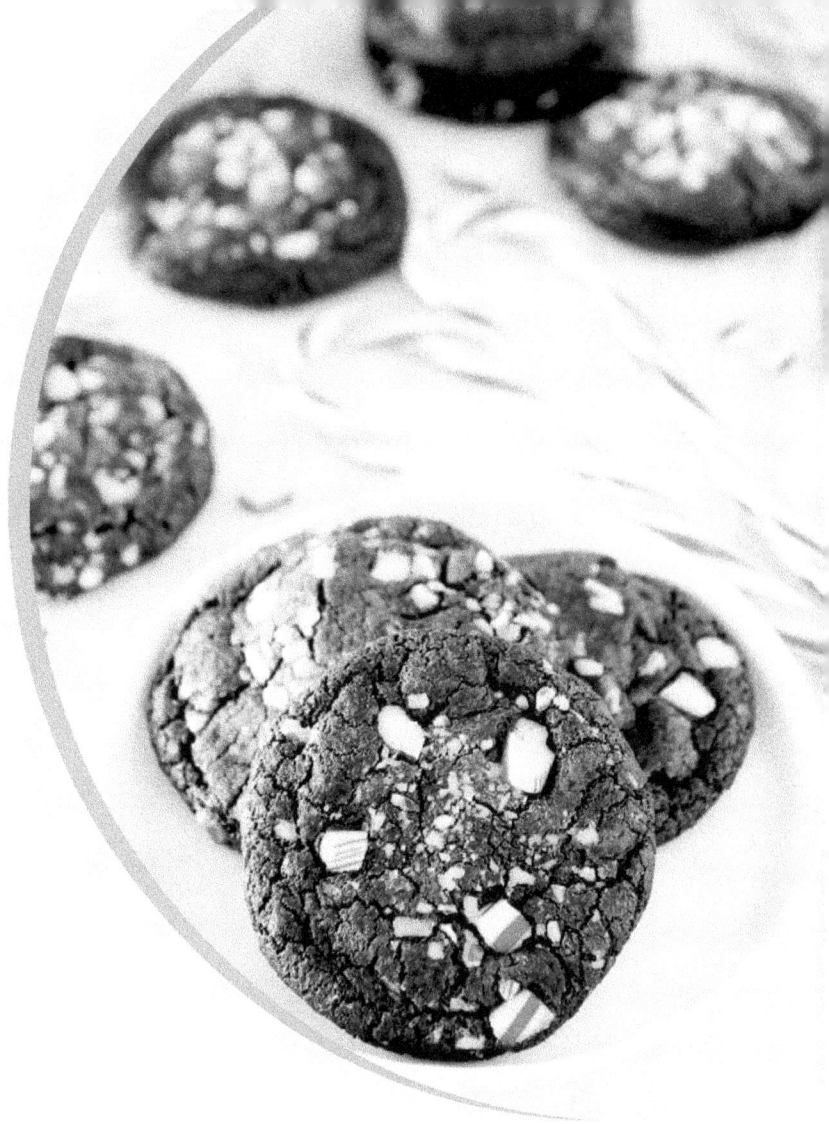

Calories 150
Carbohydrates 22 g
Protein 2 g
Sodium 67 mg
Potassium 17 mg
Phosphorus 24 mg

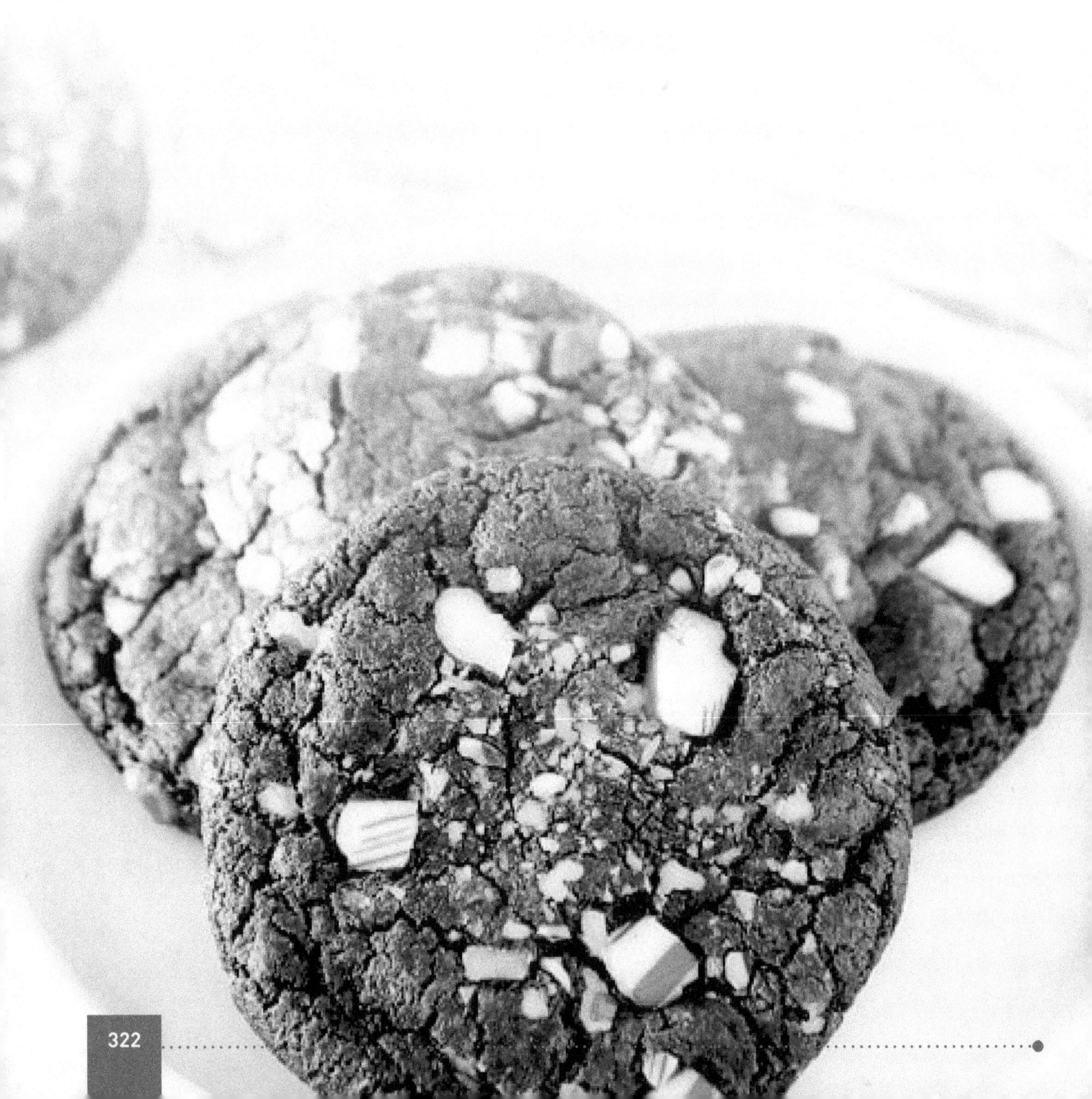

CONCLUSION

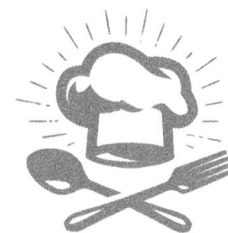

When you have chronic kidney disease, it is incredibly important to focus on promoting healthy lifestyle factors. You can't just take some medicine and get better. Instead, you have to prioritize eating a low-protein diet with the correct proportions of nutrients, exercising to maintain healthy muscles and organs, and sleeping well so that your body has the strength to function to the best of its ability. In one study on chronic kidney disease, it was found that patients who eat a healthy diet, stay physically active, maintain healthy body weight, and don't smoke can increase their longevity greatly. The participants who met all of these healthy lifestyle qualities reduced their risks of dying from the disease by sixty-eight percent compared to those who don't follow these lifestyle choices.

These same lifestyle factors have also long been shown to greatly affect heart health and diabetes, in which two-thirds of the population with chronic kidney disease also have. It is important because if your diabetes or heart health is not under control, it will put more pressure on your kidneys and increase your fatality risk. On the other hand, if you treat these conditions through a healthy lifestyle, you can greatly improve your diabetes or heart health and kidney health. Overall, you can only benefit from focusing on improving your lifestyle.

Suppose you don't yet have chronic kidney disease, but you or a family member are at risk of developing the condition. In that case, you can reduce your risk and potentially prevent yourself from developing the disease by making healthy lifestyle changes. Remember, you are more likely to develop kidney disease if you have a family history, diabetes, heart disease, or high blood pressure.

By managing the conditions associated with kidney diseases, such as diabetes and high blood pressure, you can benefit your kidney health and the health of your entire body and mind.

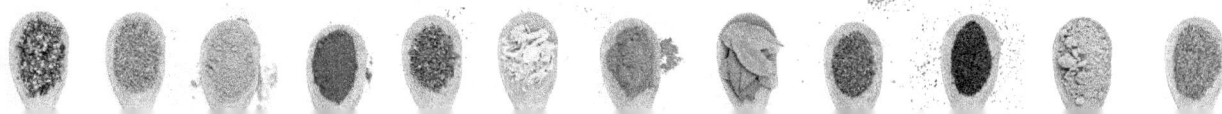

You can take to improving your kidney health is managing your blood pressure. Most people only think about the effect blood pressure has on the heart, but it also affects other organs, such as your kidneys. When blood pressure is chronically high, it causes damage to the kidneys. Therefore, you should maintain blood pressure at the goal set by your physician.

When you experience long-term stress, it greatly affects your health. Not only does stress often increase poor life choices, such as smoking, drinking, irregular sleep, and an unhealthy diet. But, chronically high stress increases blood sugar, raises blood pressure, and may lead to depression. You first need to prioritize a healthy lifestyle overall to manage your stress. Exercise, eating well, sleep, and other healthy lifestyle factors can all reduce chronic anxiety. However, you may need different methods of stress relief, as well. Try making a list of any calming activities you find helpful, such as listening to music, meditation, yoga, sketching, reading, or whatever else comes to mind. You can then use this list as inspiration when you are anxious. Whenever you find your stress increased, try completing one or two calming tasks from your list.

Excessive body weight causes your kidneys to push harder to complete their work and cause damage over time. Not only that, but excess weight also increases your risk of high blood pressure, high blood sugar, and more. Together, all of these aspects worsen kidney health, making it vital to maintain a healthy body weight to increase kidney health.

Adequate sleep and good sleep quality are important for overall physical and mental health. When you don't sleep well, it can negatively affect you in many ways, such as raising blood pressure and blood glucose. Studies have shown that adults should get seven to eight hours of solid sleep a night.

It is best to try to be active for at least thirty minutes a day. However, you should specifically try to maintain thirty minutes of moderate exercise three to four times a week. Along with moderate exercise, it is good to include some light flexibility-based exercises, which can reduce your risk of injury and make your more difficult exercises easier.

Of course, you should take any prescribed medication your doctor gives you. Whenever you see any of your doctors, make sure they all know every single medication you are taking, whether prescribed or over the counter, as well as supplements. These can affect your health in more ways than you might realize, and a simple over-the-counter supplement could negatively interact with one of your conditions or medications.

Besides giving your doctor a list of your medications, you should also talk to either your doctor or pharmacist before taking any new over-the-counter medications or supplements. These can cause many problems, which might not be listed on the label. For instance, many painkillers can damage the kidneys and should not be taken by anyone with kidney disease or injury.

As you know, diet is also an important aspect of your lifestyle so you can live better and longer.